Quality in the Manufacture of Medicines and other Healthcare Products

Quality in the Manufacture of Medicines and other Healthcare Products

John Sharp

BSc, Hon MRPharmS, CChem,
FRSC, CBiol, MIBiol, FIQA

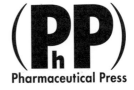

Pharmaceutical Press

Published by the Pharmaceutical Press
1 Lambeth High Street, London SE1 7JN

First published 2000

Text design by Barker/Hilsdon, Lyme Regis, Dorset
Typeset by Type Study, Scarborough, North Yorkshire
Printed in Great Britain at the University Press, Cambridge

ISBN 0 85369 431 1

A catalogue record for this book is available from the British Library

Contents

Part eight

Self-inspection/quality audit and other techniques

Preface

Although a wide variety of materials, usually of natural origin, have been used for medicinal purposes over several thousands of years, the large-scale industrial manufacture of medicines and other healthcare products is a phenomenon of only the last fifty or sixty years. The synthesis, by Paul Ehrlich in 1911, of arsphenamine (Salvarsan) and its subsequent use in the treatment of syphilis is generally taken to mark the beginning of the chemotherapeutic era. The beneficial effects of this new era on our ability to treat, cure, control and diagnose disease are both very considerable and widely acknowledged. Most notable secondary effects have been the emergence of the modern pharmaceutical industry and the consequently necessary changes in our approach to the control, assurance and management of the quality of manufactured medicines.

Prior to this modern era, medicines and the like were produced almost entirely on a very small-scale, 'cottage' basis. Many of the materials employed, if they did little good, could also cause in most cases little harm. The research, development and manufacture of synthetic compounds is not something that could be done on a multiplex cottage-industry scale. It demanded a concentration of resources into relatively few large-scale businesses. Active substances became ever-more potent and the potential hazards of quality failures in manufacture became, in consequence, increasingly serious and widespread. This has dictated the need for a most rigorous and highly organised approach to the means of ensuring the quality of manufactured medicines and other healthcare products.

This book is intended as a practical survey and critique of those means. Although considerable reference is made throughout to relevant national and international rules and regulations, it is essentially not a book about 'How to survive an inspection' or 'How to deal with the FDA'. Although it will assist in such aims, it is primarily a book on assuring/managing product quality in manufacturing as an intrinsically worthwhile exercise *per se*, from the aspects both of ensuring the 'safety, well-being and protection of the patient' and of the commercial health of the manufacturing company. It is based upon over forty years' involvement in, and concern for, the quality of manufactured medicines. It will be of interest and value to all those with similar involvement and concerns: those already working in industrial or hospital manufacturing, and pharmacy (and other) students contemplating a career in the industry. It is also hoped that it will be read with interest by community and hospital dispensing pharmacists wishing to be more aware of the issues surrounding the quality of the products that they dispense. It also covers a large proportion of the Joint (RPSGB/RSC/IoB) 'Study Guide for Qualified Persons', and of the syllabuses of the various academic bodies offering post-graduate degrees and diplomas in pharmaceutical quality assurance.

About the author

After working nearly 20 years in the Pharmaceutical Industry, variously in the practice and management of the chemical analysis, QC/QA, production and distribution of most major categories of medicinal product, and of the bulk production of a number of active substances, John Sharp joined the UK Medicines Inspectorate in 1971. He was promoted to Principal Inspector in 1972.

In addition to his inspection duties, he compiled and edited the 1977 and 1983 editions of the UK *Guide to Good Pharmaceutical Manufacturing Practice* ('The Orange Guide'), the latter later forming the basis for the EC/EU GMP Guidelines.

Since leaving the Inspectorate in 1985, he has held appointments with the Association of the British Pharmaceutical Industry (Project Manager) and has returned briefly to Industry (Technical Director, Waverley Pharmaceutical). Since 1987 he has run his own consultancy business.

He is the author of over 70 published papers, books, booklets and manuals on many aspects of pharmaceutical technology, QA/GMP, etc. (including three entire modules in the Manchester University Advanced Pharmaceutical Training series, and four modules for the ABPI NVQ Operator Training series). He has presented papers to technical, professional and academic seminars/symposia in Britain, Continental Europe, Canada, the USA, Africa and Asia. Currently he is the editor of *The Industrial Pharmacist*, a member of the Editorial Board of the *European Journal of Parenteral Science*, and a referee for the US PDA's *Journal of Pharmaceutical Science and Technology*.

John Sharp is an honours science graduate of London University, a Fellow of the Royal Society of Chemistry (and a member of the RSC's panel of assessors for Qualified Persons), an Honorary Member of the Royal Pharmaceutical Society (for services to Pharmacy in the field of GMP), a Member of the Institute of Biology, a Fellow of the Institute of Quality Assurance, an Honorary Life Member of the Parenteral Society, an Honorary Life Member of the Pharmaceutical BFS Operator's Association, a Member of the US Parenteral Drug Association (Korczynski Award for international contributions to the pharmaceutical sciences, 1996) and a member of the Harlequin FC and of Middlesex CCC.

Introduction

A major motive in writing this book has been a persistent and growing realisation that far too much that has been said and written in this general field is
either (a) largely devoted to management-speak generalities ('addressing corporate strategies', 'defining system parameters', 'prioritising cross-modular
interfaces' and the like) to the virtual exclusion of any consideration of the
nuts and bolts of what, in fact, has to be done, and how to do it, and/or (b)
concerned with describing 'how to meet the regulatory requirements', as if
this were the sole reason for being concerned about the quality of medicinal
and other healthcare products.

It cannot be denied that the issue of a broad, general, corporate strategy and approach to product quality is of crucial importance. However,
quality principles and philosophies are of little value if they descend no
further down to earth than the corporate office. Although it is essential that
senior management should foster a 'quality culture' and lead by example,
the real quality battle is more often fought, and lost or won, at a much more
basic level. Sadly it all too frequently happens that the high aims and ideals
enshrined in statements of Corporate Quality Policy, in Company Quality
Manuals and in similar devout doctrinal texts are very far from realised on
the factory floor.

As examples of the mode of thought indicated in (b) above, I have
before me as I write a brochure for an international industrial pharmaceutical conference, where one of the sessions has the sub-title 'Finding
workable solutions to today's and tomorrow's regulatory obstacles'. (Note:
'*obstacles*'.) I also have by me a book, on an important aspect of pharmaceutical technology, in which the preface indicates that its *raison d'etre* is
that the 'regulatory requirements . . . within the pharmaceutical industry are
being continually and incessantly tightened . . .'

The driving force behind, and the ethic informing, this present book is
a very different one. One of its objectives is to provide a wide-ranging survey
of the basic 'whats' and 'hows' of achieving quality in the manufacture of
medicinal and other healthcare products, although it will inevitably be necessary, as a preliminary, to explore some of the more rarefied conceptual areas.
A fundamental basis is a profound conviction that quality assurance (QA) –
and hence good manufacturing practice (GMP) – is thoroughly worthwhile
per se, and not something to be regarded merely as a means of satisfying the

requirements of any national or international regulatory body. Although it would be both pointless and foolhardy (not to say illegal) to ignore or dismiss the regulatory dimension, this book is not intended to be a handy guide to satisfying any, or every, regulatory requirement. However, it should be noted that the pursuit of the perhaps more worthy aim of ensuring maximum protection of the health and well-being of the consumer should, as a consequence, achieve regulatory objectives. Indeed, it could well be argued that if any regulatory edict requires a manufacturer to act in a manner which fails to ensure adequate consumer protection, or to take measures in excess of what is required to provide that protection, then it is the regulatory body which is at fault, and not the manufacturer. Pointless 'regulatory obstacles', and 'continually and incessantly tightened' regulatory requirements which add nothing to patient safety need to be challenged with all the force of the scientific evidence available. (A good example, and one to be followed, is provided by the Technical Report No. 25 of the US PDA on 'Blend uniformity analysis: validation and in-process testing' (PDA, 1997). In this report, the decision of US Judge Wolin in the much-vaunted case of US versus Barr Laboratories, which the FDA has, for a number of years, been using as a weapon to bludgeon the industry, is comprehensively shown to be seriously flawed, both practically and statistically.)

In its Introduction, the last truly British guide to good pharmaceutical manufacturing practice, the so-called 'UK Orange Guide' (Sharp, 1983), states in reference to good manufacturing practice (which it later, in effect, defines as the ongoing, day-to-day part of quality assurance):

> The object of GMP . . . is, initially, the assurance of the quality of the product, and ultimately the safety, well-being and protection of the patient.

An earlier draft of that guide continued with a further very pertinent comment which was deleted from the published version:

> . . . any so-called GMP measure which does not contribute directly or indirectly to those ends is an irrelevance.

So a basic philosophy underlying this book is that *pharmaceutical* quality assurance (of which, to re-emphasise, GMP is a major component and a routine manifestation) is essentially about ensuring the safety of the consumer. However, the pursuit of this fundamental ethical issue will also yield economic benefits to the manufacturer and should additionally ensure regulatory compliance. Indeed, since the aim of the regulators is to provide consumer protection on behalf of their respective governments the quality objectives of regulatory bodies and of manufacturers should be closely similar.

A number of substantial volumes, and innumerable articles, have been published on quality assurance as applied to the manufacture of goods and the provision of services generally. This present publication is concerned with the application of quality assurance to the manufacture of a more narrow, but crucially important and distinctly special range of goods, that is: the manufacture and supply of medicinal (or pharmaceutical) and related products such as medical devices and diagnostics.

That these goods are crucially important, and have a profound effect, one way or another, on human well-being could hardly be denied. That they are 'special', in both manufacturing and quality terms, to an extent which sets them apart from such other manufactured items as screws, plastics bags, balls of string or socks is a point that will shortly be argued. Indeed, another basic philosophy which informs this book is that a number of the concepts implicit in more general 'quality' dogmas may well be of doubtful value in the context of the manufacture of medicines and other healthcare products, and as such should at least be questioned.

A final motivation for writing this book has been the thought that too many volumes published in this field are simply a collection of papers, written by a number of different authors, and often showing obvious signs of being articles originally published separately, or merely 'tidied-up' notes of previously presented lectures. An advantage of such an 'edited collection' is that some of the chapters may be well written by acknowledged experts in their respective fields. Too often, many chapters are not. For better or for worse, this book is a one-man effort. It is hoped that what it may lack in specific expertise may be compensated by its coherence and singular approach. Its faults, no less than such merits as it may have, are entirely due to me. This is not to say that during over forty years working in, for and around the pharmaceutical industry, I have not benefited from advice and ideas, and had my mind prompted and provoked by many colleagues and friends. Their number is legion. Five names must however be mentioned. They are Alan Badby, Jim Chissel, Bryan Hartley, Gerry Prout and the late Mick Fidler. Although they are in no way directly responsible for this book, my grateful thanks are due to all of them for what they have taught me.

Terminological note

In this book, references will be found to the European Community (EC), the European Economic Community (EEC) and the European Union (EU) since it is difficult to decide whether or not *all* references to 'EC' (or 'EEC') should be changed to 'EU', as the EU continues to refer, on occasions, to itself as both 'EC' or 'EEC'. For example, the relevant GMP Guide is still referred-to as 'The EC Guide'; Directives are still referenced in the form 91/356/EEC, and so on. By and large, I have adopted the term 'EC'. Therefore, where appropriate, for 'EC' please read 'EU'.

References

PDA (1997). Blend uniformity analysis: validation and in-process testing. Technical Report No. 25, published as a supplement to *PDA J Pharm Sci Technol* 1997, **51** (S3).

Sharp J, ed. (1983). *Guide to Good Pharmaceutical Manufacturing Practice*, 3rd edn. London: HMSO.

Part One

Principles

1

Applications and definitions

There are no such things as applied sciences, only applications of science
Louis Pasteur (1822–1895)

A book entitled *Quality in the Manufacture of Medicines and other Health-care Products* calls for an immediate clarification of what is meant by 'quality' and by 'medicines' (or 'medicinal products').

Consideration of the concept of 'quality' and of what precisely is meant by the term when applied to this specialised range of products, is reserved for the next chapter. A chapter largely devoted to formal definitions, as derived from various statutory regulations, is potentially a touch tedious, and could hardly be considered the most stimulating start to a book. There will also be readers who are already well aware of the formal definition of the range of products with which they are routinely concerned, and for them the potential for tedium would become a reality. Perhaps more cogently, an initial chapter given over mainly to quotations from regulatory texts might well seem to be a reversal of the principle asserted in the introduction, that 'a profound conviction that quality assurance (QA) – and hence good manufacturing practice (GMP) – is thoroughly worthwhile *per se,* and not something to be regarded merely as a means of satisfying the requirements of any national or international regulatory body'. Hence the placing of the relevant definitions in an annex to this chapter.

The range of products, of which the assurance of quality is the concern of this book, includes:

- Medicinal products
- Pharmaceutical products
- Drug products
- Medical devices
- Diagnostics (*in vivo* and *in vitro*)
- Bulk pharmaceutical chemicals (BPCs)
- Active pharmaceutical ingredients (APIs).

This book also has relevance to the manufacture of foodstuffs and cosmetics/toiletries. Indeed, *Food and Drink – Good Manufacturing Practice* (IFST,

1998) bears a very strong resemblance to the last (1983) edition of the UK's guide to GMP, which is known as the 'UK Orange Guide' (Sharp, 1983).

Before turning, in the next chapter, to the consideration of 'quality', it is worth reflecting on the rather special nature of the products which are our concern.

The special nature of medicines

Medicines and the like *are* special. Medicinal products generally have a great potential for good; but, if wrongly made or wrongly used they can cause much harm. Yet no other products are consumed so totally on trust: 'Nothing of so great importance to human welfare is used more completely on faith than a medicinal product' (Taylor, 1947). Indeed, in many circumstances, the ultimate consumer (the patient) may be totally unaware of what is being consumed or if anything is being consumed at all (the patient could be unconscious).

In contrast, the purchaser (the consumer) of, say, a motor car is fully aware of what is happening and knows what a car should be like. There are a number of ways of deciding whether or not the particular model or specimen in mind is just what is needed and can be afforded. The purchaser can read the manufacturer's literature and independent reports in the consumer magazines and can discuss a potential purchase with other owners of the same type of vehicle or can hire an engineer to inspect and report. He or she can personally examine the car, and can take a test-drive. A decision can then be made whether or not to be a consumer on the basis of a substantial quantity of objective data. The same sort of considerations apply also to the potential consumer of cameras, audio/visual goods, domestic appliances and so on. The purchaser of food or drink can still reject the actual or potential purchase on grounds of appearance, odour, texture or taste. In many cases, the general consumer is also covered by guarantees or warranties.

The consumer of medicines, however, quite literally takes a medicine, in the vast majority of cases, *entirely* on trust. The average consumer of, say, an anti-inflammatory tablet will be able, usually, to decide whether or not a tablet has been supplied, and that's about all. There is no way of knowing whether it contains an anti-inflammatory substance, whether it is the right anti-inflammatory substance, whether it is the correct dosage, or whether any contaminants or degradation products are present. The ultimate consumer, the patient, is very largely not in a position to recognise that a medicine is incorrect or defective. The consumer is at one end of a chain of implicit trust which extends back through administering, dispensing, prescribing and distributing, right back to those responsible for manufacturing the product. All along the line there is an implicit trust that the manufacturer has done their job properly. The social and moral implications of this 'chain of trust' alone are sufficient to make medicines, and their manufacture and quality assurance, 'special'. Not that ethical considerations are the only constraint: in addition there are sound legal and economic reasons to reinforce these ethical imperatives. It is hardly good business to inflict damage on one's customers, or to have one's activities restrained by regulatory authorities.

Another factor which makes medicines and the like special is the problem of testing them. There are very great potential hazards if even only a small proportion of defective items or ingredients are present within a batch, and yet these might well remain undetected by anything less than 100% testing. Furthermore, it is a practical impossibility to test a product for everything that might be 'wrong' about it, in terms of formulation error, mix-up, contamination or degradation. It would thus be perfectly possible for a medicinal product to be sampled and tested against a well-founded specification and yet still fail to have the desired effect, or to be dangerous or even lethal.

A yet further 'special' factor is the profound effect that formulation changes and changes in the method of processing can have on the safety and efficacy of the end product. In a number of manufacturing industries, *ad hoc* modification of the process (as, for example, adjusting the seasoning in cookery) may be acceptable, even desirable. This is unequivocally not the case in the manufacture of medicines and other healthcare products. Some real-life examples of the ill-effects of formulation/processing changes are:

- An injectable product, in the form of a derivative of mammalian glands, dispersed in an oily vehicle was reported, on a number of different occasions (different patients), suddenly to be displaying a much more rapid onset, combined with a much shorter period, of activity. A number of ingenious theories were proposed to explain this, including a change in the mammalian species from which the glands were derived. In the event the problem was found, and conclusively proved, to be due to the purchase of a set of new, and somewhat larger, balls for the ball-mill used to mill the active substance in the oil as part of the batch manufacturing process, thus milling the powder finer than hitherto. To rectify the variation, the milling time was reduced, and a primitive (by today's standards) test specification for particle size control in the end product was established. The problem then ceased to occur (author's own unpublished personal archives).

- Significant incidence of phenytoin intoxication in an Australian city due to change of capsule filler from calcium sulphate to lactose, which increased the bioavailability of the phenytoin (Tyrer *et al.*, 1970).

- Bioavailability problems with 'Lanoxin' brand of digoxin due to change in particle size, resulting in over-digitalisation of formerly stabilised cardiac patients (Johnson *et al.*, 1973).

- Wide variation in patient reactions to generic digoxin tablets, and in assay results on samples taken from the market. Found to be due to the effects of a newly installed dust extraction system, over the powder mixer, which selectively drew the finer, lighter, digoxin powder from the heavier excipients in the powder mix (UK Medicines Inspectorate unpublished archives).

Thus, for a number of good reasons, it may reasonably be maintained that medicines and similar products are indeed 'special', in that:

1.   They are potentially very hazardous to the ultimate consumer.
2.   They are (nevertheless) usually consumed with unquestioning trust.
3.   It is more than usually difficult (if not impossible) to establish their suitability for consumption by testing alone.
4.   The safety and efficacy in use can be profoundly affected by formulation and processing changes.

Therefore, quite clearly, the approach to assuring the quality of these products needs to be an especially rigorous one.

References

IFST (1998). *Food and Drink – Good Manufacturing Practice*, 4th edn. London: Institute of Food Science and Technology.

Johnson B F *et al.* (1973). Biological availability of digoxin from Lanoxin produced in the United Kingdom. *Br Med J* **4**, 323–326.

MCA (1997). *Rules and Guidance for Pharmaceutical Manufacturers and Distributors*. London: Medicines Control Agency. Available from The Stationery Office (HMSO), London.

Sharp J, ed. (1983). *Guide to Good Pharmaceutical Manufacturing Practice*, 3rd edn. London: HMSO. Also stated *verbatim* with guidance on the detailed interpretation of these rules in MCA, 1997. (Referred to as the UK Orange Guide.)

Taylor F O (1947). Quality control. *J Am Pharm Assoc* **III** (3), March.

Tyrer J H *et al.* (1970). Outbreak of anticonvulsant intoxication in an Australian city. *Br Med J* **4**, 271–273.

Annex

Formal definitions – and discussion

Definitions of such terms as 'medicinal product', 'drug product' and 'medical device' are provided in various regulatory statutes and guidelines. Although there is a certain evident variability, taken together these formal definitions should be sufficient to indicate the general borderlines within which our specialised brand of quality assurance applies.

Medicinal product

One of the most explicit definitions of a medicinal product is given in Section 130 of the UK Medicines Act (1968) in the following way (original text somewhat abridged):

> 'medicinal product' means any substance or article (not being an instrument, apparatus or appliance) which is manufactured, sold or supplied, imported or exported for use . . . in either or both of the following ways . . .
>
> (a) use by being administered to one or more human beings or animals for a medicinal purpose;
> (b) use [in certain circumstances] as an ingredient . . . of a substance or article which is to be administered . . . for a medicinal purpose.

What this in effect says is that a medicinal product is something (other than an instrument, etc.) which is either itself administered for a medicinal purpose, or used (in circumstances to be defined) as an ingredient of something that is intended to be administered for a medicinal purpose.

This establishes that administration (actual or intended) is, in British law, an essential feature of a medicinal product. Thus, for example, *in vitro* diagnostics are excluded by this definition.

A definition of a 'medicinal purpose' is clearly now required and this is provided by the UK Medicines Act, thus:

> . . . a 'medicinal purpose' means any one or more of the following:
>
> (a) Treating or preventing disease;
> (b) Diagnosing disease . . . [or other condition];
> (c) Contraception;
> (d) Introducing Anaesthesia;

(e)   Otherwise interfering with the normal operation of a physiological function.

The UK Medicines Act also makes provisions for Ministers, as they see fit, to declare other things, not covered by this definition, to be medicinal products 'under the Act'. These provisions have been used to apply the controls exerted by the Act, in whole or in part, to surgical ligatures and sutures, certain materials used in surgical operations, contact lens solutions, intrauterine contraceptive devices, radioactive substances and cyanogenetic substances. However, most, if not all of these have since lost the status of 'medicinal products', and have been re-classified as 'medical devices' and regulated under different legislation.

The UK Medicines Act in addition states that:

> . . . 'administer' means administer . . . orally, by injection, or by introduction into the body in any other way, . . . or by external application . . . either in its (i.e. the medicinal product's) existing state, or after it has been dissolved, dispersed, diluted or mixed . . . (in or with) some other substance used as a vehicle.

There remains the clause about 'use as an ingredient'. This applies only in certain circumstances, and this part of the definition does not mean that all ingredients used in the manufacture of medicinal products are themselves necessarily 'medicinal products'. The 'certain circumstances' in which ingredients do become, themselves, medicinal products are:

> . . . one or more of the following [circumstances], that is to say:

(a)   Use in a pharmacy or hospital;
(b)   Use by a practitioner (i.e. a doctor, dentist or veterinarian);
(c)   Use in . . . a business which consists of or includes the retail sale . . . of herbal remedies.

So, as defined, the ingredients used to manufacture medicinal products on an industrial scale are not themselves 'medicinal products'. There is, however, one further complication. Having thus, in general terms, been excluded from definition as 'medicinal products', *some* ingredients in bulk form have been re-defined as medicinal products in their own right, e.g. by The Medicines (Control of Substances for Manufacture) Order, No. 1200 of 1971. Bulk materials which were in this way reinstated as medicinal products in their own right included certain antibiotics, antigens, antitoxins, antisera, insulin, toxins, vaccines, preparations of blood and a number of other biological substances. (However – see later under 'Starting materials'.)

The legal UK definition is perhaps one of the most comprehensive and it does illustrate the approach of definition by actual, intended, or purported *use*.

Definition on the basis of *use* is also adopted by the EC. For example, in the EC guide to GMP (EC, 1992), referred to here as the 'EC GMP Guide', 'medicinal product' is defined as:

> Any substance or combination of substances presented for treating or preventing disease in human beings or animals.

Any substance or combination of substances which may be administered to human beings or animals with a view to making a medical diagnosis or to restoring, correcting or modifying physiological functions in human beings or animals is likewise considered a medicinal product.

Drug product

In the US Food and Drug Association's current good manufacturing practice regulations (US FDA, 1990), hereafter referred to as the 'US CGMPs', the term 'drug product' rather than 'medicinal product' is used. It is defined (21 CFR 210.3 (b)(4)), in contrast to the EC/UK, basically in terms of *form* thus:

'Drug Product' means a finished dosage form, for example, tablet, capsule, solution, etc., that contains an active ingredient generally, but not necessarily, in association with in-active ingredients. The term also includes a finished dosage form that does not contain an active ingredient but is intended to be used as a placebo.

Products for clinical trials

This US definition of 'drug product' embraces products and materials intended for use in clinical trials. Paradoxically, in Britain and in Europe generally, products manufactured for use in clinical trials were not, for some time, subject to the same licensing and inspection requirements that applied to products intended for routine administration to patients. The implication seemed to be that clinical trial products and materials were not, officially considered to be, 'medicinal products'. At the time of writing (1998) this dubiously equivocal situation is in the process of being righted, and moves are under way in Europe to bring the manufacture of products and materials for clinical trial under the licensing and inspection regulatory umbrella, thus asserting their proper status as medicinal products. To this end, a draft directive has been issued for comment, on good clinical practice (GCP), which includes *inter alia* proposals for the licensing and inspection of the manufacture of investigational medicinal products (IMPs), i.e. products for use in clinical trials. It is also worthy of note that the EC GMP Guide, perhaps in anticipation, has an Annex (No. 13, revised December 2, 1996) on the manufacture of investigational medicinal products, which has an Introduction that in part reads as follows:

Medicinal product intended for research and development trials are not at present subject either to marketing or manufacturing Community legislation.
However . . . Member States *may* [author's emphasis] require compliance with the principles of GMP during the manufacture of products intended for use in clinical trials. It was also suggested in an EC Discussion paper (III/3044/91) in January 1991 that it is illogical for experimental products not

to be subject to the controls which would apply to the formulations of which they are the prototypes . . .

The Commission is currently preparing a draft directive on clinical trials and this first revision of the annex will be reviewed when necessary.

Pharmaceutical product

The term 'pharmaceutical product', although commonly used, is not formally defined in EC or UK legislation or guidelines. However, the Pharmaceutical Inspection Convention (PIC – now being replaced by 'PICS' – see Annex II to Chapter 3) has published the *Guide to Good Manufacturing Practice for Pharmaceutical Products* (PIC, 1989), hereafter referred to as the 'PIC GMP Guide', which is now 'harmonised with the EC Guide to Good Manufacturing Practice for Medicinal Products'. This defines 'pharmaceutical product' (somewhat inconclusively) as:

> Any medicine or similar product intended for human use, which is subject to control under health legislation in the manufacturing or importing state.

Starting materials/ingredients

The PIC GMP Guide has a single annex, originally published in June 1987, on 'Guidelines for the manufacture of active pharmaceutical ingredients (bulk drug substances)' which states, *inter alia*, that 'It is expected that the principles of GMP be observed throughout all stages of the manufacture of the active pharmaceutical ingredients'.

The EC GMP Guide (as reprinted in the MCA's orange *Rules and Guidance for Pharmaceutical Manufacturers and Distributors*; MCA, 1997) does not have any section or annex on bulk ingredients. However, in its Introduction it states:

> With regard to the manufacture of active ingredients, it was agreed that the 'Guideline for the Manufacture of Active Pharmaceutical Ingredients' published by the Pharmaceutical Inspection Convention of 6 June 1987 would be an appropriate reference for manufacturers and a basis for inspection by competent authorities.

The precise legal status of bulk ingredients (active or inactive) as 'medicinal products' (etc.), in terms of government control, licensing and inspection in the EU was, for a while, somewhat equivocal. However, in September 1997, the European Commission issued a first draft of a legislative proposal on GMP for starting materials, and inspection of manufacturers of both medicinal products and starting materials (amending Directives 75/319/EEC and 81/851/EEC).

These proposals define starting materials as:

All the constituents of a medicinal product: the active ingredient(s) and the excipients as well as intermediate products, e.g. granules. For biological products it means all of the constituents as well as the source materials.

Manufacture of starting materials is defined as including both total and partial manufacture, or importation, dividing up, packaging or presentation, including repackaging or relabelling – but wholesaling or brokering are not covered.

In summary, the effects of these proposed amendments to the two already existing directives will be:

- Licensed manufacturers and importers must only use starting materials made in compliance with GMP for starting materials (although the holding of some form of Authorisation or Licence does not seem to be proposed).
- Manufacturers of starting materials (as listed in Annex II to the proposal) must: (a) obtain prior agreement of the medicinal product manufacturer before making any change to the starting materials supplied (a very broad requirement, and it has to be wondered if it is indeed intended to apply to *any* change, no matter how trivial); (b) allow inspection by a competent authority; and (c) provide samples to the European Pharmacopoeia on request.

Within the proposals are requirements that, subject to any arrangements between the Commission and third countries, a member state, the Commission, or the European Medicines Evaluation Agency (EMEA) may require inspection of a third country starting material manufacturer, and that member states shall ensure that the starting materials (as given in Annex II to the proposals – see below) when they are for use in medicinal products, are manufactured in compliance with GMP for starting materials.

Annex II to the proposals has two 'lists' of starting materials:

- List 1 – All active pharmaceutical ingredients (APIs) and intermediates.
- List 2 – Gelatin and its derivatives; tallow and its derivatives.

The term 'intermediates' is in need of clarification. In the explanatory memorandum it is defined as applying to such things as granules intended for compression into tablets, thus providing considerable potential for confusion with 'intermediate' in a chemical synthesis sense.

Other draft proposals include requirements that:

- Member states shall inspect starting materials manufacturers whenever they consider it necessary for the purposes of implementing the revised directive, or at the request of the starting material manufacturer, another member state, the Commission or the EMEA.
- Member states shall issue an inspection report to the starting material/medicinal product manufacturer.

- Member states shall issue a GMP Certificate, if appropriate, within 90 days of the inspection. The certificates must be entered in a Community register. (A standard format is proposed, but has yet to be agreed.)
- If the starting material/medicinal product manufacturer does not comply with GMP, this must be entered in the Community register.

The proposals also state that an annex to the EC GMP Guide, for starting materials, will be published. The explanatory memorandum states that this will draw upon the PICS and WHO guidelines. In the same month (September 1997) that these proposals were issued by the European Commission, PIC/PICS issued for consultation a draft 'internationally harmonised' GMP Guide for Active Pharmaceutical Ingredients – APIs. The working party that produced this draft consisted of representatives from Canada, US FDA (2), India, Switzerland, Australia, Finland and China. Although this draft is comprehensive and highly detailed, it is unclear in places and could lead to confusion. In scope it embraces APIs for use in both human and veterinary products (including clinical trials products); the later chemical isolation and purifications steps of an API derived from biological, biotech or fermentation processes; and the point immediately prior to the API being rendered sterile (for sterile APIs). Medicinal gases, dosage forms and radiopharmaceuticals are not covered.

In this EC draft, an API is defined thus:

> ... any substance that is represented for use in a drug (medicinal product) in the manufacturing, processing or packaging of a drug, becomes an active ingredient or a finished dosage form of the drug. Such substances are intended to furnish pharmacological activity, or other direct effect in the diagnosis, cure, mitigation, treatment or prevention of disease, or to affect the structure and function of the body of man or other animals. APIs include substances manufactured by processes such as: chemical synthesis, fermentation, recombinant DNA or other biotechnology methods, isolation/recovery from natural sources, or any combination of these processes.

In the USA, the corresponding term is 'bulk pharmaceutical chemicals' (BPCs), which applies to both active and inactive ingredients; the regulatory status of such materials in unequivocal. The US FDA's *Guide to the Inspection of Bulk Pharmaceutical Chemicals* (US FDA, 1990) states:

> BPCs are components of drug products. The manufacture of BPCs should be carried out in accordance with concepts of good manufacturing practice (GMP) consistent with this guide whether or not the manufacturers are required to register under 21 CFR 207. The manufacturers of inactive ingredients may not be required to register with FDA, but they are not exempt from complying with GMP concepts, and they are not exempt from inspection . . .

Medical devices

A **device** ('medical' being implied and understood) is defined in Section 201(h) of the US Food, Drug and Cosmetic Act as:

> Any instrument or apparatus intended for use in the diagnosis, treatment, cure
> or prevention of disease in man or other animals which does not achieve any
> of its intended purposes through chemical action or metabolism in the body.

Such articles are controlled under the US Food, Drug and Cosmetic Act 21
CFR 820 'Good manufacturing practice for medical devices' which requires
inter alia that 'every finished device manufacturer shall prepare and implement a quality assurance program that is appropriate to the specific device
manufactured'.

Devices are now, however, generally excluded from statutory control
under the UK Medicines Act (see UK definition of 'medicinal product'
above), although the UK Health Department did operate a registration (as
distinct from statutory licensing) system, in connection with which a
number of quality/GMP guidelines have been issued.

The current (1999) situation in the European Community as a whole,
with regard to medical devices, is that a Council Directive concerning
medical devices (91/C 237/03) was finally implemented on 13 June 1998
with the net effect that all medical devices sold in Europe on, or after, that
date must bear a CE mark, this mark to be granted only after evaluation of
the manufacturer by a Notified Inspection Body approved by the Competent Authority.

This device directive defines a **medical device** as:

> . . . any instrument, apparatus, appliance, material or other article, including
> software, whether used alone or in combination, intended by the manufacturer
> to be used for human beings solely, or principally for the purpose of:
>
> — diagnosis, prevention, monitoring, treatment or alleviation of disease,
>   injury or handicap,
> — investigation, replacement or modification of the anatomy or of a
>   physiological process,
> — control of conception,
>
> and which does not achieve its principal intended action in or on the human
> body by pharmacological, immunological or metabolic means, but which may
> be assisted in its functions by such means.

This definition also includes the statement that medical devices are 'here-
inafter referred to as "devices" '.

An **implantable device** is defined as:

> . . . any device which is intended:
>
> — to be totally or partially introduced into the human body or a natural
>   orifice, or
> — to replace an epithelial surface or the surface of the eye
>
> . . . by surgical intervention, which is intended to remain after the procedure
> for at least 30 days, and which can only be removed by medical or surgical
> intervention.

An *in vitro* **diagnostic device** is defined as:

> . . . any device which is a reagent, reagent product, kit, instrument, equipment
> or system, whether used alone or in combination, intended by the manufacturer
> to be used solely or principally in vitro for the examination of substances

derived from the human body with a view to providing information for the detection, diagnosis, control or treatment of a physiological state, of a state of health or disease, or of a congenital abnormality.

In the USA, the position regarding *in vitro* diagnostic products is, again, unequivocal. Requirements for manufacturers of *in vitro* diagnostics are set out in 21 CFR 809, Subpart C 809.20, which requires compliance with the CMP Regulations found in 21 CFR 820. That is, for GMP/QA purposes, *in vitro* diagnostics are treated as medical devices.

References

EC (1992). *The Rules Governing Medicinal Products in the European Community, Volume IV, Good Manufacturing Practice for Medicinal Products.* (Published 1989, revised 1992.) Luxembourg: Commission of the European Communities. Available from The Office for Official Publications of the European Communities, Luxembourg. Also available from The Stationery Office (HMSO), London, and The EC Information Service, Washington, USA. Also stated *verbatim* with guidance on the detailed interpretation of these rules in MCA, 1997. (Referred to as the EC GMP Guide.)

MCA (1997). *Rules and Guidance for Pharmaceutical Manufacturers and Distributors.* Medicines Control Agency. Available from The Stationery Office (HMSO), London.

PIC (1989). *Guide to Good Manufacturing Practice for Pharmaceutical Products.* Document PH 5/89, Convention for the Mutual Recognition of Inspection in Respect to the Manufacture of Pharmaceutical Products, September 1989. Geneva, Switzerland: Pharmaceutical Inspection Convention. Available from the EFTA Secretariat, Geneva. (Referred to as the PIC GMP Guide.)

US FDA (1990). *Code of Federal Regulations, Vol. 21, Ch. 1, Part 210,* Current good manufacturing practice in manufacturing, processing, packaging or holding of drugs, general; *CFR Vol. 21, Ch. 1, Part 211,* Current good manufacturing practice for finished pharmaceuticals; *CFR Vol. 21, Ch. 1, Part 820,* Good manufacturing practice for medical devices (revised 1995). Washington: US Food & Drug Administration. (Collectively referred to as the US CGMPs.)

2

The concept of quality

Come, give us a taste of your quality
　　　W Shakespeare, *Hamlet*, Act 2, Sc. 2

Words strain . . . slip, slide, perish . . . Decay with imprecision . . .
　　　　　T S Eliot, *Burnt Norton* from *Four Quartets*, 1944

Some words are simple, easy to define, and have just the one generally accepted meaning, or perhaps a few closely related shades of meaning. 'Quality' is, emphatically, *not* one of those words. It can have a wide range of different meanings, in both everyday and in more specialised contexts. Even some of the more formal definitions specific to the field of quality assurance have often tended to confuse rather than to clarify the issue. Indeed, surprisingly, the whole general field of 'quality' – as an activity, profession, or philosophy – tends to be muddied by an excess of imprecise and poor-quality thinking (which is not limited solely to the definition and use of terms).

The meaning of 'quality'

The Oxford English Dictionary (2nd edn, 1991) takes nearly two of its large and closely printed pages to define 'quality'. It gives 26 different definitions, plus a further six as used in very specialised contexts (logic, law, grammar, acoustics, etc.). *Webster's Dictionary* (3rd International Edition) has over 20 definitions.

A number of the dictionary definitions are relevant to persons rather than things, and here alone 'quality' can have a variety of different meanings, including:

- Character or disposition;
- Capacity, ability or skill (as, for example, in the sense intended by Hamlet in the quotation above);

- A feature of a person's character, a characteristic or trait ('he has many interesting personal qualities' – note that these could be either good or bad);
- Personal excellence ('a person of quality') and rank or position in society.

Such *personal* uses, or implications, of quality do have a certain relevance to *things* which are manufactured, in that goods are often sold (i.e. marketed) and purchased, at least in part, on the basis of what might be termed 'conferred quality': a belief that the purchase and possession of Company X's quality product (i.e. a product which is perceived to be excellent or superior) will confer a degree of personal excellence/superiority on the purchaser. While such factors are significant, although not necessarily the whole story, in the sale and purchase of, for example, Rolex watches, Gucci handbags, Saville Row suits and Rolls Royce motor cars, it is doubtful if they are notably relevant to the sale and purchase of medicinal products and the like. Consumers of medicines do not usually acquire one product or brand rather than another in order to 'feel good' (in the social superiority sense). Indeed, the decision about the nature and brand of the product that is required in any given circumstance is usually made for, not by, them.

Note in passing that it is at this 'conferring interface' between the quality of things and the quality of persons that 'quality' is perhaps at its most indeterminately woolly. What one person regards as 'quality' (in both aspects) another may not. 'Quality' in this sense has a certain analogy with 'style'. What one generation regards as stylish in reference to things or persons, another will consider crude, or perhaps quaint. One would consider that Artur Rubinstein, Muhammed Ali, Sir Thomas Beecham, Duke Ellington, Denis Compton and Marilyn Monroe all had abundance of quality, in the sense of style. It was manifest in very different ways, and by no means everybody would agree. Individual views of quality, in this sense, are both variable and subjective.

In relation to *things,* rather than persons, dictionary definitions include such concepts of quality as:

- The essential nature of some thing – that which makes it what it is.
- Nature, characteristic, property or attribute.
- Excellence, superiority, high grade.
- Degree or level of excellence – comparative grade (e.g. 'top quality', 'premium quality', 'best bitter').

This is just an outline of the more general usages of the word 'quality'. It is a slippery word, and writers and speakers (unwittingly, or with possible deliberate intent) will often be found by attentive readers or listeners to slide from one meaning to another. A careful critical attitude of mind towards all utterances (including those of the author) should be adopted on the subject of quality. This is particularly necessary now the spectrum of meaning has been extended by the more specialised usage in the field of quality control

(QC) and quality assurance (QA). Clearly, if we are going to talk of 'quality' and its 'assurance' in regard to that very special group of products with which we are concerned, we need a clear, precise definition. Any ambiguity or imprecision cannot be tolerated.

Before settling upon such a definition, and in order to emphasise that there is indeed a need for an appropriately critical attitude to the concept of 'quality', here is a brief classification of the various possible meanings.

Meanings of 'quality' classified

1. Philosophical (or Platonic)

The quality of some thing is, in this sense, its essential nature or the totality of its attributes and properties (i.e. of its 'qualities' in another sense!) which make that thing what it is. It is what the Latin word '*qualitas*', from which the English word is derived, originally meant. The 'thing' may be either concrete or abstract. For example, when Shakespeare's Portia speaks of 'the quality of mercy' she is referring to the *essential nature* of mercy.

2. Quality as meaning 'property' or 'characteristic'

For example, one of the qualities of a diamond is hardness, of a beetroot that it is red, of lead that it is heavy and of aloes that they are bitter. In this sense, a quality can be good or bad, desirable or undesirable. It is possible for a quality in this sense to be experienced via the senses, e.g. by touch, sight or taste.

3. Quality as excellence, superiority or goodness

A number of products or services are promoted and sold on the grounds of their quality. 'Quality' in this context implicitly, or explicitly, means a high degree of excellence or superiority in relation to comparable or competing products or services. This type of meaning is exemplified by exhortations of the type:

- 'Do not delay, buy one of our new quality designer homes/quality special edition motor cars/quality fitted kitchens . . . (or whatever) . . . NOW!!!'
- 'Buy your meat at J. Butcher and Sons, purveyors of quality products for over a century.'
- 'Quality you can see!' (This has actually been trumpeted in an advertisement for medical devices.)

The more formal attempts that have been made to characterise 'quality' in this sense, when examined carefully, hardly shed any real light on the subject. For example:

- [Quality is] '. . . a condition of excellence implying fine quality as distinct from poor quality . . . Quality is achieving or reaching for the highest standard, as against being satisfied with the sloppy or fraudulent' (Tuchman, 1980).
- 'Quality is neither mind nor matter, but a third entity independent of the two . . . even though quality cannot be defined, you know what it is' (Pirsig, 1974).

We are forced to conclude that this concept of quality (as excellence), although very common, is an excessively vague one.

4. Quality as a degree or level of excellence

This operates as a comparison between products or services, e.g. as in 'top quality' or 'premium quality'.

5. The traditional quality control view of 'quality'

The common, more technical, view of 'quality', which probably derives from traditional inspection/measurement approaches to QC, is the one that holds that quality consists of conformity with a predetermined specification. For example, 'Quality is the degree to which a specific product conforms to a design or specification' (Gilmore, 1974).

   Just how good is end-product testing as a determinant of the quality of a *medicinal* product? This is something we have already touched upon in Chapter 1, and the answer is 'not very good at all'. There are very great potential hazards if even only a small proportion of defective items or ingredients, undetectable by anything less than one-hundred percent testing, are present within a batch. But most testing of medicinal products can only be performed on small samples, quite simply because the majority of the tests are destructive, and if the entire batch were tested there would be no product. It is also impossible to test for everything that could be 'wrong' about a product, in terms of faults in manufacture or packaging, incidence of contamination or degradation, and so on. A third consideration is that product testing is retrospective, and is based on detection rather than prevention. *If* an end-product test detects a fault (and it may not) it *might* prevent consumer hazard. It will not prevent the waste of effort, time, money and resources spent in making the defective product.

   Thus, there needs to be a rather special approach to providing QA in the manufacture of medicines and other healthcare products. This need arises from the interaction of *three important factors:*

(a)   The severe limitations of end-product testing.
(b)   The potential high hazard of a small proportion of defectives.
(c)   The low probability of detection by the consumer.

The classic, and oft-quoted, example of the fallibility of end-product testing is that of the standard pharmacopoeial sterility test. This test is based on the

Table 2.1   How the standard sterility test can fail to detect a significant contamination level

Contaminated units (%)	0.1	1.0	5.0	10.0
Chance of passing test (%)	98	82	36	12

examination of the contents of selected test units (ampoules, vials, bottles, etc.) to see if microbial growth will result in contact with sterile bacteriological growth medium. The sample size recommended for standard industrial-scale batches is 20 units. With this sample size, the chances of passing batches at various levels of microbial contamination are as listed in Table 2.1.

Thus, there are 98 chances out of every 100 of passing a batch which has one in every thousand units contaminated (and 12 chances per 100 of passing a batch in which one in every ten units are contaminated). So much for the value of sampling and testing as a means of assuring so crucial a quality characteristic as the sterility of a product intended for injection.

In this case in particular, and indeed generally, the 'traditional quality control' view of quality is just not adequate for our purposes. What about the views and wise sayings of the professional quality experts, the so-called 'gurus'? Here, surely, we will find enlightenment?

6. The professional quality expert's view

In the more general commercial environment, a whole separate 'Quality Industry' has emerged, almost as an end in itself. Certainly, from this general 'professional quality' sphere a fair amount of unfocused thinking does seem to have emerged, along of course with much that is valuable. However, of late there has been a tendency towards uncritical acceptance of all the statements of the 'general' quality experts, whether they are relevant to the special case of the manufacture of medicines/healthcare products or not. It is wise, therefore, to cultivate a critically selective view of what is truly relevant. This is a matter to which we will return. The following are some examples of definitions of 'quality' from the 'quality experts':

- 'Quality [is] conformance to requirements' (Crosby, 1979).
- 'Quality then is simply meeting the requirements' (Oakland, 1989).
- 'Quality consists of the capacity to satisfy wants' (Edwards, 1968).
- 'The total composite product and service characteristics of marketing, engineering, manufacture and maintenance through which the product and service in use will meet the expectations of the customer' (Feigenbaum, 1986a).
- 'Quality is in its essence a way of managing the organisation' (Feigenbaum, 1986b).
- [Quality] 'means best for satisfying certain customer conditions' (Feigenbaum, 1986c).
- 'Quality refers to the amounts of the unpriced attributes contained in each unit of the priced attribute' (Leffler, 1982).
- 'The totality of features and characteristics of a product or service that

bear on its ability to satisfy stated or implied needs' (ISO 8402/BS 4778, 1986/87).
- 'Quality is fitness for purpose or use' (Juran, 1974).

Some of these definitions of 'quality' are vague and/or ambiguous. For example, although from Crosby's book as a whole his intention is fairly clear, the above quotation from it is inadequate as a stand-alone definition in the absence of a definition of 'requirements'. A 'requirement' could be 'meets specification when a 0.01% sample is tested', which does not appear to be what Crosby means. A requirement could also be 'looks good but it does not matter whether it works or not'.

Oakland, in largely mimicking Crosby, embraces the same ambiguity, and perhaps underscores it by his use of the definite article ('*the* requirements'). Many other 'definitions' are completely incomprehensible.

Quality as 'fitness for purpose'

The US codes of current good manufacturing practice (CGMP) for finished pharmaceuticals (US FDA, 1990), the 'US CGMPs', refer to 'quality control' and to a 'quality control unit'. The corresponding regulations relating to medical devices (Part 820) refer to 'quality assurance' (which is defined as 'all activities necessary to assure and verify confidence in the quality of the process used to manufacture a finished device') and to a 'quality assurance program'. Despite the *process*, rather than *product*, orientation of the device regulations, it is clear that both sets of regulations are largely directed at product quality. Neither, however, appear to define just what is meant by 'quality'.

The second edition of the *Guide to Good Pharmaceutical Manufacturing Practice* (Sharp, 1977), the UK 'Orange Guide', was probably the first publication of its type to define 'quality':

> Quality – The essential nature of a thing and the totality of its attributes and properties which bear upon its fitness for its intended purpose.

The terminological debt to Juran is obvious. The initial reference to more Platonic concepts displays a recognition that it is more than usually essential that medicinal products and the like are indeed precisely what they are intended and purported to be. This definition was repeated in the third edition (Sharp, 1983).

Although it follows the UK Orange Guide in many respects, The EC guide to GMP (EC, 1992), hereafter referred to as the 'EC GMP Guide', does not offer a formal definition of 'quality' in its Glossary. However, in the first paragraph of its first chapter, 'Quality management', it states that a manufacturer:

> . . . must manufacture medicinal products so as to ensure that they are fit for their intended use . . .

It also states that a manufacturer must ensure that their products:

. . . do not place patients at risk due to inadequate safety, quality, or efficacy.

The simple 'fitness' definition of quality is one that is clear, concise and has practical value. It does not require the resolution of questions of 'excellence', 'superiority' or 'classiness'. It also has to be asked if there is a *need* for medicinal and healthcare products which are 'superior'. Surely, what is required is that they safely and effectively do the job that they are intended to do. The sort of 'extra quality' that finds expression in many consumer products hardly has a place in relation to medicines and like products. Nor does that peculiarly modern syndrome, through which the owner of a 'quality object' believes that he or she has thereby had a measure of quality bestowed upon themselves, and thus feels good about it. We have already touched upon this type of conferred 'quality-as-superiority' which often has little or nothing to do with the practical quality and utility of an object as it is. For example, the genuine, objective, intrinsic value of a time piece (i.e. its quality in 'fitness' terms) surely must primarily reside in its time-keeping accuracy. It is now possible to buy a quartz digital watch for a few pounds with an accuracy unapproached by the traditional clockwork watches of 25 years or so ago. Yet there are those who are prepared to pay thousands of pounds for a traditional (quality?) mechanical-action watch, of possibly lower accuracy, just to feel good about it. Many medicines are intended to make you feel good (or better), but not in this way.

In this present text 'quality' is to be taken to mean 'fitness for intended purpose'. A number of definitions include such additional considerations as:

• Satisfying consumers' needs.
• At a price acceptable to the consumer.

Yet with many medicines, the ultimate consumer often doesn't *know* what he or she needs. Further, it is arguable whether economic considerations do, or should, have quite the same significance as they do in relation to such things as motor cars, package holidays, washing-up liquids or hi-fi. By and large, the need in pharmaceutical manufacturing for these probably redundant add-on extras to the simple fitness for purpose criterion is at least questionable.

There are other examples of redundancy in definition. We have already mentioned the EC GMP Guide's reference to 'safety, quality or efficacy'. Earlier, the UK Medicines Act (HMSO, 1968), in its Section 19, stated the 'factors relevant to determination of an application for a licence' (i.e. for a licence to market a product) as:

• Safety.
• Efficacy.
• Quality.

However, if the quality of a medicinal product is measured by its fitness for purpose, then safety and efficacy are not separate from quality but

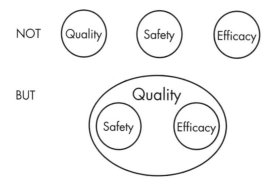

Figure 2.1 Quality definition.

are part of it. For, if a medicinal product is unsafe, and/or not efficacious, then it is not fit for its purpose. That is, quality (as defined here) must inevitably be taken to include safety and efficacy. We can depict this as in Figure 2.1.

Some texts also refer to quality *and* reliability, implying that these too are separate and distinct entities. However, if a product (particularly a medicinal product) is *un*reliable, then it is not fit for its intended purpose. Therefore reliability must also be considered as part of the overall quality and not as something which is separate or distinct from it.

Fitness for purpose in the context of medicinal products

So, what makes a medicinal product fit for its purpose? In essence when:

- *It is the right product* (made in accordance with a predetermined formula and method).
- *It is the right strength.*
- *It is free from contamination.*
- *It has in no way deteriorated or broken down.*
- *It is in the right container.*
- *It is correctly labelled.*
- *It is properly sealed in its container and protected against damage and contamination.*

That is, when it is fit to be given to, or used by, a patient in the secure knowledge and confidence that it will have the desired effects and not cause harm or damage in any way through faults in manufacture.

In principle and in concept, it all seems so very simple. However, achieving that sort of fitness for purpose, *all the time and every time*, is by no means easy, but it is what the assurance of quality in routine manufacture of pharmaceuticals is all about.

There are other facets of quality which need to be considered.

The two major aspects of quality

All efforts to manufacture goods which are fit for their intended purpose will be wasted if there is some flaw or omission in their original design which renders them fundamentally unfit or inadequate. It is thus conventional, and sound quality theory, to distinguish between two separate, but interrelated aspects of quality:

- Quality of design.
- Quality of manufacture.

(Note that the second aspect may sometimes be stated as 'quality of conformance'. 'Quality of manufacture' or even 'quality *in* manufacture' is preferred, because it avoids any possible implication that quality consists in mere conformity with a specification.)

Before a product of any sort can be manufactured to be 'fit', it must be designed (that is, researched and developed) to ensure that it will achieve its stated, desired and intended purpose. If it is not, nothing done during the manufacturing process can satisfactorily correct any fundamental and inherent flaw. The obvious corollary is that even the most quality-perfect design can be ruined by faults in the manufacturing process; that is, by failure to ensure quality of or in manufacture.

There is another side to quality of design which has sometimes been forgotten. A perfectly designed product will be of little or no value if it is not technologically feasible, or economically viable, to produce the product on a large scale. Large-scale manufacture is usually a very different proposition to the one-off or few-off of R and D, or pilot-scale production.

Some years ago, a company designed and developed an injectable product for use in critical life-or-death situations. It was a two-component system – two liquids which needed to be mixed before injection, but which were unstable when mixed, except in the very shortest term. They therefore needed to be mixed immediately before injection. The product, as designed, was a two-compartment pre-filled syringe. The two liquids were separated by a membrane, which was intended to be broken just before administration (rupture membrane/shake/inject). However, a complicating factor was that it was not possible to sterilise the product terminally. All parts (syringe components, active liquids) had to be separately pre-sterilised and then assembled and filled aseptically. It was quite possible to do this on a laboratory-bench scale, but the product was so complex that aseptic assembly (with assurance of sterility) on any commercially viable scale or rate, and with the resources then available, was just not possible. The project was abandoned.

The two aspects of quality (quality of design and quality of manufacture) therefore pose the following two questions:

1.   Is it designed to be fit?
2.   Does the design allow that fitness to be reproduced in routine large-scale manufacture?

Much (some might argue virtually all) of the 'quality of manufacture' aspect is embraced, in the healthcare field, by the requirements of GMP. It is necessary therefore to consider the relationships and interactions between quality assurance, good manufacturing practice and quality control. But first it will be necessary to consider the regulatory factor, as regulatory bodies have much to say about quality and related concepts.

References

Crosby P B (1979). *Quality is Free*. New York: New American Library, p. 15.

EC (1992). *The Rules Governing Medicinal Products in the European Community, Vol. IV: Good Manufacturing Practice for Medicinal Products*. Luxembourg: Commission of the European Communities. Available from The Office for Official Publications of the European Communities, Luxembourg. Also available from The Stationery Office (HMSO), London, and The EC Information Service, Washington, USA. Also stated *verbatim* with guidance on the detailed interpretation of these rules in MCA, 1997. (Referred to as the EC GMP Guide.)

Edwards C D (1968). The meaning of quality. *Qual Prog* October, 37.

Feigenbaum A V (1986a). *Total Quality Control*, 3rd edn. New York: McGraw-Hill, p. 7.

Feigenbaum A V (1986b). Ibid., p. xxi.

Feigenbaum A V (1986c). Ibid., p. 9.

Gilmore H L (1974). Product conformance cost. *Qual Prog* June, 16.

HMSO (1968). *The Medicines Act 1968*. London: Her Majesty's Stationery Office.

ISO 8402/BS 4778 (1986/1987) *Quality Vocabulary: Part 1, International Terms*. Available from the British Standards Institute.

Juran J M (1974). *Quality Control Handbook*, 3rd edn. New York: McGraw-Hill.

Leffler K B (1982). Ambiguous changes in product quality. *Am Econ Rev* December, 956.

MCA (1997). *Rules and Guidance for Pharmaceutical Manufacturers and Distributors*. London: Medicines Control Agency. Available from The Stationery Office (HMSO), London.

Oakland (1989). *Total Quality Management*. Oxford: Heineman Professional Publishing, p. 3.

Pirsig R M (1974). *Zen and the Art of Motorcycle Maintenance*. New York: Bantam Books.

Sharp J, ed. (1977). *Guide to Good Pharmaceutical Manufacturing Practice*, 2nd edn. London: HMSO.

Sharp J, ed. (1983). *Guide to Good Pharmaceutical Manufacturing Practice*, 3rd edn. London: HMSO. Also stated *verbatim* with guidance on the detailed interpretation of these rules in MCA, 1997. (Referred to as the UK Orange Guide.)

Tuchman B W (1980). The decline of quality. *N Y Times Magazine* 2 November, 38.

US FDA (1990). *Code of Federal Regulations, Vol. 21, Ch. 1, Part 210*, Current good manufacturing practice in manufacturing, processing, packaging or holding of drugs, general; *CFR Vol. 21, Ch. 1, Part 211*, Current good manufacturing practice for finished pharmaceuticals; *CFR Vol. 21, Ch. 1, Part 820*, Good manufacturing practice for medical devices (revised 1995). Washington: US Food & Drug Administration. (Collectively referred to as the US CGMPs.)

3

The regulatory factor: background

It is time now to write the next chapter, and to write it in the books of law
   L B Johnson (1908–1973), 36th President of the USA, speech to Congress 1963

The first thing we do, let's kill all the lawyers
   W Shakespeare, *Henry IV, Part 2*, Act 4, Sc. 2

Government health authorities are, naturally and rightly, concerned about the quality of medicines and healthcare products. It should not, however, be forgotten that the objective of quality assurance is not *primarily* the satisfaction of the demands of national or multinational regulatory bodies. It is the assurance of the safety, protection and well-being of the consumer, or patient. Ideally, in this area, regulatory and industrial aims should be closely similar, and it would seem sensible that a cooperative, rather than a confrontational relationship should be fostered.

Regulatory bodies now usually legislate for the 'two aspects of quality' (see Chapter 2) by:

(a) Some form of product registration or licensing (the US New Drug Applications, the UK Product Licence or the EC Marketing Authorisation, for example) to regulate 'quality of design'.
(b) Setting down their quality requirements for routine manufacture in the form of good manufacturing practice (GMP) regulations and/or guidelines.

If the regulations/guidelines are inadequate to ensure the necessary degree of consumer protection, then it is the regulatory authority which is mainly at fault. If regulatory demands are in excess of what is necessary, and thus inhibit innovation or stifle investment, then the regulatory body is again blameworthy. If the demands are sensible, reasonable and well-founded, and the industry responds positively, then all should be well: consumers will be protected and a good cooperative relationship may be expected to exist between the regulators and the regulated. If the industry fails to respond to reasonable quality demands, then the industry is ethically and professionally culpable and commercially stupid. In this case, the regulatory authority would also again be at fault for failing to enforce its reasonable demands.

The interaction between industry and regulations

The historical development of attitudes towards the maintenance of the quality of manufactured medicines has thus been both two-pronged and interactive: industrial/professional on the one hand, and regulatory on the other. The two 'sides' obviously interact, although at any one time it is not always entirely clear which side is leading and which is following. This has led to the concept of the regulatory/industry 'spiral stairway effect' which can (if uncontrolled) result in evermore (and unnecessarily) demanding standards (see Fig. 3.1).

Ideally, this interaction should work to the ultimate benefit of the consumer, and also provide salutary incentives to the manufacturer. Confrontation is unlikely to be beneficial, although it has not always been avoided.

The broad thrust of this historical development may also be considered to fall into three main phases. In the very early days, the sole emphasis was on 'following the recipe'. Then, in around 1880, a product was placed on the market which was claimed to be the first to have a standardised potency, confirmed by assay on each batch. (It was a Liquid Extract of Ergot.) This could well be considered as the start of the second phase which, as analytical methodology and resources developed, nourished the widespread notion that end-product testing was the all-important determinant of 'quality' – a view that took some time to die, and which has still perhaps not been entirely laid to rest. It has, however, largely been replaced by the current view that true assurance of quality can only be achieved when such testing is regarded as but part of an overall picture, and is integrated within a more general framework of a detailed understanding and appraisal of the methods and conditions of manufacture. Generally, regulatory trends have followed the same historical pattern.

It is widely believed that the USA was one of the very first, if not *the* first nation, to put in place *comprehensive* regulatory control of the quality of medicinal and other healthcare products. This, indeed, is probably true, although it is always dangerous to make sweeping unqualified assertions about who, or what, was first in any field. It is important to note the word 'comprehensive', and to remember (see Chapter 1) that quality (as defined) embraces safety and efficacy. Certainly, a wide variety of diverse elements of regulatory or other official control had been instituted in different parts of the world long before the relevant US Acts, but they are nevertheless a convenient place to start.

Regulation in the USA

The first extensive US federal law regulating medicinal (drug) products is generally considered to be the Pure Food and Drugs Act of 1906, a stimulus for which was a growing awareness of instances of adulteration, fraudulent claims and insanitary manufacturing conditions. This Act was, however, far

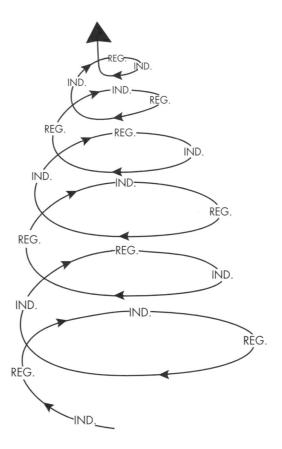

Figure 3.1   The industrial/regulatory interactive spiral staircase effect. Industry makes a technological advance or develops a new concept; regulatory agency embraces it in a new regulation or guideline; industry moves to comply, and the more advanced companies (possibly 'encouraged' by the more zealous inspectors, or possibly to out-do their competitors) 'go one better'; regulatory agency responds to this new 'state of the art' by tightening, or introducing new, requirements; industry responds accordingly . . . and so on, ever upwards and onwards on a spiral of increasingly demanding standards. Alternatively, the process may be kicked-off by the regulators, but whichever way it happens the whole effect is often stimulated by the 'experts' – the writers, speakers, seminar organisers, etc. – who purport to explain (for a fee) 'how to meet the new requirements'.
IND = industry; REG = regulatory body.

from comprehensive and was much more limited in scope than current US law. It was intended to regulate adulterated and misbranded food and drugs which might enter into interstate commerce. It did not require that the Federal Government should review a product or its labelling prior to marketing, or that evidence should be provided as to efficacy. (It is interesting, however, to note that an earlier federal law, of 1902, did in fact require pre-marketing clearance and licensing in the limited area of 'biologics'.)

In 1937 an elixir of sulphanilamide was marketed in the USA, resulting in the death of approximately one-hundred people as a consequence of diethylene glycol having been used as a vehicle. This led to the passing of the 1938 Federal Food, Drug and Cosmetic (FD&C) Act, which extended the concept of statutory pre-marketing clearance to drug products other than biologics (initially only to those placed on the market for the first time after the effective date of the Act). The major emphasis was on safety; evidence of efficacy was not required, and the federal officials who reviewed the safety data indicated their acceptance of an application simply by taking no action.

New drug applications (NDAs)

In 1962, the 1938 FD&C Act was amended to include, among other things, a requirement for evidence of efficacy as well as safety. No new drug could now legally be marketed without positive government approval of a formal application to market, called a new drug application (NDA). Requirements for the data required as evidence of safety and efficacy, assurance of product quality and labelling are set out in considerable and specific detail, and the required content of an NDA is defined at some length, to include information on, for example:

- Chemistry, method of manufacture and quality control
- Preclinical pharmacology and toxicology
- Human pharmacokinetics and bioavailability
- Clinical trial data
- Stability studies
- Statistical data
- Proposed labelling.

Abbreviated NDAs (ANDAs), containing only chemistry, manufacturing and bioequivalence data, are all that is required to market duplicates of drug products already on the market. This can only happen after a 5-year period of exclusivity given to new chemical entities has elapsed.

Quality of design regulations and CGMPs

In this fashion the amended FD&C Act regulated the quality of design aspect. Furthermore, 1962 also saw the introduction of a requirement that all drugs marketed in the USA, including those marketed without an NDA (for example, older products that had been on the market before 1938), must be manufactured in accordance with 'current good manufacturing practice' (CGMP). Any drug product not manufactured in accordance with CGMP is deemed to be adulterated (whether it has been shown to be defective or not) and 'the person who is responsible for the failure to comply shall be subject to regulatory action'. All manufacturers must register with the Food and Drug Administration (FDA), listing all the products they

make. Usually, a manufacturing facility is inspected by FDA investigators
prior to approving a new application, and all US manufacturing plants are
inspected periodically (in theory, but possibly not always in practice, at
least every 2 years). The FDA inspect foreign facilities at the time of NDA
approval, and periodically after that. An exception is where there is a reciprocal recognition agreement, as there is between the FDA and the regulatory bodies of Canada, Switzerland and Sweden. (Note: At the time of
writing, a number of other mutual recognition agreements (MRAs) are in
the early stages of implementation, notably one between the USA and the
EU.)

The 1962 amendment (the 'Kefauver-Harris amendment') also specified what was then perceived as constituting current good manufacturing
practice. It is, however, interesting to note that probably the first official
document to set down the basic principles of GMP was published in Canada
in 1957 (Canada, 1957). This document is clearly 'about GMP', although
it does not in fact use that term, which did indeed make its first 'official'
appearance in the US 1962 amendment.

The FDA regulations for current good manufacturing practice (the US
CGMPs) have been subject to various revisions and updating processes, and
are published in the US Code of Federal Regulations (US FDA, 1990).

Over the years, the FDA has also issued a series of drug and biologic
guidelines, which include guidance on such matters as clinical evaluation,
OTC drugs, biotechnology, labelling, drug master files, and various GMP
issues such as validation, aseptic processing, cleaning and computer
systems. These guidelines do not have full legal status but are intended as
guidance to compliance with the regulatory requirements, or as guidance
to their own staff on performing different types of inspection. (Examples
of FDA guidelines are listed in Annex I to this chapter.) On 3 May 1996,
the FDA published, in the Federal Register, some proposed revisions to
their CGMP regulations. At the time of writing, these proposals are still
under discussion.

The FDA have separate GMP regulations for medical devices – CFR
Vol. 21, Part 820 (US FDA, 1990). The major sections ('subparts') of these
regulations cover:

(a) General provisions, scope, definitions and quality assurance
(b) Organisation and personnel
(c) Buildings
(d) Equipment
(e) Control of components
(f) Production and process controls
(g) Packaging and labelling control
(h) Holding, distribution and installation
(i) Device evaluation
(j) Records.

The CFR Vol. 21, Part 820 regulations were last revised in 1995.

The UK regulatory scene

The earliest known written code on the quality of medicinal substances in Britain was the *Ordinances of the Guild of Pepperers of Soper Lane* in 1316, the worthy gentlemen of this Guild having taken over the distribution of the imported herbs and spices then used in medicine. Over the subsequent centuries a variety of measures were introduced by various statutory and professional bodies to regulate, and more specifically to exert control over, the quality of healthcare products and materials. The first edition of the *London Pharmacopoeia* appeared in 1618. The *Edinburgh Pharmacopoeia* appeared in 1699, and the *Dublin Pharmacopoeia* in 1807. In 1858 the Medical Act created the General Medical Council, one of the duties of which was to compile an official pharmacopoeia for the whole of the UK The first edition of the *British Pharmacopoeia* was published in 1864.

There was an Adulteration of Food and Drugs Act in 1872, and a Sale of Food and Drugs Act in 1875, but these were of limited application. In the 1920s, the increasing realisation of the problems of standardisation and of controlling the quality of biologicals and the new chemotherapeutic substances (specifically the then new arsphenamines of Paul Ehrlich) led to the Therapeutic Substances Act (TSA). This was originally passed in 1925, and was revised and amended a number of times subsequently. It applied, however, only to a limited range of substances, principally to vaccines, sera, toxins, antitoxins, antigens, arsphenamine and related compounds, insulin, pituitary hormones, and surgical sutures. Other groups of substances were added subsequently, but the TSA was never comprehensive in its coverage. It did however provide for a government licensing system, and it displayed an early recognition that (within the Act's sphere of influence at least) the competence of the workers and the conditions under which they worked were at least as important as the tests applied to the end product. Factory inspections and in-process control were therefore significant aspects of the supervision exerted by the Licensing Authority.

Among other enactments were the Pharmacy and Poisons Act of 1933, the Venereal Disease Act of 1917 and the Cancer Act of 1939. The latter two were concerned with preventing fraudulent claims of efficacy in these two conditions.

Despite this relatively long history of control (*in some form*), the overall UK regulatory situation, prior to 1968, was that while there had been this piecemeal regulation of *some* aspects of the quality of *some* medicines, and there had been legislation on poisons and drugs of addiction for many years, there was no comprehensive, integrated body of law to control the manufacture, sale, supply, advertising, etc. of *all* medicines. Furthermore, although responsible British-based pharmaceutical manufacturers had practised some form of some aspects of GMP prior to the late 1960s, there was no nationally agreed and accepted GMP code or guideline.

Comprehesive regulation

The thalidomide tragedy of the early 1960s focused attention in the UK on the lack of comprehensive medicines legislation. The immediate reaction was the setting up of an interim voluntary scheme for the assessment of all new drug data by an independent body of government-appointed experts. This system *was* voluntary and applied only to new drug substances, but the industry responded well, and it was by no means a toothless system. The Committee on Safety of Drugs (as the body of experts was then called), under its chairman Sir Derrick Dunlop, published the results of its deliberations in the *London Gazette*. Nevertheless, it became generally felt that more extensive, *statutory* control was required and the ultimate result was the passing of the UK Medicines Act of 1968. It is both one of the longest acts ever to pass through a British parliament, and one of the most extensive pieces of medicines legislation ever, anywhere. Among many other things, the new Act introduced a system of Product Licences (similar in concept to the US NDAs, and thus regulating quality of design) covering both old and new medicinal products. It also introduced a separate system for the licensing of manufacturing sites and facilities by Manufacturer's Licences. The Manufacturer's Licence system provides the framework for the statutory control of quality of manufacture.

Product and manufacturer licensing

A high proportion of the UK Medicines Act, and a great deal of the mass of subordinate legislation (that is, the implementing Regulations, or Statutory Instruments) that has been issued under it, is about product licensing. However, the conditions and requirements for the ongoing processes of manufacture and control are treated very briefly and very generally. The legal requirements for these aspects were originally stated (in no more than one-and-a-half pages) in Schedule 2 of The Medicines (Standard Provisions for Licences and Certificates) Regulations (S.I. No. 972 of 1971). Under these regulations the holder of a Manufacturer's Licence was required, for example to:

1. Provide and maintain such staff . . . as are necessary for the carrying out in accordance with his licence, and the relevant product licence, of such stages of manufacture and assembly . . . as are undertaken by him.
2. Provide and maintain such staff . . . for the handling, storage and distribution . . . as are necessary to avoid deterioration of the medicinal product.
3. Provide and maintain such staff . . . as are necessary for carrying-out in accordance with the relevant product licence any tests of strength, quality or purity of the medicinal products that he manufactures . . . [or] make arrangements with a person approved by the Licensing Authority for such tests to be carried-out. . .

GMP legislation

Under the Medicines Act, and its statutory regulations, there was little or nothing that is any more detailed or comprehensive than that. These regulations have subsequently been amended to require compliance with certain provisions of the, also relatively brief and general, 'EC GMP Directives' (91/356/EEC and 91/412/EEC); see later in this chapter. This does not alter the general proposition that GMP *regulations* in the UK are relatively sparse.

Clearly, some more substantial flesh was needed on those original very bare regulatory bones. This was provided in the form of a *guide* to GMP, rather than in GMP regulations. This guide was produced by the Medicines Inspectorate of the UK Health Department, in consultation with the industry, the professions and with all other interested parties.

The Medicines Act requires the establishment of an organisation to inspect manufacturing, warehousing and testing facilities in order to confirm compliance with the law and with the principles of GMP. This body was, and is, the UK Medicines Inspectorate which was formed in the late 1960s and became operational in early 1972. The work of this body is roughly comparable to that of the FDA investigators. However, they use as a major basis for their work not GMP regulations but the non-statutory consultative GMP guide. The first edition was published in 1971, the second in 1977 and the third and last edition in 1983 (Sharp, 1983). Due to the colour of its original cover, the guide ubiquitously became known as the 'UK Orange Guide' and has remained orange in all subsequent editions.

It is worth emphasising that the UK 'Guide' was indeed what its title suggests. That is, it is an indication of the means of attaining satisfactory standards of manufacture and control, but it states explicitly that the methods outlined are not the only ones necessarily capable of achieving those standards. In contrast to the US CGMP regulations (US FDA, 1990), the UK Orange Guide does not have full statutory force in UK legislation. However, failure to comply with its guidance without adequate justification may be considered in any proceedings under the Medicines Act. A compliance with the spirit and overall standards of the guide, rather than strict adherence to every statement, was always a feature of the UK regulatory control of manufacturing activities, and has led to a cooperative rather than a confrontational relationship between the industry and the Medicines Inspectorate. Certainly, by and large, the provisions of the UK Orange Guide were well accepted in Britain (and elsewhere) as a consensus on sensible GMP. Thus their application in the UK is largely a matter of discussion and cooperation between the Inspectorate and the industry, rather than one of one-sided enforcement by the former.

Medical devices

UK medicines legislation does not embrace medical devices, and the definition of a medicinal product given in the UK Medicines Act specifically excludes any 'instrument, apparatus or appliance'. A Medical Devices Directorate, within the UK Department of Health, from 1981 operated a registration scheme for the manufacturers of such products. Until 1985 it was restricted to manufacturers of sterile medical devices and cardiac pacemakers. From April 1985 its scope was extended to include medical equipment that relies on a power source and is intended for use in diagnosis or treatment. Orthopaedic implants were included in the scheme from December 1985, and various items of rehabilitation equipment from 1986. The current (1999) situation is that a European Council Directive concerning Medical Devices (EC, 1991a) was implemented on 13 June 1998 with the net effect that all medical devices sold in Europe on, or after, that date must bear a 'CE' mark, this mark to be granted only after evaluation of the manufacturer by a Notified Inspection Body approved by the Competent Authority.

The UK Medical Devices Agency, in the past, issued a series of documents on quality systems/good manufacturing practice requirements, against which applicants for registration were assessed, including:

- Guide to good manufacturing practice for sterile medical devices and surgical products (1990).
- Quality systems for implantable cardiac pacemakers.
- Guide to good manufacturing practice for medical equipment.
- Guide to good manufacturing practice for orthopaedic implants.
- Quality systems for dental materials.

GMP and other regulatory matters in Europe generally

In Europe as a whole, the mid–1960s and 70s were fertile times for the development and spread of regulatory concepts. In the wake of the thalidomide disaster, a number of countries introduced, or tightened, their regulatory systems for medicinal products, and formed their own inspectorates to assess and monitor manufacturing operations.

However, the enacted regulations and published guidelines produced by the various European Health Authorities during this period tended in most cases to place major emphasis on measures to examine, evaluate and control the 'quality, safety and efficacy' of drug substances (particularly new drug substances, or new presentations of existent drugs). In contrast, in some countries the assurance of quality by the observance of good practices in the ongoing, day-to-day processes of manufacture received notably less attention, at least as far as any formal published GMP guidelines are concerned. (Put simply, and in US terms, many countries awarded greater importance to NDAs than GMPs.)

(The author's personal opinion is that this is a reflection of the fact that ministers, officials and administrators, and many of their advisers, find the dangers of thalidomide-type incidents easier to grasp, and readily concede the need to protect against these dangers. Perhaps surprisingly to those who have been actively involved in manufacture, the just-as-real hazards of 'bad manufacturing practices' are *not* so obvious to those who have not had this practical experience and involvement. To illustrate the point: by the mid–1970s many European countries had some form of medicines regulatory law in place. Yet when, in 1981, the author prepared a comparison of the then available European Community guides and certain other national and international GMP guides and regulations (as background material for an EEC Working Group set up to consider a European GMP Guide), he found that only four European national GMP guidelines were available. These were from Denmark, France, Italy and the UK. Of these, only two were documents of any size and substance – those from France and the UK. Since 1981, other national European GMP guidelines have been published (e.g. in Holland and Greece), as have substantially revised and enlarged editions of the UK and French guides. And there is now the EC GMP Guide (EC, 1992), to which we will shortly return.)

One of the first European initiatives to formalise an industry view of what constituted GMP was the preparation, in 1968, by the European Pharmaceutical Industries Association (EPIA), of a Basic Code of Pharmaceutical Manufacturing Practices. This was commended by the members of EPIA, including the Association of the British Pharmaceutical Industry (ABPI), to their member companies 'as a source of guidance on the minimum standards which are desirable in pharmaceutical manufacture'. Although in comparison with later guides on GMP, the EPIA document appears very rudimentary, it none the less articulated some of the basic philosophies of pharmaceutical manufacture and control which were already generally accepted and practised by the better and more responsible manufacturers.

It is of interest to note that, at about the same time as the EPIA was drawing up its GMP Code, the World Health Organisation (WHO) was also elaborating a guideline on GMP which it was hoped would find international acceptability as a basic standard for worldwide use. The WHO guidelines were adopted by the World Health Assembly of 1969 and a number of states enshrined the WHO guidelines verbatim in their national legislation. Most notable of these until its accession to the Pharmaceutical Inspection Convention (PIC – see Annex II to this chapter) was the then Federal Republic of Germany. In a very similar fashion to the EPIA Guide, the WHO guide did not purport to be a comprehensive treatise on GMP, and it certainly did not contain anything like the detailed advice of some of the later guides – notably the UK, French, and European Community Guides. What the WHO guideline did do was to provide a very basic outline of the minimum steps required to set up a manufacturing facility which would be capable of producing medicines to a standard acceptable to WHO. As such, it formed a basis for the WHO Certification Scheme for Essential Drugs.

The increase in medicines legislation and control inevitably led to the institution of various inspectorates to assess and monitor the suitability of pharmaceutical manufacturers (the UK Medicines Inspectorate was one of these). This, and the ever-expanding nature of the market, led to consideration of agreements on the mutual recognition of inspectorates. One such agreement was the Pharmaceutical Inspection Convention (PIC) which produced its own GMP guidelines (see Annex II to this chapter).

UK and EC authorisations

Member states of the European Community (EC) are required to implement a system of what are termed 'marketing authorisations', which are closely comparable to the UK Product Licences and the US NDAs. Quality of manufacture is regulated within the Community by a parallel system of 'manufacturing authorisations', closely similar in nature, content and application to the former UK Manufacturer's Licences. It is illegal to sell or supply medicinal products within the Community that have not been granted a marketing authorisation and which have not been manufactured, tested and approved for release at a facility (or facilities) which is subject to a manufacturing authorisation. The granting of a manufacturing licence involves, among other things, inspection by agents of the relevant national health authority to monitor compliance with good manufacturing practice.

The EC GMP Guide

The first move towards harmonisation of GMP requirements in the EC were made in the early 1980s when a working group of the European Commission's Pharmaceutical Committee was first set up to look at the feasibility of producing a Community Guide to GMP. Armed with the comparison of various existing guidelines/regulations mentioned above, this working party set about preparing a draft guide for consultation. This was eventually published in summer 1987 and was fully reviewed by industry both at a national and European level. The draft drew most heavily on the UK Orange Guide (Sharp, 1983), and to a lesser extent on the French guidelines on GMP, the *Bonnes Pratiques de Fabrication* (BPF). Consultation with the European industry continued through the early part of 1988 and the final document was published in January 1989, with an annex on the manufacture of sterile medicinal products. In January 1992, the document was reprinted, with a few textual amendments, and issued with a number of additional annexes on more specific topics, for example, on the manufacture of biological medicinal products, radiopharmaceuticals and medicinal gases. In 1993, the UK Medicines Control Agency issued, as a fourth edition of the UK Orange Guide, the full text of the EC GMP Guide, plus other material, under the title *Rules and Guidance for Pharmaceutical Manufacturers*. In 1997, the MCA issued a fifth edition, under the title *Rules and Guidance for Pharmaceutical Manufacturers and Distributors*. This latest edition (MCA, 1997), in addition to the full text of the EC GMP Guide (EC, 1992) plus a total of 14 more specific annexes, contains the texts of the two GMP Directives (91/456/EEC and 91/412/EEC) on products for human use and for animal use, respectively. It also contains the UK Standard Provisions for Manufacturer's Licences, the Code of Practice for Qualified Persons, UK Guidance on Certificates of Analysis, the UK Standard Provisions for

Wholesale Dealer's Licences and guidance on the appointment and duties of the Responsible Person, the Directive 92/25/EEC on Wholesale Distribution, the EC Guidelines on Good Distribution Practice, and a note on the UK Defective Medicines Report Centre.

An EC directive requires the acceptance by every member state of reports on pharmaceutical manufacturers prepared by other member states. In effect, a mutual recognition of inspections within member states has been introduced. There is a provision for one member state to question the content of a report prepared by another member state, but the criteria upon which such questioning can be based have yet to be clarified.

EC Directive 91/356/EEC (EC, 1991b) made compliance with stated broad general principles of GMP mandatory. Again, in a process closely comparable to that which had already existed in the UK, compliance with general GMP principles is mandatory. A non-statutory guideline provides detailed guidance on how to comply, whilst recognising that there may well be acceptable alternative methods.

Regarding regulation of medical devices in the European Community, as noted in Chapter 1 there is an EC Device Directive, which lays down *inter alia* requirements for design, specification, labelling, testing, quality assurance and quality systems.

It would be beyond the scope of this chapter to consider in detail all other regulations and/or guidelines worldwide. They occur widely, at various levels of detail and complexity. For example, there are now over 25 national or international GMP guides, codes or regulations. The most noteworthy are perhaps the US CGMPs, the Australian Code, the Canadian GMPs, the French BPF, the UK Orange Guide, the Japanese document, the EC Guidelines and the ASEAN (Association of South East Asian Nations) Guidelines. The World Health Organisation has also recently published a revised and much enlarged edition. In terms of extent of worldwide copying or imitation (in whole or in part), it is probably true to say that the UK Orange Guide is the one which has been the most influential, outside the Americas.

References

Canada (1957). *Manufacture, Control and Distribution of Drugs.* Specifications Board, Supply and Services, Canada.

EC (1991a). Commission proposal for a council directive concerning medical devices. *Commission Directive 91/42/EEC,* COM(91) 287 final-SYN 353. Available from The Office for Official Publications of the European Communities, Luxembourg.

EC (1991b). *Commission Directive 91/356/EEC.* Laying down the principles and guidelines of good manufacturing practice for medicinal products for human use. Available from The Office for Official Publications of the European Communities, Luxembourg.

EC (1992). *The Rules Governing Medicinal Products in the European Community,*

Vol. IV: Good Manufacturing Practice for Medicinal Products. Luxembourg: Commission of the European Communities. Available from The Office for Official Publications of the European Communities, Luxembourg. Also available from The Stationery Office (HMSO), London, and the EC Information Service, Washington, USA. Also stated *verbatim* with guidance on the detailed interpretation of these rules in MCA, 1997. (Referred to as the EC GMP Guide.)

MCA (1997). *Rules and Guidance for Pharmaceutical Manufacturers and Distributors.* London: Medicines Control Agency. Available from The Stationery Office, London.

Sharp J, ed. (1983). *Guide to Good Pharmaceutical Manufacturing Practice,* 3rd edn. London: HMSO. (Referred to as the UK Orange Guide.)

US FDA (1990). *Code of Federal Regulations, Vol. 21, Ch. 1, Part 210,* Current good manufacturing practice in manufacturing, processing, packaging or holding of drugs, general; *CFR Vol. 21, Ch. 1, Part 211,* Current good manufacturing practice for finished pharmaceuticals; *CFR Vol. 21, Ch. 1, Part 820,* Good manufacturing practice for medical devices (revised 1995). Washington: US Food & Drug Administration. (Collectively referred to as the US CGMPs.)

Annex I

Some relevant FDA guidelines

The US CGMPs are set down in various parts of the US Code of Federal Regulations (US FDA, 1990). FDA *guidelines* do not have full legal status but are intended as guidance to compliance with the regulatory requirements, or as guidance to their own staff on performing different types of inspection. FDA guidelines of particular relevance include:

- Guideline on Sterile Drug Products Produced by Aseptic Processing
- Guideline on the General Principles of Process Validation
- Guide to Inspection of Bulk Pharmaceutical Chemical Manufacturing
- Guidelines for Drug Master Files (DMFs)
- Good Automated Laboratory Practice
- Stability Testing of Biotechnological Products
- General Principles of Software Validation
- Manufacture, Processing or Holding of Active Pharmaceutical Ingredients
- Guideline on Validation of Analytical Procedures for Pharmaceuticals
- Guidance on the Validation of Chromatographic Methods
- Medical Devices: Validation and Routine Control of Ethylene Oxide Sterilisation.

The following are primarily aimed at the FDA's own inspectors (or 'investigators'), but become available for general consumption under the US Freedom of Information (FOI) Act:

- Guide to Inspection of Active Pharmaceutical Ingredient Manufacturers
- Guide to Inspections of Foreign Pharmaceutical Manufacturers
- Guide to Inspections of Foreign Medical Device Manufacturers
- Guide to Inspection of Computerised Systems in Drug Processing
- Guideline for the Manufacture of In-Vitro Diagnostic Products
- Guide to Inspection of Dosage Form Drug Manufacturers
- Guide to Inspection of High Purity Water Systems
- Guide to Inspection of Lyophilization of Parenterals
- Guide to Inspection of Microbiological Quality Control
- Guide to Inspection of Oral Solid Dosage Forms

- Guide to Inspection of Oral Solutions and Suspensions
- Guide to Inspection of Pharmaceutical Quality Control Laboratories
- Guide to Inspection of Sterile Drug Substance Manufacturers
- Guide to Inspection of Topical Drug Products
- Guide to Inspection of Validation of Cleaning Processes.

Copies of most, if not all of these documents can be obtained from the Executive Secretariat, CDER, 7500 Standish Place, Rockville, MD 20855, USA. Fax +1 (301) 594 1118 or the Office of Regulatory Affairs, The US Food and Drug Administration, 5600 Fishers Lane, Rockville, MD 20857, USA.

Reference

US FDA (1990). *Code of Federal Regulations, Vol. 21, Ch. 1, Part 210,* Current good manufacturing practice in manufacturing, processing, packaging or holding of drugs, general; *CFR Vol. 21, Ch. 1, Part 211,* Current good manufacturing practice for finished pharmaceuticals; *CFR Vol. 21, Ch. 1, Part 820,* Good manufacturing practice for medical devices (revised 1995). Washington: US Food & Drug Administration. (Collectively referred to as the US CGMPs.)

Annex II

The Pharmaceutical Inspection Convention (PIC)

In 1960, a European Free Trade Association (EFTA) was formed to reduce trade barriers between its members. EFTA was, and is, a different organisation from the European Community. The original EFTA countries were the Scandinavian countries, plus Austria, Switzerland and the UK.

One document from EFTA which is of relevance in our present context, is the international agreement entitled the 'Convention for the Mutual Recognition of Inspections in Respect of the Manufacture of Pharmaceutical Products'. This is usually referred to more briefly as 'The Pharmaceutical Inspection Convention' or PIC.

This Convention was ratified in 1971, between the then members of EFTA. Fundamentally, it is an agreement between the health authorities of the member states that they will, on request, and subject to the agreement of the manufacturer(s) concerned, exchange information obtained during their own national inspections of manufacturing sites. The importing authority could then appraise this information in relation to their own national requirements. Thus, whilst inspections across the various national boundaries were not precluded by the Convention, the need to carry out such inspections was expected to be much reduced, and that indeed proved to be the case.

Although the Convention was originally framed within EFTA, membership has never been restricted solely to EFTA countries. It was, and still is, open to any member of the United Nations that can satisfy the officials of PIC that they have adequate medicines legislation, and a properly functioning medicines inspectorate. Some of the original members of EFTA, including the UK, have later left to join the EC, but have remained as members of PIC. Thus PIC, whilst still receiving administrative support from the Geneva offices of EFTA virtually took on a separate life of its own.

Officials of the Convention meet regularly, in an attempt to ensure common standards, and representatives of all member states meet at seminars (several days) around twice a year. The published papers of these seminars provide a useful source of information. (Copies are obtainable from the EFTA Secretariat, Geneva.)

The Convention has also published its own formal statement on GMP, the original, quite brief, *Basic Standards of GMP*. This has been supplemented over the years by the separate publication of more detailed, specific Guidelines on:

- Handling of Starting Materials
- Manufacturing and Analysis under Contract
- Sterile Products
- Good Control Laboratory Practice
- Manufacture of Active Ingredients.

The similarity of many of these guidelines to the corresponding sections of the UK Orange Guide (Sharp, 1983) is a mark of the influence that the Orange Guide has had in Europe generally.

The membership of PIC has grown steadily, and the number of requests for information exchange increases every year. It is interesting to note that the UK accounts for the overall highest number of requests, both for information required and for information supplied.

However, in 1997 the PIC was in the process of being replaced by PICS (Pharmaceutical Inspection Co-operation Scheme) since some aspects of PIC were in conflict with European Community Law. Until all PIC members become members of PICS, both organisations will operate in parallel. Current membership of PICS comprises Australia, Belgium, Czech Republic, Denmark, Finland, France, Hungary, Iceland, Ireland, Liechtenstein, Netherlands, Norway, Romania, Slovak Republic, Spain, Sweden, Switzerland and the UK.

The main functions of PICS are very similar to those of PIC, and include:

- Mutual acceptance of GMP inspections.
- Exchange of GMP inspection reports.
- Training of GMP inspectors (seminars and joint inspections).
- Promotion of international harmonisation of GMP.

Suggested further reading

Appelbe G E, Wingfield J (1997). *Dale and Appelbe's Pharmacy Law and Ethics*, 6th edn. London: The Pharmaceutical Press. [Covers UK/EC legislation.]

Griffin J P, ed. (1989). *Medicines Regulation Research and Risk*. Belfast: Queens University.

Walker S R, Griffin J P, eds (1989). *International Medicines Regulations*. Kingston-upon-Thames: Kluwer Academic Publishers.

Wells F O, ed. (1990). *Medicines Good Practice Guidelines*. Belfast: Queens University. [Especially chapter on 'Good pharmaceutical manufacturing practice' by M Murray.]

Reference

Sharp J, ed. (1983). *Guide to Good Pharmaceutical Manufacturing Practice*, 3rd edn. London: HMSO.

4

QC, QA and GMP: their nature and inter-relationships

I'll make assurance double sure, and take a bond of fate
W Shakespeare, *Macbeth*, Act 4, Sc. 1

Control procedures must encompass all things that may influence the quality of the completed medicinal preparations; they must permit inquiry into every phase of purchasing, manufacturing, packaging, storage and labelling . . .
Frank O Taylor, *J Am Pharm Assoc* **III** (3), March 1947

This chapter will consider what is meant by the terms 'quality control', 'good manufacturing practice' and 'quality assurance' and how they relate one to the other. As a means of illustrating the range of differing views, and in an attempt to clear up confusion, reference will be made to a number of previously published texts. The quotes are for illustrative purposes only.

Since the term 'quality control' has perhaps the longest history of use, it is convenient to turn first to this term.

Quality control: historical interpretations

A considerable number of books have been published which have 'quality control' in their title, or which are explicitly or implicitly about this topic. It is instructive to compare what it is the authors of some of these volumes regard as constituting 'quality control'. The following are just some examples.

Essentials of Quality Control by Huitson and Keen (1965)

This is a brief volume which is entirely concerned with applications of the mathematics of probability and distribution theory, that is, it is an introduction to *statistical* quality control. It includes chapters on:

• Graphical frequency distributions

- Distribution theory
- Control charts for variables
- Sampling inspection schemes
- New developments in quality control.

This last chapter is very short, and is concerned only with a very brief mention of 'cusum' (cumulative sum) control charts (a 'new development'!), and with recommending a number of books on statistical techniques and methods.

A Practical Approach to Quality Control by Caplen (1988)

This is a substantial volume (c. 350pp), which largely, but in rather more detail, covers similar ground to that covered above. Over 70% of the book is about the statistics of sampling and inspection, sampling plans, frequency distributions, control charts (of various types), etc. This largely mathematical treatment is, however, embedded in a broader discussion of more general 'quality' issues, and the text *does* consider such things as:

- Quality of design
- Vendor appraisal
- Quality circles
- Quality audits
- Design and implementation of quality control systems.

There is a final, very short, chapter on 'quality assurance' which is mainly concerned with a brief review of various British (BS) and International (ISO) Quality Assurance Standards. It does, however, contain the following encapsulation of the evolution of the Quality Assurance concept:

> Increasingly, what was once the inspection department is being developed into the quality assurance department, with a quality manager or quality director in charge. Quality assurance is responsible for overall surveillance of everything to do with quality throughout the Company. Thus it is concerned with the quality aspects of sales, research, design, development, pre-production, material, plant, tooling, operators, inspectors, manufacture, storage, packaging, transit, installation, commissioning, customer comments and complaints.

Nevertheless, *in essence* this is a book (and a useful one) on the statistical control of quality by sampling, inspection, and control charts, although it will be noted that in the passage quoted above, Caplen draws a distinction between 'quality control' and 'quality assurance'. He also refers to a Quality Assurance *Department*.

Right First Time – Using Quality Control for Profit by Price (1989)

This book provides a very simple treatment of the sort of statistical quality control techniques covered by Huitson & Keen and Caplen. In the first of its two parts, it covers the subject in a considerably more elementary fashion than either of the other two above publications. The much shorter Part Two (Quality and People) discusses more general, even philosophical, issues. This book has acquired almost cult status among many 'quality professionals', and 'right first time' has become something of a catchphrase.

Total Quality Control by Feigenbaum (1986)

This was originally published in the early 1950s. A substantial proportion of the book is about those statistical aspects which have already been mentioned in connection with the books above. Feigenbaum introduces a new and distinct concept (total quality control), which is defined as:

> Total quality control is an effective system for integrating the quality-development, quality-maintenance and quality-improvement efforts of various groups in an organisation so as to enable marketing, engineering, production and service at the most economical levels which allow for full customer satisfaction.

Although the larger part of the book deals with frequency distributions, sampling tables and control charts, it does also cover:

- Quality management
- Quality systems
- Productivity
- Product design and development
- Systems engineering
- Quality information feedback
- Organisation for quality
- Training for quality.

Feigenbaum interestingly traces 'the evolution of total quality control' as follows:

- *Pre- and early 1900*: 'Operator quality control', i.e. one, or a few operators were responsible for the manufacture of the entire product, and was/were therefore solely responsible for its quality.
- *Early 1900s–1920s*: 'Foreman quality control'.
- *1920s–1940s*: 'Inspection quality control', i.e. quality control by random (non-statistical) or 100% inspection.
- *1960s–1970s*: 'Total quality control'.

Feigenbaum also predicts that the '1980s and beyond' will be the era of a new phase: 'Total Quality Management'. Before proceeding, a few general points are worth noting:

1. The validity of any account of the evolution of a concept will depend on what is meant by the terms involved, i.e. one could be talking about a merely semantic, rather than an actual or practical, evolution.
2. Terms, fads and fashions are less important than the genuine assurance

of the quality of products (particularly of medicinal products) by whatever means or techniques.

3.   Whatever the respective merits (or otherwise – and none is entirely without merit) of the volumes thus far considered, they all have something in common. The authors all largely proceed on an assumption of the use of the techniques and methods which they propose in the engineering, parts-manufacturing, hardware fabrication and similar industries. They do not consider application, or relevance, to the very special case of the manufacture of medicines and other healthcare products.

Much of what has been said and written about 'general quality control' varies considerably in its viewpoint, which is rarely strictly pharmaceutical. However, one text that appears to be concerned specifically with the control of quality of pharmaceuticals is the following.

The Pharmaceutical Quality Control Handbook by Bryant (1989)

This book is claimed by the publisher to 'present a standardised quality control system for pharmaceutical manufacturing', and to be a 'blueprint for quality'. The author states that what he has done is to 'simplify the concepts of a workable, standardisable quality control system'.

The first chapter is headed 'What is quality control', and the author states:

> One dictionary entry for *quality control* gives us the following definition: an aggregate of activities (as design analysis and statistical sampling with inspection for defects) designed to ensure adequate quality in manufactured products.

Bryant also adds that '. . . for pharmaceuticals, "quality control" is also the name of the department which performs this function,' and he also states, 'Quality control is an after-the-fact testing of materials to determine if they have, in fact, met the requirements.'

The book is essentially a discussion of some aspects of good pharmaceutical manufacturing practice. The significant point, however, is that qualitatively and quantitatively, it is based on a *wholly different* concept of quality control as compared with the other books we have discussed.

Is it true then that *pharmaceutical* quality control is different from 'more general' quality control? Is there perhaps a formal or even a legal definition of 'quality control' in the special context of the manufacture of medicines?

The US regulations for current good manufacturing practice (US FDA, 1990) define 'quality control unit' as 'any person or organisational element designated by the firm to be responsible for the duties relating to quality control' (21 CFR Ch. 1, Part 210.210.3 (15)). 'Quality control' is not formally defined, but the intended meaning may be inferred from Part 211, 211.22 which states *inter alia* that:

(a)   There shall be a quality control unit that shall have the responsibility and authority to approve or reject all components, drug product containers, closures, in-process materials, packaging material, labelling, and drug products, and the authority to review production records to assure that no errors have occurred, or if errors have occurred, that they have been fully investigated . . .

(c)   The quality control unit shall have the responsibility for approving or rejecting all procedures or specifications impacting on the identity, strength, quality and purity of the drug product . . .

The UK Medicines Act 1968 uses the word 'quality' (albeit undefined) but not the phrase 'quality control'. The term was, however, used in regulations made under the Act in 1971 (HMSO, 1971a,b).

These regulations do refer to 'quality control' and to 'the person . . . in charge of quality control' without defining the term. Careful reading of the regulations and other related documents published at around the same time leaves an impression that, to those responsible for drafting these regulations, 'quality control' meant 'testing samples to check compliance with a predetermined specification'.

QC and QA: modern interpretations

One of the most influential publications on quality control is by J M Juran. In *Juran's Quality Control Handbook* (Juran & Gryna, 1988) there is a definition of what quality control in fact *is*, in a glossary at the end of the volume. It is defined as:

> The operational techniques and the activities used to fulfil the requirements of quality.

In this same glossary, quality assurance is defined as:

> All those planned or systematic actions necessary to provide adequate confidence that a product or service will satisfy given requirements for quality.

The handbook contains a whole section on quality assurance, in which it states:

> 'quality assurance' is the activity of providing the evidence needed to establish confidence, among all concerned, that the quality function is being effectively performed.

Much earlier, Juran states:

> It is convenient to have some short name to represent the activities, departmental and company-wide which collectively result in product quality. In this handbook that short name is the 'quality function'.

Some may find that, taken together, these definitions from the one source tend to confuse rather than clarify.

Clearly, there is also considerable divergence among authors in defining the meaning of 'quality control'. These resolve into three main types:

1.   Quality control as the application of statistical methods and techniques to the selection and carrying out of tests and measurements on samples ('engineering QC', or 'statistical QC').
2.   Quality control as an overall 'systems approach', in which statistical methods are the tools, but not the totality, of the enterprise.

3.   Quality control as mere testing of samples in the laboratory (i.e. for 'Quality Control Department' read 'Analytical Lab').

Type 3 above is an extreme expression of a position which might be described as the 'old, traditional industrial pharmaceutical' view. It was a view that was still to be encountered well into the 1970s, but has long since been abandoned by the more enlightened pharmaceutical manufacturers. Nevertheless, in the early 1970s more than one UK pharmaceutical company (faced with the need to comply with the then new Medicines Act) implemented 'quality control' by the simple expedient of painting out 'Chief Analyst' or 'Head of Analytical Department' on the laboratory manager's door, and replacing it with 'Quality Control Manager'.

QC and QA in the context of medicines

There had, of course, been stirrings towards more acceptably 'modern' views much earlier. A prime example is the paper entitled simply 'Quality control' (Taylor, 1947), from which the quotation at the head of this chapter is derived. Despite the title of his paper, Taylor writes about what he terms 'control procedures'. Side-stepping the semantics, what he was in fact discussing was something very like quality assurance, around 30 years before the time when, according to some experts, quality assurance actually hit the pharmaceutical industry.

Taylor's work deserves to be regarded as a landmark paper. In addition to the points made in the quotation at the head of this chapter, he also refers to the quality implications of research, development and distribution activities.

Up to the mid-1970s, considerable semantic, conceptual and practical confusion reigned in the UK and the rest of Europe over the precise meaning of 'quality control' in the context of medicinal and other healthcare products, and (in consequence) over how it related to the newer concept of quality assurance. There was further confusion over how both, in turn, stood in relation to good manufacturing practice. For example the international Pharmaceutical Inspection Convention (PIC) held a seminar in Berne in 1974 under the title 'Manufacture and quality control under contract' (PIC, 1974) which inevitably raised the question: 'While it is obviously both possible and acceptable (given certain conditions) to contract-out all or part of a manufacturing operation, is it even possible to contract-out Quality Control, or may only analytical testing be done under external contract?' That question was answered, at least by implication, by some speakers who refrained from mentioning 'quality control' at all and talked only of 'contract analysis', or 'contract analytical control'. The matter was further debated at a subsequent PIC seminar in Copenhagen the following year on 'The manufacturer's quality control department' (PIC, 1975).

The inter-relationship between QC, QA and GMP

The issue was finally resolved by the publication of the second edition of the UK Orange Guide to good pharmaceutical manufacturing practice (Sharp, 1977), which in addition to defining quality as 'fitness for intended purpose', gave the following definitions of quality assurance, good manufacturing practice, and quality control.

> Quality Assurance –
> . . . Is the sum total of the organised arrangements made with the object of ensuring that products will be of the quality required by their intended use. It is Good Manufacturing Practice plus factors outside the scope of this Guide (such as original product design and development).
>
> Good Manufacturing Practice –
> . . . Is that part of Quality Assurance aimed at ensuring that products are consistently manufactured to a quality appropriate to their intended use. It is thus concerned with both Manufacturing and Quality Control procedures.
>
> Quality Control –
> . . . Is that part of Good Manufacturing Practice which is concerned with sampling, specification and testing, and with the organisation, documentation and release procedures which ensure that the necessary and relevant tests are, in fact, carried out, and that materials are not released for use, nor products released for sale or supply, until their quality has been judged to be satisfactory. ('Quality Control' is sometimes used in the sense of the organisational entity which has responsibility for these functions.)

That this resolution of the confusion over definitions has met with general satisfaction was attested by the acceptance of these definitions by a Working Party of the European Organisation for Quality Control (EOQC 1978) as 'the most adequate definitions', and by their near word-for-word adoption in the EC GMP Guide (EC, 1992), and in other national and international GMP guides. The same definitions were adopted in the 3rd edition of the UK Orange Guide (Sharp, 1983).

The logic of the inter-relationships between the three terms, or concepts, may be illustrated as in Figure 4.1.

Quality assurance

Quality assurance is the all-embracing concept. Its influence should extend from original product research, design and development on the one hand; through materials purchase, receipt and control, onwards through batch manufacturing, packaging, testing, control and storage; and finally through distribution, dispensing and use on the other hand.

Put simply, GMP could be said to be the large middle segment of the above sequence – from the ordering and receipt of materials (ingredients and packaging materials) through to distribution. At each of two boundaries of

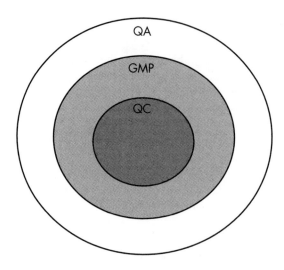

Figure 4.1   QA/GMP/QC inter-relationship.

this 'middle segment', routine GMP considerations merge with the broader and more general concepts of QA. The boundaries occur where full-scale manufacturing procedures have to be derived from the R and D work, and where full-scale manufacturing formulas and production methods have to be established. The boundaries also occur at a point in the chain from manufacturer's warehouse, through wholesale, retail, prescribing, dispensing and administration to patients.

Figure 4.2 is an attempt to develop the simple illustration (Fig. 4.1) of the inter-relationships into a more detailed indication of the areas over which QA, GMP and QC exercise, jointly and severally, their influences. Thus, QA is shown as embracing the entire spectrum from research to administration to patient. GMP considerations must come into play at some stage in the 'scale-up' phase, and retire from the scene (at least as far as the industrial-scale manufacturer is concerned) at some stage in the distribution chain.

Quality control is then shown having involvement with materials control, with in-process control in both product manufacture and packaging, in end-product testing and release (or rejection), and with checking on the quality of stored goods or materials.

On the left of the diagram (at X), feedback/-forward aspects of in-process, control and their relationships with batch recording, end-product testing and release (or rejection) are indicated.

The sequence illustrated is:

1. First, design the product (R&D, pharmacology, clinical trials, etc.).
2. Scale-up process, design plant, install equipment and develop relevant documentation (formulas, manufacturing methods, material and product specifications, maintenance schedules, etc.).
3. Validate process(es) – as scaled-up.
4. Make and package product (with trained staff, using confirmed quality

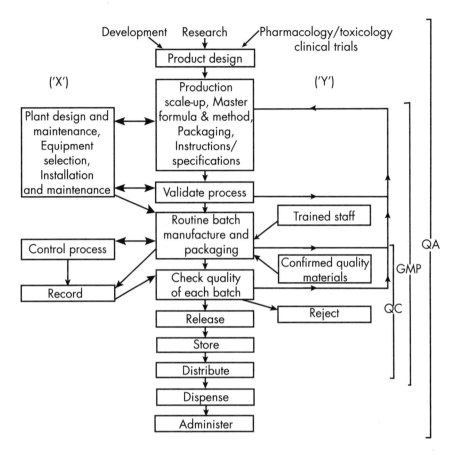

Figure 4.2   The overall QA function.

materials, following validated processes, and in accordance with the
pre-established formulas and methods).
5.   While doing so, carry out in-process checks and controls.
6.   Adjust process as necessary.
7.   Record all process details.
8.   Record details of in-process checks/controls.
9.   Test end product against established specification.
10.   Make release/reject decision on the basis of:
   •   End-product test results.
   •   Review of batch manufacturing and batch packaging records.
   •   Review of in-process control records.
   •   All other information relevant to the quality of the product.

On the right-hand side of the diagram (at 'Y') a series of interconnected feedback loops is shown:

•   Having designed and 'written-up' a production-scale process, validate
   it.

- If necessary, revise process/procedures as a result of the validation exercise.
- Validate revised process.
- Move to routine manufacture using validated process.
- If experience of routine manufacture indicates the need, revise basic process/procedures (and return through validation loop).

Other internal and external feedback loops are, of course, possible.

The 'make release/reject decision' is possibly the critical phase. Thereafter the product goes into storage and becomes available for distribution, dispensing, and administration. So, what factors need to be taken into account before the decision is taken to release a batch of product for sale?

The formal answer to that question is to be found in the joint 'Code of Practice for Qualified Persons' (by the Royal Pharmaceutical Society, Institute of Biology, and Royal Society of Chemistry), which has been reprinted in the MCA's *Rules and Guidance for Pharmaceutical Manufacturers* (MCA, 1997) to which we have already referred. This Code states *inter alia* that before certifying a batch prior to release the QP should always ensure that the following requirements have been met:

5.1 The Product (PL) and the Manufacturer's Licence (ML) requirements for the medicinal product have been met for the batch concerned.

5.2 The principles and guidelines of good manufacturing practice as laid down in Directive 91/356/EEC (Human) or Directive 91/412/EEC (Veterinary) and interpreted in the 'EC Guide to GMP' have been followed.

5.3 The principle manufacturing and testing processes have been validated.

5.4 All the necessary checks and tests have been performed and account taken of the production conditions and manufacturing records.

5.5 Any planned changes or deviations have been notified in accordance with a well-defined reporting system before any product is released. Such changes may need notification to and approval by the MCA.

5.6 Any additional sampling, inspection, tests and checks have been carried out or initiated, as appropriate, to cover planned changes or deviations.

5.7 All necessary production and QC documentation has been completed and endorsed by supervisors trained in appropriate disciplines.

5.8 Appropriate audits, self-inspections and spot checks are being carried out by experienced staff.

5.9 All relevant factors have been considered including any not specifically associated with the output batch directly under review (e.g. sub-division of output batches from a common input, factors associated with continuous production runs).

5.10 The legal requirements regarding imported products have been fully met.

This passage encapsulates a number of significant elements of QA/GMP. It should also destroy, once and for all, any remaining illusions that the quality (and hence 'release-worthiness') of a batch of product can be evaluated on the basis of end-product test results alone. (Further information of the nature, functions and legal status of the 'Qualified Person' is given in Chapter 11.)

Having established the relationship between GMP and QA, the next chapter will consider the various topics which, in combination, form the corpus of GMP, which is in effect the routine, day-to-day application of quality assurance in the manufacture of medicines and other healthcare products.

A final thought on the material of this chapter. While it will be apparent that it is perfectly rational to refer to 'quality control', as is common, in the sense of a process and of a department or organisational unit, it does not make good sense to refer to a 'Quality Assurance Department'. To do so displays a limited view of the true nature of quality assurance, which is an all-embracing concept, or philosophy, not to be restricted to the activities of any one functional department or unit. The entire company, in a very real sense, should be capable of being regarded as one large 'Quality Assurance Department', with the aim of delivering quality.

These thoughts are an entirely logical consequence of the definition and discussion of quality assurance in this book, and in other texts. However, such thoughts will not dissuade a number of companies from having a 'Quality Assurance Department', and it is probably not disastrous for them so to do – provided that the overall concept is understood, and followed in practice.

References

Bryant R (1989). *The Pharmaceutical Quality Control Handbook*. Oregon: Aster Publishing Corp.

Caplen R H (1988). *A Practical Approach to Quality Control*, 5th edn. London: Hutchinson Business Books.

EC (1992). *The Rules Governing Medicinal Products in the European Community, Vol. IV: Good Manufacturing Practice for Medicinal Products*. Luxembourg: Commission of the European Communities. Available from The Office for Official Publications of the European Communities, Luxembourg. Also available from The Stationery Office (HMSO), London, and The EC Information Service, Washington, USA. Also stated *verbatim* with guidance on the detailed interpretation of these rules in MCA, 1997. (Referred to as the EC GMP Guide.)

EOQC (1978). Quality control – technical problems. Report of a seminar, Zürich, 1978. Berne: EOQC.

Feigenbaum A V (1986). *Total Quality Control*, 3rd edn. New York: McGraw-Hill.

HMSO (1971a). The Medicines (Application for Product Licences and Clinical Trial and Animal Test Certificates) Regulations. *SI. No. 973*. London: HMSO.

HMSO (1971b). The Medicines (Application for Manufacturer's Licences and Wholesale Dealers Licences) Regulations. *SI. No. 974*. London: HMSO.

Huitson A, Keen J (1965). *Essentials of Quality Control*. London: Heinemann.

Juran J, Gryna F, eds (1988). *Juran's Quality Control Handbook*, 4th edn. New York: McGraw-Hill.

MCA (1997). *Rules and Guidance for Pharmaceutical Manufacturers and Distributors*. London: Medicines Control Agency. Available from The Stationery Office (HMSO), London.

PIC (1974). Manufacture and quality control under contract. Collected papers of a PIC seminar in Berne, Switzerland, July 1974. Geneva: EFTA Secretariat.

PIC (1975). The manufacturer's quality control department – structural and functional aspects. Collected papers of a PIC seminar in Copenhagen, Denmark, June 1975. Geneva: EFTA Secretariat.

Price F (1989). *Right First Time – Using Quality Control for Profit.* Aldershot: Gower Press.

Sharp J, ed. (1977). *Guide to Good Pharmaceutical Manufacturing Practice,* 2nd edn. London: HMSO.

Sharp J, ed. (1983). *Guide to Good Pharmaceutical Manufacturing Practice,* 3rd edn. London: HMSO. Also stated *verbatim* with guidance on the detailed interpretation of these rules in MCA, 1997. (Referred to as the UK Orange Guide.)

Taylor F O (1947). Quality control. *J Am Pharm Assoc* **III** (3), March 1947.

US FDA (1990). *Code of Federal Regulations, Vol. 21, Ch. 1, Part 210,* Current good manufacturing practice in manufacturing, processing, packaging or holding of drugs, general; *CFR Vol. 21, Ch. 1, Part 211,* Current good manufacturing practice for finished pharmaceuticals; *CFR Vol. 21, Ch. 1, Part 820,* Good manufacturing practice for medical devices (revised 1995). Washington: US Food & Drug Administration. (Collectively referred to as the US CGMPs.)

5

The essentials of GMP: UK/EC and USA GMPs compared

Comparisons are odorous
  W Shakespeare, *Much Ado About Nothing*, Act 3, Sc. 5

Worldwide, there are now around 30 different official (national and supra-national) statements on good manufacturing practice (GMP). These have been published variously as guides, codes and regulations. Possibly the major world influence, over the longest period, has been the US regulations for current GMPs (US FDA, 1990). It is also probably true to say that outside the American continent and since the late 1970s, the primary source for official bodies in the process of framing statements on GMP has been the UK *Guide to Good Pharmaceutical Manufacturing Practice* (Sharp, 1983), also referred to as the **Orange Guide**. One publication, massive in the spread of its application, which clearly demonstrates this influence is the European Community GMP guide (EC, 1992) – a review of which is pro-vided by Sharp (1989). Thus, the documents that are most relevant to this chapter, in addition to the original UK Orange Guide, are:

- *Code of Federal Regulations*, 21 CFR Ch. 1, Parts 210/211, by the US Food & Drug Administration. Referred to here as the **US CGMPs** (US FDA, 1990).
- *Good Manufacturing Practice for Medicinal Products*, Volume IV of *The Rules Governing Medicinal Products in the European Com-munity*, by Commission of the European Communities. Published 1989; reprinted with additional annexes 1992. Referred to here as the **EC GMP Guide** (EC, 1992). Note, this EC guide is also available in the UK, incorporated *verbatim*, together with other material, in the Medicine Control Agency's *Rules and Guidance for Pharmaceutical Manufacturers and Distributors* (MCA, 1997).

So, what are the basic elements of GMP, which as we have described is the routine, day-to-day application of industrial pharmaceutical quality assur-ance? A convenient summary of the main elements of GMP for pharma-ceuticals is to be found in EC Directive 91/356/EEC. The basic, legally enforceable, principles of GMP which it lays down are given below. (Directive 91/341/EEC, which for all practical purposes is identical to Directive 91/356 apart from its cross-references, lays down the same principles for veterinary medicines.)

Basic principles of GMP as laid down in EC Directive 91/356/EEC

Quality management

The manufacturer shall establish and implement an effective pharmaceutical quality assurance system, involving the active participation of the management and personnel of the different services involved.

Personnel

1. At each manufacturing site, the manufacturer shall have competent and appropriately qualified personnel at his disposal in sufficient number to achieve the pharmaceutical quality assurance objective.
2. The duties of managerial and supervisory staff, including the qualified person(s), responsible for implementing and operating good manufacturing practice shall be defined in job descriptions. Their hierarchical relationships shall be defined in an organisation chart. Organisation charts and job descriptions shall be approved in accordance with the manufacturer's internal procedures.
3. Staff referred to in paragraph . . . shall be given sufficient authority to discharge their responsibilities correctly.
4. Personnel shall receive initial and continuing training including the theory and application of the concept of quality assurance and good manufacturing practice.
5. Hygiene programmes adapted to the activities to be carried out shall be established and observed. These programmes include procedures relating to health, hygiene and clothing of personnel.

Premises and equipment

1. Premises and manufacturing equipment shall be located, designed, constructed, adapted and maintained to suit the intended operations.
2. Lay out, design and operation must aim to minimise the risk of errors and permit effective cleaning and maintenance in order to avoid contamination, cross contamination and, in general, any adverse effect on the quality of the product.
3. Premises and equipment intended to be used in manufacturing operations which are critical for the quality of the products shall be subjected to appropriate qualification.

Documentation

1. The manufacturer shall have a system of documentation based upon specifications, manufacturing formulae and processing and packaging

instructions, procedures and records covering the different manufacturing operations that they perform. Documents shall be clear, free from errors and kept up to date. Pre-established procedures for general manufacturing operations and conditions shall be available, together with specific documents for the manufacture of each batch. This set of documents shall make it possible to trace the history of the manufacture of each batch. The batch documentation shall be retained for at least one year after the expiry date of the batches to which it relates, or at least five years after the certification referred to in article 22 (2) of Directive 75/319/EEC whichever is the longer.

2. When electronic, photographic or other data processing systems are used instead of written documents, the manufacturer shall have validated the systems by proving that the data will be appropriately stored during the anticipated period of storage. Data stored by these systems shall be made readily available in legible form. The electronically stored data shall be protected against loss or damage of data (e.g. by duplication or back-up and transfer onto another storage system).

Production

The different production operations shall be carried out according to pre-established instructions and procedures and in accordance with good manufacturing practice. Adequate and sufficient resources shall be made available for the in-process controls.

Appropriate technical and/or organisational measures shall be taken to avoid cross contamination and mix-ups.

Any new manufacture or important modification of a manufacturing process shall be validated. Critical phases of manufacturing processes shall be regularly revalidated.

Quality control

1. The manufacturer shall establish and maintain a quality control department. This department shall be placed under the authority of a person having the required qualifications and shall be independent of the other departments.

2. The quality control department shall have at its disposal one or more quality control laboratories appropriately staffed and equipped to carry out the necessary examination and testing of starting materials, packaging materials and intermediate and finished products testing. Resorting to outside laboratories may be authorised in accordance with article 12 of this Directive and after the authorisation referred to in article 5b of Directive 75/319/EEC has been granted.

3. During the final control of finished products before their release for sale or distribution, in addition to analytical results, the quality control department shall take into account essential information such as the production conditions, the results of in process controls, the examination of the manufacturing documents and the conformity of the products to their specifications (including the final finished pack).

4. Samples of each batch of finished products shall be retained for at least one year after the expiry date. Unless in the Member States of

manufacture a longer period is required, samples of starting materials (other than solvents, gases and water) used shall be retained for at least two years after the release of the product. This period may be shortened if their stability, as mentioned in the relevant specification, is shorter. All these samples shall be maintained at the disposal of the competent authorities.

For certain medicinal products manufactured individually or in small quantities, or when their storage could raise special problems, other sampling and retaining conditions may be defined in agreement with the competent authority.

Work contracted out

1. Any manufacturing operation or operation linked with the manufacture which is carried out under contract, shall be the subject of a written contract between the contract giver and the contract acceptor.
2. The contract shall clearly define the responsibilities of each party and in particular the observance of good manufacturing practice by the contract acceptor and the manner in which the qualified person responsible for releasing each batch shall undertake his full responsibilities.
3. The contract acceptor shall not subcontract any of the work entrusted to him by the contract giver without the written authorisation of the contract giver.
4. The contract acceptor shall respect the principles and guidelines of good manufacturing practice and shall submit to inspections carried out by the competent authorities as provided for by Article 26 of Directive 75/319/EEC.

Complaints and product recall

The manufacturer shall implement a system for recording and reviewing complaints together with an effective system for recalling promptly and at any time the medicinal products in the distribution network. Any complaint concerning a defect shall be recorded and investigated by the manufacturer. The competent authority shall be informed by the manufacturer of any defect that could result in a recall or abnormal restriction on the supply. In so far as possible, the countries of destination shall also be indicated. Any recall shall be made in accordance with the requirements referred to in Article 33 of Directive 75/319/EEC.

Self inspection

The manufacturer shall conduct repeated self inspections as part of the quality assurance system in order to monitor the implementation and respect of good manufacturing practice and to propose any necessary corrective measures. Records of such self-inspections and any subsequent corrective action shall be maintained.

Thus do the health authorities of the European Community sum up the major elements of GMP and lay down the *minimum* legal GMP requirements for all pharmaceutical manufacturers in all member states of the EC.

Guidance on the detailed interpretation of these principles is to be found in the EC GMP Guide (EC, 1992) as reprinted in *Rules and Guidance for Pharmaceutical Manufacturers and Distributors* (MCA, 1997).

The main body of the text of the EC GMP Guide is presented in nine chapters, approximately (but not precisely) in line with the principles of the corresponding directive, as set out above. The chapters in the EC GMP Guide are:

- Chapter 1 Quality management
- Chapter 2 Personnel
- Chapter 3 Premises and equipment
- Chapter 4 Documentation
- Chapter 5 Production
- Chapter 6 Quality control
- Chapter 7 Contract manufacture and analysis
- Chapter 8 Complaints and product recall
- Chapter 9 Self inspection

Annexes to the EC GMP Guide

The nine chapters listed above are followed by 14 annexes as follows:

1. Manufacture of sterile medicinal products
2. Manufacture of biological medicinal products for human use
3. Manufacture of radiopharmaceuticals
4. Manufacture of veterinary medicinal products other than immunologicals
5. Manufacture of immunological veterinary medicinal products
6. Manufacture of medicinal gases
7. Manufacture of herbal medicinal products
8. Sampling of starting and packaging materials
9. Manufacture of liquids, creams and ointments
10. Manufacture of pressurised metered dose aerosol preparations for inhalation
11. Computerised systems
12. Use of ionising radiation in the manufacture of medicinal products
13. Good manufacturing practice for investigational medicinal products
14. Manufacture of products derived from human blood or human plasma.

Basic principles of GMP as set out in the UK Orange Guide (1983)

A collation of the various 'principles' which head the first nine, major, sections of the 1983 edition of the UK Orange Guide, provides another useful general GMP overview, perhaps for comparison with the principles given in the EC GMP Guide.

1. Quality

There should be a comprehensive system, so designed, documented, implemented and controlled, and so furnished with personnel, equipment and other resources as to provide assurance that products will be consistently of a quality appropriate to their intended use. The attainment of this quality objective requires the involvement and commitment of all concerned, at all stages.

2. Personnel and training

There should be sufficient personnel at all levels with the ability, training, experience and where necessary, the professional/technical qualifications and managerial skills appropriate to the tasks assigned to them. Their duties and responsibilities should be clearly explained to them and recorded as written job descriptions or by other suitable means. Training should cover not only specific tasks but Good Manufacturing Practice generally and the importance of personal hygiene.

3. Documentation

Documentation is a prime necessity in Quality Assurance. Its purposes are to define the system of control, to reduce the risk of error inherent in purely oral communication, to ensure that personnel are instructed in the details of, and follow, the procedures concerned, and to permit investigation and tracing of defective products. The system of documentation should be such that the history of each batch of product, including the utilisation and disposal of starting materials, packaging materials and intermediate, bulk and finished products, may be determined.

4. Premises and equipment

Buildings should be located, designed, constructed, adapted and maintained to suit the operations carried out in them. Equipment should be designed, constructed, adapted, located and maintained to suit the processes and products for which it is used. Building construction, and equipment lay-out, should ensure protection of the product from contamination, permit efficient cleaning and avoid the accumulation of dust and dirt.

5. Manufacture

Manufacture should follow previously defined procedures which are known to be capable of yielding finished products which are those intended and which conform to their specifications. Special attention must be paid to labels and labelling throughout the entire production cycle.

6. Recovered materials

Material may be re-worked or recovered by an appropriate and authorised method, provided that the material is suitable for such reprocessing, that the resultant product meets its specification and there are no significant changes in product quality. Documentation should accurately record the reworking processes carried out.

7. Complaints procedures and product recall

The full significance of a complaint may only be appreciated by certain responsible persons, and then possibly only with the knowledge of other related complaints. A procedure must therefore exist to channel complaint reports appropriately.

A complaint, or otherwise reported product-defect, may lead to the need for a recall. Any action taken to recall a product suspected or known to be defective or hazardous, should be prompt and in accordance with a pre-determined plan. The procedures to be followed should be specified in writing and made known to all who may be concerned.

8. Good control laboratory practice

It is essential that control laboratories should have appropriate facilities, with properly trained, managed and motivated staff, in order that reliable results may be obtained from any analytical or other test procedure, whether its nature is chemical, physical, biological or microbiological. Steps should be taken to ensure the reliability of the laboratory's own systems and test methods.

9. Manufacture and control of sterile medicinal products

Sterile products should be manufactured with special care and attention to detail, with the object of eliminating microbial and particulate contamination. Much depends on the skill, training and attitudes of the personnel involved. Even more than with other types of medicinal product, it is not sufficient that the finished product passes the specified tests, and in-process Quality Assurance assumes a singular importance.

This chapter has, thus far, been concerned with providing a general summary of the basic elements of GMP. It is time now to attempt to draw a comparison, against that background, between the two major official statements on GMP: the UK/EC guidelines and the US regulations.

GMP guidelines/regulations: UK/EC vs USA

Legal status

Here, at the outset, is a crucially important basic difference between the EC GMP Guide and the US CGMPs.

The EC GMP Guide is not a directive or a regulation. EC statutory requirements for GMP in the manufacture of human medicines are set out in Directive 91/356/EEC. The EC GMP Guide is, as its title indicates, a *guide* to the more detailed interpretation of the statutory regulations. In passing it is of interest to note that the UK Orange Guide specifically declared (Preface):

> It has no statutory force, and should not be regarded as an interpretation of the requirements of any Act, Regulation or Directive. Its purpose is to recommend steps which should be taken . . . by manufacturers of medicinal products with the object of ensuring that their products are of the nature and quality intended.

The EC Guide does not carry quite so unequivocal a statement, but it does declare in its Introduction:

> It is recognised that there are acceptable methods, other than those described, in the Guide which are capable of achieving the principles of Quality Assurance. The Guide is not intended to place any restraint upon the development of any new concepts or new technologies which have been validated, and which provide a level of Quality Assurance at least equivalent to those set out in this Guide.

The adoption of flexible, mutually agreed GMP guidelines helps to avoid the potential for confrontation between industry and the inspecting body. Compliance with the spirit and overall standards of GMP, rather than insistence on rigid adherence to every point of detail and the enforcement of an inflexible set of rules, has usually been a feature of the UK regulatory control of manufacturing activities, and this in turn has led to cooperation rather than confrontation. Evidence so far suggests that this is/will be the European approach. (It needs to be noted that for such an approach to be both acceptable and successful, an appropriately qualified and trained Inspectorate, with relevant practical industrial experience, is both implicit and essential.)

In contrast, the US CGMPs have unequivocal legal status (and this has inevitable effects on the approach to regulatory inspection of manufacturers – see the Annex to this chapter).

The US CGMPs are presented as part of the Code of Federal Regulations. In section 210.1 (b) it is stated:

> The failure to comply with any regulation set forth in this part and in Parts 211 through 226 of this chapter in the manufacture, processing packing or holding of a drug shall render such drug to be adulterated . . . and such drug, as well as the person who is responsible for the failure to comply shall be subject to regulatory action.

The US CGMPs have full 'every word' legal status within the USA. In Europe, and elsewhere outside the USA they have, of course, no legal status at all. However, their economic force and influence is considerable, and any manufacturer wishing to export to the USA will be required by the relevant US inspecting body (the Investigators of the FDA) to comply with the CGMPs. Failure to comply (or to be 'in violation' as they say) will result in failure to tap the valuable US market, i.e. approval to sell in the USA will be withheld or withdrawn.

The US CGMPs for finished pharmaceutical products consist of Part 210 'General', which deals with such matters as status, applicability and definitions of terms, and Part 211, which contains the core requirements. Part 211 has 11 subparts:

A. General provisions
B. Organisation and personnel
C. Buildings and facilities
D. Equipment
E. Control of components* and drug product containers and closures
F. Production and process controls
G. Packaging and labelling control
H. Holding and distribution
I. Laboratory controls
J. Records and reports
K. Returned and salvaged drug products

*'Component', in the context of the US CGMPs means 'any ingredient intended for use in the manufacture of a drug product', and 'drug product' means 'a finished dosage form . . .'

As a complete, detailed, point-by-point comparison of the EC GMP Guide with the US CGMPs would be tiresome, the following is intended only as a summary of significant differences and similarities.

Personnel

The EC GMP Guide, reflecting the mandatory requirement (Directive 91/356/EEC/11.1) for the independence of quality control, states that 'the heads of production and quality control must be independent from each other'. The US CGMPs do not appear specifically to require this separation of responsibility and authority, although it is perhaps implicit in the statements on the responsibility and authority of the quality control unit which appear in 211.22. In any event, this separation does seem to be standard practice in US pharmaceutical manufacturing companies.

Both documents stress that there should be an adequate number of appropriately qualified, trained and experienced personnel.

The EC GMP Guide requires that 'the manufacturer must have an organisation chart' and that 'people in responsible positions should have specific duties recorded in written job descriptions, and adequate authority to carry out their responsibilities'.

Both indicate the need for initial and ongoing training, in both GMP and in specific task-related skills and knowledge.

Both documents require hygienic personal practices and the wearing of suitable protective clothing.

The US CGMPs require that 'persons shown . . . to have an apparent illness or open lesions which may adversely affect . . . drug products shall be excluded from contact with components . . . containers, closures, in-process materials, and drug products'. The EC GMP Guide has a similar requirement, and also requires that 'all personnel should receive medical examination on recruitment', to be repeated thereafter 'when necessary'. Manufacturers are also required to see that there are 'instructions ensuring that health conditions that can be of relevance to the quality of products come to the manufacturer's knowledge'.

The EC GMP Guide states 'eating, drinking, chewing or smoking, or the storage of food, drink, smoking materials or personal medication in the production or storage areas should be prohibited'. Such matters are not covered explicitly in the US CGMPs.

The US CGMPs accept the use of consultants 'advising on the manufacture, processing, packing etc.' The EC GMP Guide states that 'normally key posts should be occupied by full-time personnel'.

Buildings/premises

In general, the requirements of both documents are quite similar.

While in the EC GMP Guide the need for the segregation of various different types of operation or activity is indicated, the US CGMPs spell out 10 different types of 'defined area'.

One surprising aspect of the US CGMPs is that although there is a requirement for a separate area for aseptic processing (with special requirements for walls/floors/surfaces, air supply, environmental monitoring, disinfection, etc.), this does not appear to be required for other forms of sterile production. (This may be due to a different meaning of the word 'aseptic' in American English.)

In general, the EC GMP Guide covers all, or most of, the points in the US CGMPs in more or less similar terms. The special requirements for sterile products manufacture are not detailed in Chapter 3 'Premises and equipment', but are covered (far more extensively than in the US CGMPs) in the special Annex 1 (as revised in January 1997).

Additional points specifically mentioned in the EC GMP Guide include: prevention of contamination from external environment; segregation of animal houses, maintenance workshops, and toilet facilities; general requirements for walls, floors and ceilings; and appropriate working conditions in terms of lighting, temperature, humidity and ventilation.

Equipment

A number of the points made are similar in both documents, at least in terms of general requirements (design, construction, location, cleaning and maintenance).

The CGMPs include, in Subpart D, statements on 'automatic mechanical and electronic equipment' (211.68) which embrace requirements for 'computers and related systems', and a section (211.72) on 'fiber-releasing filters'. The former is covered, in somewhat more detail in Annex 11 of the

EC Guide. The EC GMP Guide further requires that 'measuring, weighing, recording and control equipment should be calibrated and checked at defined intervals by appropriate methods' and records maintained.

Ingredients and packaging materials

(The US CGMPs refer to ingredients (or 'starting materials') as 'components', and packaging materials as 'drug product containers and closures'.)

Overall, on these aspects the two documents are similar in content, but rather different in emphasis. The CGMPs cover documentary aspects under Subpart E, 'Control of components and drug product containers and closures'. Because of the detailed coverage in the separate chapter on documentation, the EC GMP Guide is more specific on materials specifications and records. The US CGMPs are rather more detailed on sampling of these materials than the EC GMP Guide, but lack the particular emphasis of the latter on the need to guard against mislabelling by material suppliers (see EC Annex 8).

Production and process controls

The relevant sections are Subpart F of the US CGMPs and Chapter 5 of the EC GMP Guide. The latter includes packaging, which is accorded a separate subpart (Subpart G) in the CGMPs. It also includes a four-paragraph section on validation, to be compared with occasional references in the CGMPs.

Overall, requirements are basically similar, although the CGMPs give a number of examples of the types of in-process controls to be exercised, and is also different in requiring 'time limits for the completion of each stage of manufacture'. Section 211.115 of Subpart F consists of two paragraphs on 'reprocessing'. The EC GMP Guide has, in Chapter 5, a six-paragraph section on 'rejected, recovered and returned materials'.

Packaging and labelling

The relevant portion of the US CGMPs is Subpart G, 'Packaging and labelling control'. Sections 211.122 'Materials examination and usage criteria', 211.125 'Labelling issuance' and 211.130 of this subpart are broadly similar in content and emphasis to the sections on packaging materials (5.40 to 5.43) and on packaging operations (5.44 to 5.57) in the EC GMP Guide.

The relatively lengthy section of Subpart G of the CGMPs is concerned with 'tamper-resistant packaging requirements for over-the-counter (OTC) human drug products'. This is all very sound and reasonable stuff, but some might question whether this is strictly a GMP issue.

The control laboratory

The requirements for laboratory controls, as set out in Subpart I of the US CGMPs, are broadly similar to the guidance given in Chapter 6, 'Quality control', of the EC GMP Guide, as amplified by the other sections and chapters to which it refers.

Subpart I, Section 211.166 of the US CGMPs goes into some considerable detail on stability testing; the EC GMP Guide does not, although the matter is covered elsewhere in other guidelines and regulations. (It might be argued that although a sound stability testing programme is of crucial importance, it is not part of the day-to-day process of manufacture and therefore does not come within the scope of GMP.)

Documentation/records

These are both covered in considerable detail, but with differences of emphasis, in the EC GMP Guide Chapter 4 'Documentation' and US CGMPs Subpart J 'Records and reports', respectively.

Other topics

The final subpart of the US CGMPs is Subpart K 'Returned and salvaged drug products'. These aspects are covered in the section on 'rejected, recovered and returned materials' (5.61 to 5.65) of the EC GMP Guide.

The EC GMP Guide deals with a number of topics which are either not covered at all, or covered only relatively briefly, in the US CGMPs. (See, for example, EC Chapter 7 'Contract manufacture and analysis' and Chapter 9 'Self inspection', and a number of the 14 annexes which have already been listed.)

Concluding remarks

In general, there are a number of similarities in terms of the content of the US and EC documents. However, there are certain differences; a striking contrast is the very detailed separate treatment in the EC Guide of sterile products manufacture, as compared with a few paragraphs, scattered through various subparts of the CGMPs.

There are a number of differences of emphasis. Two important broad distinctions may be drawn:

1. The EC GMP Guide is usually more detailed where it has common ground with the US CGMPs, and in addition covers topics not considered in the latter.
2. The US CGMPs are explicitly a set of legally enforceable regulations, written in a style, and with an emphasis, that reflects this. The EC GMP Guide is indeed a guide, and is overtly patient-safety orientated. This difference has significant implications in the approach to the regulatory

control of medicines manufacture, in the USA as compared with in the UK/EC.

It is perhaps in the differences in the implementation and enforcement of good manufacturing practice, and in inspection practices, that the most striking contrasts lie; this is an issue discussed in the annex to this chapter.

References

EC (1992). *The Rules Governing Medicinal Products in the European Community, Vol. IV: Good Manufacturing Practice for Medicinal Products.* Luxembourg: Commission of the European Communities. Available from The Office for Official Publications of the European Communities, Luxembourg. Also available from The Stationery Office, (HMSO) London, and The EC Information Service, Washington, USA. Also stated *verbatim* with guidance on the detailed interpretation of these rules in MCA, 1997. (Referred to as the EC GMP Guide.)

MCA (1997). *Rules and Guidance for Pharmaceutical Manufacturers and Distributors.* London: Medicines Control Agency. Available from The Stationery Office, London.

Sharp J, ed. (1983). *Guide to Good Pharmaceutical Manufacturing Practice,* 3rd edn. London: HMSO. Also stated *verbatim* with guidance on the detailed interpretation of these rules in MCA, 1997. (Referred to as the UK Orange Guide.)

Sharp J (1989). The EC Guide – a review. *Manuf Chem* Sept. 1989.

US FDA (1990). *Code of Federal Regulations, Vol. 21, Ch. 1, Part 210,* Current good manufacturing practice in manufacturing, processing, packaging or holding of drugs, general; *CFR Vol. 21, Ch. 1, Part 211,* Current good manufacturing practice for finished pharmaceuticals; *CFR Vol. 21, Ch. 1, Part 820,* Good manufacturing practice for medical devices (revised 1995). Washington: US Food & Drug Administration. (Collectively referred to as the US CGMPs.)

Annex

Approaches to the GMP inspection of pharmaceutical facilities

Many major European states have a body of inspectors with a responsibility to their respective national health authorities for the inspection of pharmaceutical manufacturing plants, to monitor compliance with relevant national law and with (at least) local perceptions of GMP.

By definition, this applies in all member states of the Pharmaceutical Inspection Convention (PIC). It is a condition of membership that member states have national medicines legislation, and a medicines inspectorate. Before an applicant nation is admitted to membership of PIC it must demonstrate to officials of the Convention that it enforces and maintains comparable standards of GMP; that is, that its industry complies with the PIC basic standards, which have now been harmonised with the EC GMP Guide. (For a discussion of PIC, see Annex II to Chapter 3.)

It is implicit in various official statements from the European Community that all members do (or at least *should*) have a body of pharmaceutical plant inspectors. For example the Introduction to the EC GMP Guide to GMP states:

> A system of Manufacturing Authorisations issued by Member States ensures that all the licensed products are only manufactured by licensed manufacturers whose activities are regularly inspected by the Competent Authorities. Manufacturing Authorisations are required by all pharmaceutical manufacturers in EEC whether the products are sold in EEC or exported.

Thus it may be *assumed* that at least 21 European nations (i.e. the EC and European PIC States combined) operate a system of pharmaceutical plant inspections. Whether or not style, approach, competence, experience, training, legal powers, etc. are closely comparable across the board is still perhaps a matter for some conjecture. A commonality in all these aspects has always been an aim of PIC, and after nearly 20 years of existence it is reasonable to assume that it has, at least to some extent, achieved that aim.

However, in terms of what a pharmaceutical manufacturer might expect from a visit from an inspector of a European State, the question of comparability (or otherwise) of European standards and styles is one that is difficult to resolve. For, with one exception, European inspectorates have not regularly and routinely inspected outside their own national boundaries. The exception is the UK Medicines Inspectorate.

The UK Medicines Inspectorate

The UK Medicines Inspectorate was formed in 1971, as a direct consequence of the implementation of the licensing provisions of the 1968 Medicines Act.

The Medicines Act confers right of entry (Section 111) 'at any reasonable time' by 'any person duly authorised in writing' in order to:

- Ascertain whether there has been any contravention of the Act or Regulations.
- Verify any statement made in an application.
- Inspect any substance, article, label, leaflet, plant or equipment.
- Examine records and documents and take copies.
- Seize and detain any substance or article.
- Take samples.

This is provided that any such substance, article, label, record, document, etc. appears to the authorised person to be a medicinal product, or is intended to be 'used in connection with a medicinal product'.

The above summarises the legal powers of the UK Medicines Inspectorate. Taken in combination with the regulations on standard provisions for the holders of Manufacturer's Licences, the net effect is that UK medicines inspectors, in addition to exercising these specific powers, are also concerned with observing, monitoring and investigating compliance with the principles of GMP.

That the UK Medicines Inspectorate is not just another inflexible policing force is a reflection of the relationship between the Government and the Industry (and it is worth recalling that, under the UK National Health Service, the Government is the Industry's single biggest customer), and nature and background of the British inspector.

There is nothing in any act or regulation which offers a definition or a specification for a medicines inspector. From the start, however, the recruitment policy was to require a formal qualification in pharmacy, chemistry or other relevant discipline, and a minimum of 5 years' experience of production management or quality management in the pharmaceutical industry. Note that inspectors were required to have had at least 5 years' experience of the *management* of production and/or quality at some level within the industry, as well as being appropriately academically/professionally qualified. The adoption of flexible GMP guidelines (as distinct from rigid regulations) virtually *demands* inspectors of this type. They are, furthermore, encouraged to aim for constructive dialogue with the companies they inspect, rather than engage in a one-sided, or confrontational, policing exercise. UK inspectors expect and enjoy discussion. They do not merely ask, they are happy to be asked, questions. Unhelpful 'yes/no' answers to their questions may not be interpreted as legal caution, but as lack of detailed knowledge or competence.

In the UK, the major portion of the Inspectorate work is related to Manufacturer's Licences (MLs). Initial applications for MLs are routed via the Inspectorate, who then schedule an inspection.

Once an ML has been granted, frequency and extent of ongoing inspection and monitoring is a matter for internal planning and scheduling by the Inspectorate's own management, via its structure of Regional Principal Inspectors and Area Inspectors.

A separate section of the agency handles Product Licence (PL) applications (or variations to PLs, etc.). However, applicants for PLs are required to describe methods of manufacture and control, and if the PL assessors feel that these aspects should be investigated 'on the ground', they can, and do, ask for an inspection.

As far as inspection outside Britain is concerned, the UK Inspectorate of course has no legal powers. However, suitable provision is made in Section 19(3) of the Medicines Act. All imported products (as well as those made in Britain) must be covered by a Product Licence. Section 19(3) indicates that in relation to medicinal products which are imported, the UK Licensing Authority may, *inter alia*, require:

> An undertaking, given by the manufacturer of any such products to permit the premises where they are, or are to be, manufactured . . . to be inspected by or on behalf of the Licensing Authority.

In practice, this undertaking is normally requested and usually given (if it is not, then the licence is not granted).

This then, is the section of the Act under which the Inspectorate operates outside Britain. In such circumstances, they have no legal powers, and the overseas manufacturer could still refuse to allow entry. (It has happened, with embarrassing consequences for the manufacturer, and the UK importer.) With the enlargement of PIC and the development of the EC, the overseas inspection workload of the UK Medicines Inspectorate is decreasing.

In the UK it is normal practice (i.e. in the majority of cases where there is no reason to suspect any breach of the law) for inspectors to give advance notice of their intention to visit and inspect. One or two inspectors spending several days (rather than the weeks or months which are common with the US FDA) on site is the norm. Having established that there are no major changes in relation to licensable activity (e.g. changes in products manufactured, in equipment or facilities used, in personnel, etc.), or recorded any changes that have taken place, inspectors will then audit the site (premises, equipment, personnel, documentation, etc.) for compliance with GMP. In all cases there will be special attention to any problems noted on a previous visit. Thereafter, the audit may cover the whole site generally, or concentrate on specific aspects or activities. Following the inspection, the inspectors will inform the company of their findings at a final summary or 'wrap-up' session, which roughly corresponds to the US FDA 'exit interview'. At this stage written comments are not left with the company, but the inspectors will seek oral comment from the company as to the steps they propose to take to correct any deficiencies noted. Here there is the opportunity for the company to express its views on whether or not the inspector's comments are reasonable and justified. In the majority of cases, this is all conducted on a professional dialogue, non-confrontational basis, with oral agreement on plans for action and timescales. In these circumstances the next step will be for the inspector to send a letter to the manufacturer, setting out his or her previously expressed views in writing and seeking written confirmation of action taken or proposed. At the same time the inspector will compile a report, which will be submitted to, and approved by, a senior officer and then held for follow-up action, with the correspondence with the company.

Other more legally stringent actions are available if necessary, e.g. revocation or suspension of the Manufacturer's Licence in whole or in part (whereupon it becomes illegal to manufacture), refusal to grant a licence if it is a new application, or prosecution via the courts for contravention of the Medicines Act. Such actions are now rare in the UK. They were more common in the early 1970s. Decisions on revocation or suspension are not made and actioned by the inspector acting alone, but only after consideration by a committee of relevant experts – pharmaceutical, medical, legal and administrative. In all such cases, the manufacturer has rights of appeal.

However, there is an additional power whereby, when 'it appears to the Licensing Authority in the interests of safety' a licence may be suspended with immediate effect for a period not exceeding 3 months.

FDA and FDA investigators

The official body in the USA concerned with regulating the manufacture, sale, supply and distribution of medicinal products is the US Food and Drug Administration (FDA), which operates under the aegis of the US Food, Drug and Cosmetic (FD&C) Act. As the Act implies, the FDA is concerned with products and materials in addition to those intended for medicinal purposes.

The FDA does not operate a system precisely analogous to the UK manufacturer's licence or the EC manufacturing authorisation. It does, however, operate a product approval system comparable to the UK product licence or the EC marketing authorisation. This is the New Drug Application (NDA) system. Before a product may be marketed in the USA an NDA must be submitted to the FDA, supported by data on safety and efficacy, and describing methods of manufacture and control and their validation. Variants on the NDA include the New Animal Drug Application (NADA), the Investigational New Drug Application (INDA – approval required before commencing clinical trials), the Abbreviated New Drug Application (ANDA – mainly used for generic products) and a Supplemental Application (used to amend an NDA after it has been approved).

Despite the very considerable influence (for better or worse) that it exerts, it is important to stress that the FDA, their regulations, and their system of NDAs (etc.) have no legal status outside the USA. Outside the USA their force is an economic one, and a powerful one it is. The US market for medicinal products is huge and lucrative.

A company in Europe (or elsewhere) wishing to export product to the USA must obtain an NDA approval. This renders the applicant liable to a pre-approval inspection by FDA investigators. Failure at such an inspection (that is, to be found 'non-compliant' with, or 'in violation' of the CGMPs) can result in failure to obtain NDA approval. Failure at any subsequent, post-NDA approval inspection can result in withdrawal of the product from the US market. This can mean the loss of a lot of money. The trepidation such inspections cause have led some industrialists to comment that FDA stood for 'fear, doubt and anxiety'. (With disarming quaintness, an FDA official has claimed they really stood for 'friendly, delightful and agreeable'.)

It is important to be aware of the economic power of the FDA, and of the differences in their background, style and approach as compared with, for example, the UK Medicines Inspectorate.

In the sphere of GMP compliance, the UK Inspectorate has operated in the context of broad, brief basic statutory GMP principles (the 'Standard Provisions' and now the Directive 91/356/EEC) supplemented by detailed non-statutory Guidance (the UK Orange Guide, and now the EC Guide), around which they aim to build a constructive dialogue. The FDA investigators have 'Current Good Manufacturing Practice Regulations' and fundamentally are looking for 'violations' of those regulations.

A further fundamental difference needs to be noted. In the USA there is a Freedom of Information Act. Thus investigators' reports, with a bare minimum of censoring, are freely available to all who care to apply for a copy, within or without the USA. On the other hand, UK medicines inspectors, as indeed are government workers (and armed forces) generally, are subject to the Official Secrets Act. Information gained during the course of their duties, at home or overseas, is officially secret and there are severe penalties for revealing it. There are also additional penalties for revealing information, under the Medicines Act itself. The relationship between inspector and inspected will obviously be coloured by the awareness of confidentiality on the one hand, and that everything can (and will) become public knowledge on the other.

In contrast to the UK Inspectorate, who are all subject to minimum requirements on recruitment for qualifications and previous experience, FDA investigators are not necessarily academically or professionally qualified in any of the relevant fields. Nor will they necessarily have had any relevant industrial experience. Both these factors tend to colour their style and approach.

Because of their background and experience, UK inspectors tend to understand, and even sympathise with, practical problems and difficulties. They expect and encourage a two-way professional dialogue.

The medicines inspectors of the UK MCA are usually relaxed, confident and approachable. A few years ago a small number of FDA personnel were found guilty of accepting bribes. This clearly hurt the moral majority. Possibly as a partial consequence, some FDA investigators can be oversensitive, defensive, and 'by the book' doctrinaire. There are signs, however, that the FDA is aiming for a more benign image.

It is not usual in UK companies for legal staff to be present during an MCA inspection. A number of US companies have their lawyer present (for

FDA) and some have said that they have instructions that FDA investigators must be accompanied at all times, even when they go to the toilet.

It is difficult to determine how many investigators work for the FDA, for many work, some of their time, on matters other than medicines manufacture. By comparison with the number of MCA inspectors (around 20) they are many. Over one hundred of them are licensed to carry guns. They have been known, in the USA, to have four or more investigators on one site for over 3 months (cf. MCA normal *maximum* of two inspectors for 4 or 5 days), so they clearly have the resource to enable them to do that.

The FDA place a massive majority emphasis on review of documentation, with rather less attention to the site/facilities/equipment/activity/personnel reviewing 'leg work' of the MCA.

US writers and speakers tend to talk of '*The* GMPs' almost as if the written word of the law (rather than its spirit or intention) was all-important, whereas British interest focuses on good manufacturing practice *per se*. A famous FDA investigation of the E Lilly (Indianapolis) plant (several investigators for a few *months*) yielded a 90-page '483'. (Form 483 is the FDA form which they hand manufacturers at the exit interview and which list violations and/or where the company is non-compliant.) Of those pages, 89 concerned violations detected in documents and only one page dealt with 'plant observations'. Such a bias is unlikely in a UK inspection.

Perhaps the final word on this topic can be derived from a statement from the European Commission Working Party on Control of Medicines and Inspections (January 1995):

> The task of an inspector is not limited to the disclosure of faults, deficiencies and discrepancies. The inspection should connect an observation with assistance in making the necessary improvements. An inspection should normally include educational and motivating elements.

Such an approach is not generally characteristic of the FDA.

6

Quality assurance beyond GMP: the wider aspects and the cost of quality

The general (as distinct from specifically pharmaceutical) quality experts conventionally consider that quality has two main components, which they term:

1. Quality of design.
2. Quality of conformance ('to that design' being implied).

As discussed in Chapter 2, the alternative term 'quality of manufacture' is probably preferable to 'quality of conformance', in order to avoid any implication that the quality of a manufactured product can be assured by merely testing for conformance to a specification.

Good practice beyond manufacturing

Thus, overall quality depends upon the fitness for purpose of the product as originally designed. That is upon whether or not it is intrinsically fit for its intended purpose; and then upon the way that 'designed fitness' is retained, and maintained, in routine day-to-day production.

Mere compliance with a specification alone is not an adequate determinant of the quality of medicinal and similar products. So, bearing in mind the definitions given in the UK Orange Guide and EC GMP Guide, if good manufacturing practice (GMP) is subtracted from quality assurance (QA), what have we left?

GMP is about QA in day-to-day production, i.e. it is concerned with quality of manufacture. As in more general quality assurance, pharmaceutical QA also reaches beyond that. It, too, embraces 'quality of design' and it also extends beyond routine manufacture in another direction. The quality of manufactured medicines needs also to be assured in warehousing, transportation, wholesaling, dispensing, administration and use of the product. Having accepted that GMP is a part of QA (and is, in fact, concerned with the assurance of quality of manufacture), what are these other non-GMP factors? What QA functions exist beyond GMP? That is, if QA–GMP = X, then what constitutes X?

Quality aspects of R&D

'Design', in the more general industrial sense, may be taken to mean what we normally term 'research and development' (R&D), and here there are two main elements, that is:

1. The research and development of the active drug substance.
2. The development of the formulation of that substance into a dosage form suitable for presentation to a patient.

It could perhaps be considered that these two elements respectively represent chemical R&D, and pharmaceutical R&D. It might be better, however, to avoid such a compartmented line of thinking and to regard the overall exercise as a multidisciplinary team effort, with the emphasis on *team*. Furthermore, in the best interests of quality assurance, there should not be a discontinuity between R&D on the one hand and routine manufacture and quality control on the other. Questions on the following aspects need to be considered, in a cooperative, coordinated manner during the R&D phase, and not left until full-scale production is under way:

- Bulk manufacture (chemicals and dosage forms).
- Sources.
- Specifications and test methods for materials.
- In-process controls.
- Product test-methods, specifications.
- Stability studies.
- Manufacturing hazards and precautions.
- Finished package format and materials.

The principal objective of pharmaceutical R&D is to find (invent or discover) active compounds which either present an entirely new therapeutic potential for the treatment of previously untreatable, or inadequately treated, diseases, or which are believed to have some benefit or advantage in comparison with substances already available to treat an existing disease or condition.

The new active substance may be derived from natural sources. It may be a synthetic molecular modification of a naturally occurring compound, or it may be a chemical modification of a synthetic substance already known to have therapeutic value. It could be the result of a theoretical consideration of molecular structure/therapeutic activity relationships, or it could have been a product of biotechnology/genetic engineering. It could be a matter of chance observation (penicillin is a classic case) or it could be the discovery of hitherto unsuspected advantageous effects in a substance under investigation for an entirely different therapeutic purpose.

Whatever its source, a new compound must pass through various stages of pharmacological, toxicological and clinical screening, and here there is a high rate of attrition. Up to 10 000 new compounds are synthesised for every new medicinal product which reaches the market. It is, however, during this very costly phase that the basic fitness, the quality of design, of the new product is established; not merely the fitness of the active compound to achieve its intended purpose, but also the preservation and promotion of that fitness in and by the dosage form which will be administered to the patient. It avails nothing if a potentially valuable new therapeutic agent has its activity negated, diminished or compromised by interference from excipients, or because of an inappropriate formulation. Here we enter upon such areas as drug design, formulation and biopharmaceutics which are outside the scope of this book. It must be remembered, however, that all these aspects bear crucially upon the quality of the product – its fitness for its intended purpose. Here we encounter another quality issue which is perhaps different from any encountered in other industries. That of the inherently undesirable effects of medicinal compounds, and of risk/benefit analysis.

In the manufacture of virtually all other types of product, faults in quality of design could be attributable to inadequacies in the designers themselves, or in the facilities (including time) available to them; to pressures placed upon them; or to compromises consciously accepted in order to deliver a product 'down to a price', rather than 'up to a quality standard'. All these factors could (note 'could', not necessarily 'do') affect the quality of design of a medicinal product. There is, in addition, the possibly unique problem of inherent side effects. It has been said that all drug substances which have 'effects' also have 'side effects', of variable degrees of severity. One of the objectives of all the pharmacological, toxicological and clinical screening is not only to determine activity and efficacy, but also to establish the nature and extent of any side effects. It is on the basis of such information that a decision can be made (by producer/marketer and regulatory authority) on whether the anticipated benefits outweigh the risks, and thus justify the marketing of the product for administration to patients.

These are all aspects which demand the most scrupulous attention by the manufacturer, and which are reviewed in detail by regulatory authorities for Marketing Authorisations.

Scale-up

Having established that a substance, formulated into a given dosage form, has a desirable level of therapeutic activity, combined with an acceptable level of patient-risk, it then becomes necessary to scale-up the laboratory-level process, possibly via pilot-scale, through to full-scale manufacture.

Problems of scale-up need to be addressed both in the manufacture of the bulk active substance, and in the manufacture and packaging of the dosage form. Here, too, routine test methods and specifications, in-process controls, etc. need to be further developed, modified and refined.

Good laboratory practice (GLP) and good control laboratory practice (GCLP)

There have been two possible interpretations of the term 'good laboratory practice' (GLP). It has been taken to refer either to good practice in pharmacological and toxicological research and testing laboratories, or to good practice in manufacturers' QC laboratories. It has become conventional to use 'good laboratory practice' in reference to the pharmacological and toxicological laboratories and to use 'good control laboratory practice' (GCLP) in the context of manufacturers' QC laboratories. GCLP is discussed in some detail later in Chapter 16.

Just as reliable results cannot be expected from analytical and/or microbiological testing laboratories unless good practices are followed, so too must good practices be followed in pharmacological and toxicological laboratories if their results are to be relied upon.

Similar principles as we have already considered when discussing the basic principles of GMP apply to GLP, the major issues being:

1. Management commitment and control.
2. Suitable premises.
3. Appropriately qualified and trained staff.
4. Properly maintained and calibrated equipment.
5. Written operating procedures.
6. Assurance that written procedures are followed.
7. Proper recording systems.
8. Adequate data storage.

Compliance with GLP, and inspection by national inspectorates to monitor and ensure compliance, are required under European directives:

1. Council directive on the harmonisation of laws, regulations and administrative provisions relating to the application of the principles of good laboratory practice and the verification of their application for tests on chemical substances (Directive 87/18/EEC).
2. Council directive on the inspection and verification of good laboratory practice (Directive 88/320/EEC).

Considerations similar to those relating to GLP also apply to the conduct of clinical trials in humans. The EC has issued guidelines on good clinical trial practice (GCTP) (*Good Clinical Practice for Trials on Medicinal Products in the EC*, Vol. III of *The Rules Governing Medicinal Products in the European Community*; EC, 1990), which are concerned with both the protection of those on whom the trials are conducted, and on the integrity and reliability of the data thus generated.

Annex 13 to the EC GMP Guide (EC, 1992), as reproduced in MCA, 1997, is on the 'manufacture of investigational medicinal products', i.e. it is concerned with GMP in the manufacture of products and materials intended for use in clinical trials. At the time this Annex 13 was published, compliance with GMP in the manufacture of products for clinical trials was not mandatory in the European Union. However, more recently (early 1998) a final draft of an EC Directive on good clinical practice has been issued for comment. This is a comprehensive document which encompasses both GCP *per se* and GMP in the manufacture of investigational medicinal products. The draft has seven chapters:

- Chapter I. Scope and definitions
- Chapter II. Protection of trial subject
- Chapter III. Commencement of a clinical trial
- Chapter IV. Manufacture, import and labelling of investigational medicinal products
- Chapter V. Compliance
- Chapter VI. Clinical safety reporting
- Chapter VII. General provisions.

Chapter I is concerned with clinical trials, including multicentre trials, on human subjects, using medicinal products as defined in Directive 65/65/EEC. It requires all clinical trials to comply with good clinical practice. There is a definition of an 'investigational medicinal product' as:

> a pharmaceutical form of an active substance, or placebo, being tested or used as a comparator in a clinical trial, or an already licensed medicinal product when it is used, or assembled (manufactured or packaged in a way different from the authorised form) or when used in a non-authorised indication, or to gain more information on its authorised use.

The provisions of Chapter IV have the most direct relevance to the subject of this book. Article 10.1 of Chapter IV requires manufacturers and importers of investigational medicinal products to hold an Article 16 Authorisation (as per Directive 75/319/EEC). In the UK that means a full Manufacturer's Licence or, for products imported from third countries, a Wholesale Dealers (Import) Licence, and this will be a new requirement in the UK.

Article 10.2 of Chapter IV of the Draft EC Directive states that Chapters IV and V of Directive 75/319/EEC shall apply to the manufacture, import and labelling of investigational products. The effect of this provision, in the UK, will be that manufacturers and assemblers of investigational medicinal products will have to hold a Manufacturer's Licence, and importers a Wholesale Dealers (Import) Licence, with all the requirements and 'standard provisions' which attach to the holding of such licences, e.g. suitable staff, premises, equipment and 'control facilities', compliance with the principles and guidelines of GMP, being subject to regulatory inspections, and having the services of a Qualified Person (QP). The duties, responsibilities, qualifications and experience of the QP must be as set out in Articles 22, 23 and 24 of Directive 75/319/EEC. (For a discussion of the nature and role of a QP in the rather special European sense, see Part Three: Personnel.)

The stated date for the full implementation of the EC Investigational Medicinal Product Directive, in its final agreed form, is 1 January 1999.

Summary of quality aspects in R&D

These may be summarised as a sequence, thus:

1. 'Discover' new drug substance.
2. Establish identity, molecular formula and structure etc.
3. Evaluate therapeutic potential vs. risks/toxicity (note GLP).
4. If substance appears promising, commence studies into developing substance into 'usable' dosage form(s).
5. At same time start development of quality test methods, standards and specifications.
6. Carry out clinical trials (note GCTP).
7. Establish final dosage form and package (complete with specification and test methods for all ingredients and packaging materials).
8. Commence stability studies on formulated and packaged product.
9. Scale-up of both active substance and dosage form manufacture and packaging.
10. In the light of (9) above, further refine, or modify as necessary, material and product test methods, specifications and controls.
11. Commence routine manufacture, ensuring that the designed quality is maintained batch after batch after batch, by the application of GMP.

Distribution, wholesale and beyond

'QA less or without GMP' is not concerned just with R&D (i.e. with aspects of quality before batch manufacture begins); there is also the question of what happens to those batches of product after they have been manufactured and packaged.

The crucial issue must surely be of the quality of the product as it is administered to the patient. Once a product has been packaged and passed from a manufacturer's own released product storage area it still has to face a number of potentially quality-hazardous steps before it achieves its ultimate objective. It needs to be transported, often to and then from, a wholesale dealing establishment. It needs to be dispensed, and it needs to be administered to, or taken by, the patient, all without hazard to the quality as designed and as (one hopes) maintained throughout the manufacturing and packaging process.

Quite obviously finished products must be stored and transported under conditions which will minimise the possibility of deterioration, contamination, breakage, spillage, etc. Where special storage conditions (e.g. temperature, humidity, light) are required, steps need to be taken to ensure that such conditions are indeed provided, and maintained. Steps need also to be taken to ensure that any identification, status- or batch-numbering labelling is not lost or mixed up.

Good practice in wholesale distribution

The issue of legal requirement and good practice by wholesale dealers is covered in the following three publications, all of which are reprinted in

Rules and Guidance for Pharmaceutical Manufacturers and Distributors (MCA, 1997):

- The UK *Standard Provisions for Wholesale Dealer's [sic] Licences.*
- Directive 92/25/EEC, *Wholesale Distribution of Medicinal Products for Human Use.*
- EC *Guidelines on Good Distribution Practice of Medicinal Products for Human Use* (Directive 94/C 63/03).

Good practice in dispensing

The dispensing of products to patients provides a further opportunity for mix-up, contamination, and/or mislabelling. One would not of course wish to suggest that dispensing pharmacists would, or even could, be responsible for any of those sorts of things, but it is a sound general QA principle to assume that if a mistake can happen then, given a chance, it ultimately will, and thus to aim to eliminate the possibility altogether. Approximately 400 million prescription items are dispensed per year in the UK alone. We commonly talk of 'human error' in terms of a 'one in a million chance'. Let us assume that the average pharmacist is 10 times less prone to error than the ordinary mortal, and that therefore he or she has only a 1 in 10 million chance of making a mistake. That would still equate to 40 dispensing errors per year in the UK. Whether or not that figure approximates the actual annual number of dispensing errors per year it is not possible to say. Why not, therefore, abandon the 'traditional' dispensing methods altogether, so that the dispenser cannot possibly count, measure or weigh out the wrong product or the wrong quantity, or contaminate the product in handling, etc.?

Patient packs

Certainly the wisdom has been questioned of expecting a manufacturer to produce a product under strict standards of hygiene and control and to package it in a container system tried and tested with regard to compatibility, product-protection and security, only to have that container breached, the contents re-handled, repackaged (in a product/container/ closure system which usually has *not* been the subject of suitability and stability studies) and relabelled. A response to this, in recent years, has been various attempted moves towards original pack, or patient pack dispensing, where the manufacturer provides a product in packages of a size and design suitable to be given direct to a patient (with just the addition of the legally required pharmacist's dispensing label) and containing a sufficient number, weight or volume for a defined course of treatment. This is a concept which has long been the norm in a number of European countries. It is slowly developing in the UK, but 'slowly' is perhaps the operative word.

Good practice in administering medicines

The final potential hazard to product quality is the patient, and/or the person who administers the product to him or her. Research has shown that the way patients take their medicine, in terms of amount, timing, conditions, manner, precautions and so on, often falls short of the ideal. A current move to improve this situation is the provision (along with patient packs) of patient information leaflets, designed to make patients better informed about their medicine, and to take it better.

The wider implications of GMP/quality

The Introduction in the 1983 UK Orange Guide states:

> The object of GMP . . . is, initially, the assurance of the quality of the product, and ultimately the safety, well-being and protection of the patient.

Sadly, it has not always been seen in that way, and one has encountered company training manuals which state, in effect, 'we have GMP and GMP training, because if we do not, we will be in trouble when the inspector calls'. Another narrow view is to consider that GMP is something which involves only Production and QC Departments. Yet another is exemplified by the 'blurbs' for new items of manufacturing equipment which describes them as 'complying with GMP' – when all that is often meant is that the equipment is relatively easy to clean.

If an appropriately wider view is taken, it will be seen that there are interactions between GMP considerations and many other sections or functions within a manufacturing company. These include:

- Personnel/recruitment policies
- Training/motivation
- Engineering/maintenance
- Production planning/sales forecasting
- Inventory policy and levels
- Factory design and layout
- Warehousing systems/materials handling
- Product range and variety
- Documentation
- Regulatory affairs
- Finance/costing ('the cost of quality').

All these functions bear upon, and are affected by, GMP – a conclusion which may be thought of as not unlike a basic philosophy of the so-called 'total quality management' (TQM). It is, however, a view that some pharmaceutical industry people have been expressing for a number of years.

A number of the topics or functions listed above will be discussed later. Some are worthy of further comment now.

Engineering and maintenance

The importance of the engineering and maintenance functions hardly needs re-stating. Quite simply, equipment and services need to be properly installed, commissioned, and maintained in order to ensure optimum, consistent performance, and hence consistent product quality. There is no longer any room for the traditional divide, the apparently unbridgeable gulf, between Engineering on the one hand and Production on the other. Engineers need to be fully aware of the special requirements and disciplines of medicines manufacture, and no less do production people need to understand that engineers are (or should be) a beneficial necessity rather than a necessary evil.

Production planning

The basic data required for production planning include:

1.   A forecast of anticipated sales.
2.   A knowledge of current stock levels.
3.   Company policy on inventory levels.
4.   Plant capacity.

In other words, you need to know what stocks you expect to sell, what you have got, what are the optimum stock levels you wish to hold, and the capacity you have to produce those stocks.

These factors all interact one with another. They also interact significantly with quality considerations. Poorly planned production (either through bad forecasting, inadequate stock data, failure to consider plant capacities, or through incompetence, or disregard of the wider realities) can have serious effects on quality. If excess production is planned, a strain will be placed on manufacturing and storage capacities, with resultant congestion, prevention of smooth work flows, and ultimate problems of stability and shelf-life. If too little production is planned to meet demand, the result will be chaos-inducing panic production and rescheduling, which is inimical to the planned, orderly approach that is the essence of GMP.

Inventory levels

Inventory policy will also have quality effects. To minimise holding costs it is sound sense to keep inventory to a low but workable level. If the level is set too low, then 'panic-production' could be a constant feature, as will congestion if it is set too high in relation to available storage space.

Decisions on inventory policy will also affect stock levels and lead times for materials, and thus whether or not sufficient materials are available in sufficient time for examination, release and use. The quality implications are obvious.

The cost of quality

These are just a few examples of the quality implications and interactions of and with other functions. Others will be discussed. There is also the question of cost.

Some have raised the question of the cost of QA/GMP, and whether that cost is justified. This is a pointless question, which displays a complete lack of understanding of what GMP and QA are all about.

Quality is intrinsic to the making of medicines. It is not, or it should not be, regarded as an extra on-cost for the manufacturer. Neither is it something, inherently undesirable, imposed upon the manufacturer from without by officials of some regulatory body.

To speak of the cost of quality is like talking of the 'additional' cost of making a motor car with a steering wheel and brakes. Quality is not an 'optional extra'. Quality is central to the business of making medicines; its very heart. The test of the validity of any quality measure is 'does it ultimately contribute to the safety, well-being and protection of the patient'? If it does not then it is an unnecessary expense, for indeed it is not about quality, or at least it is not about quality with a purpose.

Cost-effective GMP

There are, in fact, cost-benefits. Good plant layout, smooth work flows, efficient documentation systems, well-controlled processes, good stores layouts and stores records – these are all good manufacturing practices. They are also good practice from a managerial and economic viewpoint.

Ensuring properly trained, well-directed, well-motivated staff with a full understanding of what they are doing is good manufacturing practice. It is also good, cost-effective management, since staff will be happier, work better and produce more. Not only that, they will produce more of better quality.

The smooth flowing, planned approach which is essential to GMP, combined with efficient documentation systems, can result in a significant reduction in work-in-progress and hence in inventory holding costs.

Such things demonstrate the positive cost-benefits of QA/GMP. To these must be added the avoidance of the cost of quality failure, e.g. the cost of waste, of rework, of recall, of consumer compensation and of loss of company reputation.

Cost/benefit analysis

The cost/benefit implications may be summarised as in Table 6.1.

GMP/QA is not an 'on-cost'. It is not even just 'free'. It is a contribution to profit. It has been said, with some justice, that:

> Good manufacturing practice is also good management practice leading to good manufacturing profit.

The effects of QA/GMP, and the interactions with other functions within the total manufacturing organisation are many and varied. We all need to be

Table 6.1   How the cost of quality equates to a contribution to profit

Cost of quality =
[Cost of A] – [Cost of B] – [Pay-back from C] = **Profit**

A	B	C
Staff	Scrap	Improved morale
Training	Rework	Motivation
Systems	Complaints	Faster throughput
Documentation	'Chaos'	Higher productivity
Equipment	Lost sales	Increased sales
Maintenance	Recalls	Lower inventory
Calibration	Close-down	
Sampling		
Testing		
In process control		
Validation		
Auditing		

aware of this, and ensure that these various interfaces are complementary and creative, and not antagonistic or destructive. GMP should not be considered as something extrinsic to, or imposed upon, manufacturing activities, but as something which is central and basic, and which has cost-*benefits*.

References

EC (1990). *The Rules Governing Medicinal Products in the European Community, Vol. III: Good Clinical Practice for Trials on Medicinal Products in the EC.* Luxembourg: Commission of the European Communities. Available from The Office for Official Publications of the European Communities, Luxembourg. Also available from The Stationery Office (HMSO), London, and The EC Information Service, Washington, USA.

EC (1992). *The Rules Governing Medicinal Products in the European Community, Vol. IV: Good Manufacturing Practice for Medicinal Products.* Luxembourg: Commission of the European Communities. Available from The Office for Official Publications of the European Communities, Luxembourg. Also available from The Stationery Office (HMSO), London, and The EC Information Service, Washington, USA. Also stated *verbatim* with guidance on the detailed interpretation of these rules in MCA, 1997. (Referred to as the EC GMP Guide.)

MCA (1997). *Rules and Guidance for Pharmaceutical Manufacturers and Distributors.* London: Medicines Control Agency. Available from The Stationery Office (HMSO), London.

7

The quality movement, 'quality gurus', TQM and ISO 9000

. . . and all that jazz
  Anon, mid 20th century

Wisest men have erred. . . . And shall again, pretend they ne'er so wise
  John Milton, *Samson Agonistes*, 1671, line 210

Anyone who observes the world around them, with even half an eye, cannot fail to notice that there is abroad a sort of mystical quality cult. 'Quality' is used, in a variety of senses, as a selling point for a wide variety of goods and services. Companies proudly claim to be certified to a Quality Standard. The effects of this 'quality movement', have not invariably been good. For example, despite all the worthy attempts to give the term 'quality' a precise meaning in the industrial manufacturing context, the word continues to be misunderstood and misused. Worse, it is now being abused to the extent that it has been battered out of all meaningful recognition. Those who have any knowledge of industry as a whole will have noted the ornate displays in reception areas of framed 'quality policy' statements. These are often written by the directors and fulsomely declare the company's undying and total commitment to quality. Such effusions are impelled by the ISO 9000 series, which require a statement of company quality policy, and will often be found to be totally belied by what is to be seen on the shop floor. Some months ago there appeared, in the national press, a notice from a major motor-car manufacturer headed 'Important Quality Announcement'. It stated that its 'on-going quality assurance programme' had identified a potentially hazardous fault in the steering mechanism of a particular range of models (already on the road) which it was recalling for check-up. This is not quality assurance. It is rather an attempt at lending a spurious air of respectability to an abject quality *failure*.

The use and abuse of 'quality'

Closer to home, a multinational company, which engages in the manufacture of medicinal products, recently issued to its suppliers a document headed 'Quality Statement'. On examination, this turned out to be a statement of the terms and conditions under which the company will pay for goods supplied. This is followed by a statement of over ten different conditions under which they will **not** pay – and that if they do, it will take two months. What on earth has this got to do with quality, one wonders?

More recently a major foodstuffs manufacturer has announced in the press that as a result of its 'commitment to quality and safety' it is recalling some of its products which, apparently, are dangerously defective. This displays not a commitment to quality, but a hopeless inadequacy of quality commitment.

Some of the blame, at least indirectly, for these sort of perversions of 'quality', where a virtue can be made out of failure, must be laid at the door of the proponents of the quality movement and of the quality image. Go through the motions, get certified, stick-up the slogans and quality policy statements, and you are made! This is just not good enough where medicinal and other healthcare products are concerned.

Steps of the quality masters

Much of the original motivating force behind the general quality movement derives from the so-called 'quality gurus' and their (to some) sacred utterances. Although to many the clarity and precision of their thought and expression is not always of the highest quality, it nevertheless has to be accepted that, in industry at large, their influence has been considerable. Juran and Deming, for example, are frequently credited with the success of the post-war Japanese industry, and the replacement of its previous shoddy image by a reputation for high quality.

This considerable influence has probably been more apparent in industries other than pharmaceuticals. But medicines *are* different. They impose special quality demands. Because of this, the pharmaceutical industry has tended rather to plough its own quality furrow. Nevertheless, anyone concerned with, or about, the quality of manufactured products should know something of the philosophies of the gurus (who largely seem to be American), and there may even be things to be learned from them. Let us consider just the top triumvirate of Deming, Juran and Crosby, who have each summed up their respective quality philosophies as a series of 'points' or 'steps'

Walter E Deming

Deming's (1982) much-quoted '14 points' are:

1. Create constancy of purpose towards improvement of product and service.
2. Adopt the new philosophy: we can no longer live with commonly accepted levels of delays, mistakes, defective workmanship.
3. Cease dependence on mass inspection: require instead statistical evidence that quality is built-in.

4. End the practice of awarding business on basis of price tag.
5. Find problems: it is management's job to work continually on the system.
6. Institute modern methods of training on the job.
7. Institute modern methods of supervision of production workers: the responsibility of foremen must be changed from numbers to quality.
8. Drive out fear, so that everyone may work effectively for the company.
9. Break down barriers between departments.
10. Eliminate numerical goals, posters and slogans for the workforce that ask for new levels of productivity without providing methods.
11. Eliminate work standards that prescribe numerical quotas.
12. Remove barriers that stand between the hourly worker and his rights to pride of workmanship.
13. Institute a vigorous programme of education and retraining.
14. Create a top management structure that will push every day on the above 13 points.

Joseph M Juran

Juran (1974) has proposed '10 Steps to quality improvement'. These are summarised as:

1. Build awareness of the need and opportunity for improvement.
2. Set goals for improvement.
3. Organise to reach the goals (establish a quality council, identify problems, select projects, appoint teams, designate facilitators).
4. Provide training.
5. Carry out projects to solve problems.
6. Report progress.
7. Give recognition.
8. Communicate results.
9. Keep score.
10. Maintain momentum by making annual improvement part of the regular systems and process of the company.

Philip B Crosby

The third of the trinity of most frequently quoted gurus is Crosby. He also has set forth his 14 steps to quality improvement (Crosby, 1979). They are:

1. Make it clear that management is committed to quality.
2. Form quality improvement teams with representatives from each department.
3. Determine where current and potential quality problems lie.
4. Evaluate the cost of quality and explain its use as a management tool.
5. Raise the quality awareness and personal concern of all employees.
6. Take actions to correct problems identified through previous steps.

7. Establish a committee for the zero defects programme.
8. Train supervisors to carry out their part of the quality improvement programme.
9. Hold a 'zero defects day' to let all employees know that there has been a change.
10. Encourage individuals to establish improvement goals for themselves in their groups.
11. Encourage employees to communicate to management the obstacles they face in attaining their improvement goals.
12. Recognise and appreciate those who participate.
13. Establish quality councils to communicate on a regular basis.
14. Do it over again to emphasise that the quality improvement programme never ends.

It is, of course, unreasonable to form a definitive judgement on the value, or otherwise, of the works of Deming, Juran and Crosby on the basis alone of these condensed versions of their own summaries of their respective philosophies. But they do give a flavour of the sort of intellectual world they inhabit. One important factor, at least, emerges – they all place marked (indeed major) stress on *people* and their management, motivation and training. Compare:

- 'The quality of a product ultimately depends on the quality of those producing it' (Sir Dereck Dunlop, 1971).
- 'It is impossible to over-emphasise the importance of people, at all levels, in the Assurance of the Quality of medicinal products', from the Introduction to the UK Orange Guide (Sharp, 1983).

In a nutshell, for medicinal products to be fit for their purpose, it is essential that the people involved in making them should themselves be fit for that purpose.

Total quality management (TQM)

This emphasis (or perhaps re-emphasis would be a better term) on the importance of people in the assurance of quality is one of the major thrusts behind the concept of total quality management. TQM is very much a current 'in' topic (there will be others). A difficulty is, however, in stating in a precise, concise and simple way just what TQM in fact is. Perhaps the best known British book on the subject is Oakland's *Total Quality Management*. Although Oakland states that 'TQM is the new way of managing for the future', he does not appear to provide a precise statement of what it is, or what in fact makes it new, or different from (or better than) for example, 'total quality control', 'quality assurance', or the philosophies of various other gurus. He says (Oakland, 1989):

> TQM . . . is a way of managing the whole business or organisation to ensure complete customer satisfaction at every stage, internally and externally . . . TQM is an approach to improving the effectiveness and flexibility of a business as a whole. It is essentially a way of organising and involving the whole organisation . . . TQM is a method for ridding people's lives of wasted effort by involving everyone in the process of improvement.

But he does not provide a simple statement of what this 'way', this 'approach', or this 'method' is. Perhaps it is intended to be deduced from a reading of the book as a whole – which still leaves at least one reader with a feeling of 'What's new?' Oakland also says that his book 'is about how to manage in a total quality way', which opens up the question 'What is "total quality"?', as distinct, for example, from ordinary, common or garden quality? One is also left to wonder whether TQM is about:

1. The management of total quality (whatever that is), or
2. The totality of quality management, or
3. Management that is total in its quality.

Perhaps all one can do in this context is to attempt to extract what appears to be some of the basic constituent elements of TQM. These seem to be:

- Proper definition of 'quality'.
- Commitment by all to attaining that quality (as defined).
- Making quality attainment a (if not *the*) major basis for the management structure of the company.
- Ensuring quality of design.
- Using statistical techniques to control and measure quality.
- Training.
- Motivation.
- Teamwork.
- Documentation.

Features of TQM

So, one might well ask, 'Is there anything about this that is new?' Apart from a few changes of flavour, not much it would seem. Certainly not much in terms of what has long been perceived within the pharmaceutical and related industries as essential prerequisites for the attainment of quality. Perhaps TQM (whatever it is) will at least serve as a reminder that mere perception is not sufficient. It is the *implementation* of what is perceived as necessary which is important. This realisation can be assisted by what seem to be some of the basic concepts of TQM, which include:

1. *Management awareness.* Moving from archaic management/organisational structures which regard quality activities and personnel management as relatively insignificant 'extras'; moving even from a more enlightened position where quality (and its control/assurance/

management, call it what you will) is considered as a major factor and a top function in the company structure, to a position where it is *the* major factor and function.

2. *Quality training.* Moving from an archaic position where workers are 'trained' by 'sitting with Nellie' and doing what they are told; moving even from a more enlightened position where some form of training (both in specific skills and in general quality concepts and applications) is given on some form of regular and formal basis, to a situation where training and retraining is a permanent and comprehensive 'way of life'.

3. *Employee commitment.* Moving from an archaic position where workers at all levels are required merely to do unquestioningly as they are instructed, with no indication of the 'whats' and 'whys'; moving even from a more enlightened position where at least the views of supervisory personnel are considered to be of value, to a position where *all* personnel in *all* departments (not just those working directly on the product) are considered to have something useful to contribute to the quality of the product.

4. *Teamwork.* Encouragement of teamwork, and of a sense that a team is not just a worker and his or her immediate colleagues, but that each of these mini-teams is but part of 'the team', the company as a whole, the principal objective of which is product quality.

5. *Internal customer concept.* Identification of the customer and understanding precisely what he, she or it wants – AND – extending the concept of 'the customer' to embrace internal as well as external customers. An external customer is a customer outside a company, to whom the company is supplying goods or services. An internal customer is a department, section or person within a company to whom or to which another department, section or person within that same company is supplying materials, goods or services. (Awareness of the identity and specific requirements of not only external, but also internal customers is a particularly characteristic flavour of TQM.)

British Standards on quality and the ISO 9000 Series

In the early 1970s the British Standards Institute issued a series of guides on quality assurance. In 1979 a British Standard, BS 5750 'Quality Systems', was published. In this the principles of QA, as at the time perceived by BSI, were set out as *specifications* rather than as recommendations, as in the earlier guides.

In 1987 a 'new' BS 5750 was published. This was identical to the English version of the International Standards Organisation's (ISO) 9000 Series of Quality Systems Specifications. In 1994 this series of standards was reissued, with amendments, by BSI as the BS EN ISO 9000 series.

Inspecting organisations have been set up (including one by BSI itself) in order to provide for the certification of manufacturers of their compliance with the Standard(s). These certifying organisations need to be accredited by BSI, which also publishes lists of companies which have been certified as meeting one or other of the various parts of the Standard.

Some, but not all, believe that certification to BS 5750/ISO 9000 is a peak indication of 'quality standing', for want of a better phrase. There have also been a number of instances of potential importers requiring the prior BS 5750/ISO 9000 certification of potential British exporters. Furthermore, there are grounds for believing that the Medicines Inspectorate of the UK MCA is distinctly 'pro-5750/ISO 9000': witness its March 1994 announcement that it has itself been certified, as a service, to BS 5750/ISO 9000. Therefore, whatever we may think of it, it is necessary to examine this British/ISO Standard in a little more detail.

A fundamental point must be established: BS 5750/ISO 9000 is not specifically about quality assurance *in the manufacture of medicines*. It is intended as a general specification for quality systems in the provision of *any* product or service. However, it is very clear from a reading of its various sections that it has been written very much from an engineering and/or hardware fabrication point of view, and considerable and continuous mental adjustment is necessary to relate it to the manufacture of medicines and the like. It is also about having 'quality systems', and there are those who would argue that it would be possible to comply with BS 5750/ISO 9000 (i.e. by having a 'quality system') and still produce poor quality products.

Summary of BS/ISO 9001

There are a number of parts to the Standard. The principal parts are Parts 1, 2, and 3, which have the following titles:

- **BS EN ISO 9001:** 'Quality systems model for quality assurance in design, development, production, installation and servicing'
- **BS EN ISO 9002:** 'Quality systems model for quality assurance in production, installation and servicing'
- **BS EN ISO 9003:** 'Quality systems model for quality assurance in final inspection and test'

ISO 9002 is little more than a reduced version of ISO 9001, repeating many of its elements and omitting others. ISO 9003 is a further (much) reduced version of ISO 9002.

There are a number of additional BSI/ISO publications in the '9000' family, for example:

- **ISO 9000-1:** 'Quality management and quality assurance standards'. This is available in four separately issued parts:
  - Part 1: Guidelines for selection and use
  - Part 2: Generic guidelines for the application of ISO 9001, ISO 9002 and ISO 9003

    — Part 3: Guideline for the application of ISO 9001 to the development, supply and maintenance of software
    — Part 4: Guide to dependability programme management

- **ISO 9004:** 'Quality management and quality system elements'. This is available in eight separately issued parts:

    — Part 1: Guidelines
    — Part 2: Guidelines for services
    — Part 3: Guidelines for processed materials
    — Part 4: Guidelines for quality improvement
    — Part 5: Guidelines for quality plans
    — Part 6: Guidelines on quality assurance for project management
    — Part 7: Guidelines for configuration management
    — Part 8: Guidelines on quality principles and their application to management practices

There are a number of other associated BS/ISO, publications, for example, BS 4778 Part 1/ISO 8402 'Quality vocabulary – international terms' in which a number of items of quality terminology are defined in English, French and Russian.

The main substance of ISO 9001 is its Section 4 'Quality system requirements'. This sets out 20 quality system elements, numbered 4.1 to 4.20. Briefly summarised (in italics), these requirements are given below. Against each summary appears a comment (non-italicised) on where or how the corresponding requirements appear in pharmaceutical guidelines/legislation. ('OG' = The UK Orange Guide (1983); 'ECG' = The EC GMP Guide (1992); 'EC Directive' = The EC GMP Directive 91/356/EEC.)

ISO 9001 Section 4.1 Management responsibility

Management is required to 'define' and document its policy and objectives for, and its commitment to, quality and to *ensure that this policy is understood, implemented and maintained at all levels.* (cf. OG Sections 1 and 2, ECG Chapters 1 and 2 and EC Directive.)

Responsibility, authority and relationships of all relevant personnel shall be defined. (Again, see OG Sections 1 and 2, ECG Chapters 1 and 2 and EC Directive.)

'In-house' requirements for inspection, test and monitoring, for 'design review' and quality audits shall be 'identified', and adequate resources and trained personnel shall be provided. Design reviews and quality audits shall be carried-out by persons independent of those responsible for actual manufacture. (All basic principles of GMP, in OG and ECG, and of UK and EC Legislation.)

There shall be a 'management representative' responsible for 'ensuring that the requirements of this International Standard are implemented and maintained. (cf. OG, and ECG Chapters 1 and 2, and UK and EC Legislation regarding Production and QC Management, and the 'Qualified Person'.)

The quality system shall be subject to 'management reviews'. (See OG 1.4 and ECG 9 on self-inspection, and EC GMP Directive 356, Article 14.)

ISO 9001 Section 4.2 Quality systems

The supplier shall establish and maintain a documented quality system . . . including (a) the preparation of . . . procedures and instructions; (b) the effective implementation of the . . . procedures and instructions. (Generally implicit and specifically explicit in OG and ECG and in all other UK and EC regulations, directives and guidelines – all in greater and more explicit detail.)

ISO 9001 Section 4.3 Contract review

Not always relevant to medicines manufacture. Where contract manufacture of medicinal product is involved, see the more detailed and explicit clarification of requirements in OG 14, and ECG 7, and also Article 12 of EC GMP Directive. (Note however, that it is possible to regard a Product Licence or Marketing Authorisation as a carefully reviewed contract with the authorities.)

ISO 9001 Section 4.4 Design control

This whole aspect is covered in greater, and more specifically, relevant detail in UK and EC legislation on requirements for Product Licences or Marketing Authorisations.

ISO 9001 Section 4.5 Document and data control

Including approval/issue, changes/modifications, etc. (All requirements of ISO 9000 are covered in much greater detail in OG 3 and ECG 4 under 'Documentation'. See also EC Directive.)

ISO 9001 Section 4.6 Purchasing

This section of BS/ISO 9001 is concerned with verification of the quality of purchased-in materials, and the assessment of subcontractors. All aspects are covered in greater and more specifically relevant detail in OG and ECG.

ISO 9001 Section 4.7 Control of purchaser supplied product

See comments under Section 4.6 above.

ISO 9001 Section 4.8 Product identification and traceability

BS/ISO requires this 'where appropriate'. (Full product and batch identity and traceability at all stages is a fundamental requirement of all GMP guides, codes, and all national and international medicines legislation.)

ISO 9001 Section 4.9 Process control

This section of BS 5750 is concerned with the control of processes which 'directly affect quality', to include:

1.   Documented instructions on 'manner of production', use of equipment, working environment, compliance with standards.
2.   Monitoring and in-process control of processes and procedures.
3.   Approval of processes and equipment 'as appropriate'.
4.   'Criteria for workmanship'.

All these aspects are covered in greater and more specifically relevant detail in GMP guidelines and regulations.

ISO 9001 Section 4.10 Inspection and testing

This section is concerned with:

•   Verification by inspection and testing of the quality of incoming materials and products.
•   The quality of products in-process.
•   The quality of the end product.
•   Maintaining inspection and test records.

All this is (again) covered in much greater and more specifically relevant detail in the UK/EC GMP guidelines and in regulations.

ISO 9001 Section 4.11 Inspection, measuring and test equipment

This section is concerned with:

•   The maintenance and calibration of test equipment.
•   Ensuring that measurements that need to be made are in fact made.
•   Using instruments and devices 'of the accuracy and precision necessary'.
•   Maintaining records of equipment calibration and maintenance.

(See OG 4.36 and 8.5–8.9, and ECG 3.40, 3.41.)

ISO 9001 Section 4.12 Inspection and test status

ISO 9000 here requires indication of status (of product only it appears) by means of marks, tags, labels, segregation, etc. This section also requires that records be kept that shall 'identify the inspection authority for the release of conforming product.' (Re. Status OG/ECG require clear status (e.g. 'quarantine', 'on test', 'released', 'rejected', etc.) not only of product, but also of ingredients, packaging materials, intermediates, recovered or recalled goods, and equipment. Formal signed release of product by an authorised person (i.e. a 'Qualified Person') is, of course, a UK and European statutory requirement.)

ISO 9001 Section 4.13 Control of non-conforming product

This section requires procedures which will ensure that product 'that does not conform to specified requirements is prevented from inadvertent use or installation', with documented control over 'evaluation, segregation and (where practical) disposition of non-conforming product'. (Such requirements are an inherent part of GMP guidelines. It is a legal responsibility of the 'Qualified Person' not only not to release product which does not conform to specification, but also to confirm that it has been manufactured in accordance with the method, and using the materials, as specified in the Marketing Authorisation, i.e. Product Licence.)

This same section of BS 5750 also sets out requirements for disposition of non-conforming product, some of which are not applicable to medicinal products (e.g. non-conforming product 'may be . . . accepted with or without repair . . . or re-graded for alternative applications . . .', etc.). The possibility of rework is mentioned (cf. more detailed treatment in OG 6, and ECG 5.61–5.65).

ISO 9001 Section 4.14 Corrective and preventive action

This section requires written procedures for investigating causes of non-conforming product and for taking corrective action (e.g. in response to customer complaints). (Since a major thrust of GMP guidelines and regulations is that non-conforming product will not be released it follows inevitably that corrective action will and must be taken. Should faulty product get to the market, this is covered in detail by guidelines on complaints and recall, OG 7 and ECG 8, and in Statutory Requirements regarding recall as, e.g. Directive 91/356/EEC, Article 13.)

ISO 9001 Section 4.15 Handling, storage, packaging, preservation and delivery

This section contains brief general statements about preservation of product quality during handling, storage, packaging and delivery, all aspects of which are covered in much greater and more specifically relevant detail in the GMP guides.

ISO 9001 Section 4.16 Control of quality records

Covered in much greater detail in the 'Documentation' sections, OG 3 and ECG 4.

ISO 9001 Section 4.17 Internal quality audits

Similar requirements are set out in OG 1.4, with more detailed coverage in ECG 9. Self-inspection is a statutory EC requirement under Article 14 of Directive 91/356/EEC.

ISO 9001 Section 4.18 Training

Requires that training needs shall be 'identified', and that relevant training should be given. (cf. OG 2 and ECG 2. Furthermore '. . . initial and continuing training in the theory and application of the concept of quality assurance and good manufacturing practice' is a statutory requirement under Article 7(4) of Directive 91/356/EEC.)

ISO 9001 Section 4.19 Servicing

This section is relevant to contracts under which a manufacturer has undertaken to service the goods he has supplied, and therefore is hardly applicable to the supply of medicinal products.

ISO 9001 Section 4.20 Statistical techniques

The supplier is required to *identify the need for statistical techniques required for establishing, controlling and verifying process capability and product characteristics*, and to *establish and maintain documented procedures to implement and control the statistical techniques identified.*

Assessment of the BS/ISO 9000 system

Thus it would appear that, in terms of specific requirements (as distinct from some of its generalities), ISO 9001 contains little that is not an established and accepted requirement (usually expressed in greater and more explicit detail) of good pharmaceutical manufacturing practice/pharmaceutical quality assurance, and/or of relevant medicines legislation. In such circumstances, it is difficult to understand those within the industry (one hopes a minority) who appear to hail the ISO 9000 system as a new advance on what we have, and have been applying, already. No doubt ISO 9000 does represent a considerable advance in a number of other industries, where quality concepts and practices have been, and often still are, rudimentary in the extreme. Without appearing complacent, the pharmaceutical industry, because of the crucial, literally life-or-death, implications of the quality of its products, may well have more to teach other industries about quality assurance than it has to learn from them.

There is another strange feature of ISO 9000 which runs counter to any claim that it enshrines a modern 'systems' view of QA, as distinct from outmoded 'inspect and test' approaches. It is worthy of note that, measured in terms of lines of print, the major weight (some 29% of the entire text of ISO 9001) considers matters to do with inspection. The next highest percentage coverages are design control (c. 10%) and management responsibility (c. 9%).

A further aspect of ISO 9000 concerns the supply of goods to, rather than by, the pharmaceutical industry. For example, BSI have published a series of 'Pharmaceutical Supplier Codes of Practice' which have been 'compiled by members of the Pharmaceutical Quality Group in conjunction with BSI Quality Assurance'. (The Pharmaceutical Quality Group describe themselves as a 'group of pharmaceutical quality executives . . . incorporated within the Institute of Quality Assurance and the British Quality Association.')

To clarify any ambiguity, it needs to be stressed that these Codes of Practice apply to suppliers of goods *to* manufacturers of pharmaceuticals, not to the manufacturers *of* pharmaceuticals themselves. Three of these Codes have been issued (on the manufacture of pharmaceutical raw materials, of contact packaging materials, and of printed packaging and labelling materials) and have been, variously, endorsed by the Association of the British Pharmaceutical Industry (ABPI), the Proprietary Association of Great Britain (PAGB), the Institute of Packaging, The Chemical Industries Association and the British Plastics Federation. All were produced in consultation with the UK Medicines Control Agency (MCA). They thus have a high degree of official blessing. The Codes of Practice are stated to 'amplify the requirements of BS 5750: Part 2, and shall only be read and applied in conjunction with it'. Together with BS 5750: Part 2, they define a uniform organisational and quality management system for suppliers, and will 'ensure consistency in the assessment of their capabilities to satisfy the requirements of the pharmaceutical industry'.

The last word on the relevance of ISO 9000 is best left to Dr Gert Auterhoff who, in a paper on quality assurance in the pharmaceutical industry, made a detailed 'comparison of regulatory provisions in drug legislation with the ISO Standard series 9000 to 9004' (Auterhoff, 1993). He reached the following principal conclusions:

1. 'A comparison . . . shows that the comprehensive statutory provisions . . . (regulating the pharmaceutical industry) not only cover the ISO 9000 series . . . but that they go even further . . .'
2. 'ISO 9000 series only covers essential requirements. . . . However essential requirements alone are not sufficient for many sectors, amongst them the pharmaceutical industry . . .'
3. 'In discussions about . . . the introduction of the ISO 9000 series in the pharmaceutical industry, the fact is often ignored that this industry has been observing and applying GMP rules for more than twenty years and that pharmaceutical manufacture and quality control have always been subject to detailed statutory and technical impositions.'
4. '. . . the quality elements of the ISO 9000 series are nothing new to our industry: they rather reflect everyday practice.'

References

Auterhoff G (1993). Quality assurance in the pharmaceutical industry. *Drugs Made Germ* **36** (1), 12–19.

Crosby P B (1979). *Quality is Free*. New York: New American Library.

Deming W E (1982). *Quality, Productivity and Competitive Position*. Cambridge, MA: MIT Center for Advances Engineering Study.

EC (1992). *The Rules Governing Medicinal Products in the European Community, Vol. IV: Good Manufacturing Practice for Medicinal Products*. Luxembourg: Commission of the European Communities. Available from The Office for Official Publications of the European Communities, Luxembourg. Also available from The Stationery Office (HMSO), London, and The EC Information Service, Washington, USA. Also stated *verbatim* with guidance on the detailed interpretation of these rules in MCA, 1997. (Referred to as the EC GMP Guide.)

Juran J M (1974). *Quality Control Handbook*, 3rd edn. New York: McGraw-Hill.

Oakland J S (1989). *Total Quality Management*. Oxford: Heinemann.

Sharp J, ed. (1983). *Guide to Good Pharmaceutical Manufacturing Practice*, 3rd edn. London: HMSO. Also stated *verbatim* with guidance on the detailed interpretation of these rules in MCA, 1997. (Referred to as the UK Orange Guide.)

Part Two

Premises and equipment

8

Premises and contamination control

The conclusion . . . is fallacious, being based upon licensed premises
Flann O'Brien (1911–1966)

The most important single factor in the assurance of the quality of medicinal and other healthcare products is the quality of the people who manufacture them. Nevertheless, in purely practical terms, essential prerequisites are a building for those people to work in, and equipment for them to work with.

Clearly, the premises and equipment used to manufacture medicinal products will have an important bearing on the quality of those products. Although relatively few employees will experience, or will have experienced, direct involvement in the design, construction and layout of a completely new factory of any size or complexity, it is useful (indeed, important) for all those interested in the quality of medicinal and similar products to have an insight into the ways in which buildings used to manufacture those products can have a bearing on product quality.

Requirements for a pharmaceutical production facility

The MCA's *Rules and Guidance for Pharmaceutical Manufacturers and Distributors* (MCA, 1997), in its reproduction of the EC GMP Guide (EC, 1992), states:

> Premises and equipment must be located, designed, constructed, adapted, and maintained to suit the operations to be carried out. Their layout and design must aim to minimise the risk of errors, and permit effective cleaning and maintenance in order to avoid cross-contamination, build-up of dust and dirt and, in general, any adverse effect on the quality of products.

Similar statements appear in other GMP guides, codes and regulations. The US CGMP regulation (21 CFR 211.42) states *inter alia*:

> (a)   Any building or buildings used in the manufacture, processing, packing

or holding of a drug product shall be of suitable size, construction and location to facilitate cleaning, maintenance and proper operations.

(b) Any such building shall have adequate space for the orderly placement of equipment and materials to prevent mix-ups between different components, drug product containers, closures, labelling, in-process materials or drug products, and to prevent contamination. The flow of components, drug product containers, closures, labelling, in-process materials and drug products through the building, or buildings shall be designed to prevent contamination.

(c) Operations shall be performed within specifically defined areas of adequate size.

Note: the term 'component' in the context of the US CGMPs (US FDA, 1990) means 'ingredient' or 'starting material', and not a package component.

Sub-paragraph (c) then gives a list of the required 'separate or defined areas', which include areas for:

1. Receipt, identification, storage and withholding from use of components, containers, closures and labels, pending sampling testing or examination before release.
2. Holding rejected materials ('components'), containers and labels before disposition.
3. Storage of released components, containers etc.
4. Storage of in-process materials.
5. The various different manufacturing operations.
6. Packaging and labelling.
7. Quarantine storage of products awaiting release.
8. Storage of released products.
9. Control and laboratory operations.
10. Aseptic processing.

Note: 'Aseptic processing', in this context, *may* be intended to refer to all sterile products' manufacturing, not just the manufacture of those products where some form of aseptic handling is required.

Siting and building considerations

A manufacturing building, with equipment installed, could be viewed as a 'black box' (Fig. 8.1) into which are fed:

1. Raw and packaging materials (and/or part-processed products).
2. People ready to work.
3. Services (air, heat, light, power, water, etc. plus any additional support systems for (2) above).

And from which will emerge:

1. Finished products (and/or part processed products).
2. People leaving after their days work.
3. Waste, scrap, rubbish and effluent.

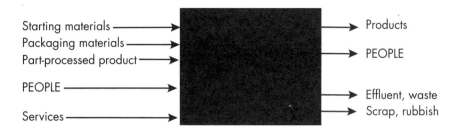

Figure 8.1   The manufacturing building 'black box'.

A primary consideration, therefore, for the siting and building of the factory is that it must be possible (and, preferably, conveniently possible) to feed materials, people and services to the site, and then to distribute products issuing from it as well as to dispose of waste, effluent, etc. (People having been persuaded to come and work in this 'box' will presumably find no greater difficulty in persuading themselves to leave it at the end of a day's work.)

Factors influencing the selection of a location for the construction of a manufacturing factory include:

- Ease of access *to* the site for and by:

    — People (i.e. proximity to centre(s) of human habitation, and thus labour availability).
    — Materials suppliers.
    — Services (water, electricity, gas, etc.).

- Climate: prevailing wind direction (and thus the potential for airborne contamination), extremes of temperature (which can bear upon product stability), and rain, snow and fog, which will affect ease of access.
- Local building restrictions, and restraints on use, and disposal, of toxic, inflammable, or explosive materials.
- Local fire safety regulations.
- Availability of development grants, which may on the one hand mean that more money can be spent on building and equipping the factory to high quality standards, yet on the other may be negated by lack of availability of suitable labour.

Within the 'black box', there will be various flow-patterns. These flows will be principally of materials and products, and of personnel. Materials will be received, held pending test, released for use, held in store, dispensed for manufacture and processed into products which are then packaged, tested, and held in quarantine pending release, and then stored pending distribution.

Alongside material and product flow-patterns, and indeed allowing or causing them to happen, are personnel flows, as people arrive for work, change into suitable protective clothing, carry out work, take breaks, change back to outdoor clothes and leave for home.

In addition to the material/product and personnel flows there will be flows of air of differing qualities (plain, conditioned, filtered), the flow of various services through pipework, ducting and conduit, and the disposal flows of waste, defective or contaminated material, and of rubbish, sewage and other effluent.

Functional aspects

Thus, the basic factors (all of which have quality implications) bearing upon the design, structure and layout of a manufacturing facility may be summarised as:

- Location.
- Building structure.
- Internal surface finishes.
- Size, scale and complexity of manufacturing operations.
- Protection: from weather, pests, dust, dirt.
- Security: *not* just an economic issue; break-ins can cause contamination and mix-up.
- Space: sufficient for *orderly* manufacture and storage and to avoid congestion and chaos.
- Internal layout

    — Smooth work flow

        – unidirectional
        – minimum of cross-over
        – minimum of back-track

    — Segregation of different types of operation/products.
    — Grouping together of similar operations.

- Lighting, heating, ventilation.
- Installation of services/fittings.
- Drains/waste disposal.
- Buildings maintenance.

Other strong influencing factors will be the company's marketing strategies, and its inventory and physical distribution policies.

An issue which dominates thinking about pharmaceutical premises, to an extent matched in few other industries, is the need (a) to avoid contamination of materials and products, either one by another ('cross-contamination') or by extraneous matter, and (b) to prevent mix-ups of ingredients ('starting materials' or 'components'), products and packaging materials. This dominant, almost over-riding, concern bears powerfully upon the issues of siting, design, structure, layout, surface finish, ventilation and waste disposal. It is therefore both useful and convenient to consider the question of contamination now, before proceeding to consider further aspects of building location, structure, design and layout.

Contamination types and sources

The word 'contamination' is a general term, covering a range of different substances. Simply put, it is material in the wrong place. Broadly, it is possible to classify the various potential forms of contamination into two main types:

- Living (or 'viable').
- Non-living (or 'non-viable').

The hazard that any contaminant represents will depend on its precise nature, and where it is found.

Living, or viable, contamination

While it would be quite reasonable to regard a tadpole, or a shark, swimming about in a vat of liquid product as a viable contaminant, the term is generally taken to refer not to such macro-organisms, but to micro-organisms – such things as bacteria, moulds and fungi, yeasts and viruses.

Micro-organisms

Single micro-organisms cannot, of course, be seen with the naked eye, but only with the aid of microscopes. As a simple illustration of the size of a single bacterium, it would take around a million of them to cover the head of a pin. Therein lies the major problem with micro-organisms. There can be many millions of them present on a surface, or in a liquid, without there being any obvious indication that they are there. However, they (and their effects) can be seen when a great many of them are growing together to form a colony, or when for example they are growing on food, turning it rotten.

As a further illustration, think of a one-litre bottle or bag of intravenous infusion fluid. When made it should look clear and bright. Even if only a few micro-organisms are present at first, under the right growth conditions they could grow and multiply very rapidly. Yet even if there are 1 million micro-organisms present in every millilitre (that is, 1000 million in the litre bottle), then only the very keenest eyesight will be able to detect the very, very faint cloudiness caused in the liquid. For the average pair of eyes to be able to detect just a very faint milkiness, 10 million micro-organisms would need to be present per ml, or 10 000 000 000 (10 thousand million) in the whole litre.

Like all living things, micro-organisms grow, feed and reproduce. Many have no built-in means of locomotion, but can be transferred from one place to another by air or liquid currents – or by the movement of a host organism, for example a person. Some can move in liquids, or on wet surfaces, by the beating of short cilia or whip-like flagellae. Some aerobic organisms, or aerobes, respire using oxygen in a manner analogous to that of mammals. In contrast, some (the anaerobes) cannot grow at all in the presence of oxygen. On the other hand, most micro-organisms can survive without oxygen for quite a long time. Three things that they all must have in order to grow and reproduce are moisture, food and warmth. A lack of these three essentials will not necessarily kill micro-organisms. However, they will not be able to flourish, grow and reproduce without them. Micro-organisms are remarkable survivors under the most trying conditions, but if moisture, food and warmth are removed (that is, if things are kept dry, clean and cool (or cold)), a good step will have been made towards controlling spread, even if they have not been killed or completely removed. Even extremes of cold will not kill them; it just keeps them under control. That is, it stops them growing and multiplying.

As for what micro-organisms can use for food, although some individual types (or species) are very selective over what they can feed on (for example a specific sugar or a specific protein), across the range of micro-organisms as a whole an amazing variety of substances is used for food. Obviously, they can live on things like meat, fruit, milk, bread and jam. Many feed on what might be termed just plain muck. Some have been known to use the most unlikely things as food such as aeroengine fuel, and disinfectants.

Bacteria reproduce by the simple process of each individual cell dividing itself in half. Under good conditions, that is when they have moisture food and warmth, they can divide in this way once every 20 minutes. So, in 20 minutes one bacterium becomes two bacteria, in 40 minutes four, in an hour eight, and so on. In 12 hours there will be over two million million descendants of the original organism.

Some bacteria can cause disease, from the minor to the very serious, as can some moulds, yeasts and viruses, but by no means all micro-organisms are harmful. In fact, in normal circumstances the great majority of them are quite harmless to fit people. A number are very useful. For example they are needed to make beer, wine, bread, cheese and yoghurt. Some live normally, and quite naturally, in our gut. We provide them with shelter, food, warmth and moisture. In return they help us with our digestion. Others break-down dead plants and animals and thus help to recycle nutrients in the soil. We could not survive without them.

But others are indeed pathogenic – causing diseases, from the most minor illnesses to those which cause death. Others can spoil food, and break down things like medicinal and cosmetic creams, lotions and other liquids. Even micro-organisms that are normally harmless can be a danger if administered to people who are already ill, and normally quite innocuous organisms can be lethal if administered to patients, in sufficient quantity, by injection.

Thus, as far as possible, micro-organisms should be kept out of, and off, medicinal products and medical devices of all types. Products that are intended to be injected, or used in the eye, on open wounds, or inserted into body cavities, tissues or blood vessels must be sterile, that is, completely free from all living organisms.

Liquids to be taken by mouth, in addition to being 'spoiled' by micro-organisms can also infect a patient swallowing the liquid. Liquids, creams and ointments, intended for application to the skin surface, if contaminated with micro-organisms, can, in addition to the spoilage risk, cause skin infections. It should be noted that skin diseases are not necessarily just slightly irritating, trivial matters. They can be very serious, even lethal, and a number of the active substances that are used in skin preparations to treat inflammation, rashes, etc. can have the effect of suppressing the normal immune response to bacterial infection. The presence of organisms in such products could thus represent a doubly serious patient hazard.

Even with dry products taken orally, such as tablets and capsules, there have been cases of serious illness in patients taking products infected with bacteria. Certain moulds (which can grow on tablets) can produce some very toxic substances.

It is important always to remember that people taking medicines are usually doing so because they are already ill, and thus their resistance to infection may well be lower than normal.

It is thus crucially important that manufacturing premises are built, laid-out, surface-finished, serviced, maintained and drained so as to minimise the harbouring and proliferation of micro-organisms.

Non-living contamination

In addition to those living (viable) forms of contamination there are also the non-living forms. These can further be classified into two main groups: active contamination, and inert (or inactive) contamination (see Fig. 8.2).

Active non-living contamination

By 'active' is meant chemically active, or having some activity when introduced into the human (or other animal) body.

That is still not the whole story. There are still other special forms of contaminating substances which must be guarded against when making

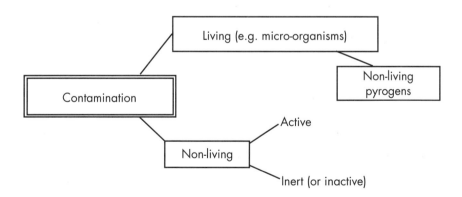

Figure 8.2 Categories of possible contamination found in pharmaceutical manufacture.

products for injection. These are called pyrogens (or 'bacterial endotoxins' – for practical purposes the terms may be regarded as virtually synonymous).

Examples of active non-living contamination are:

- Powder, dust or crystals from other batches of product, or residues of other solutions, suspensions or creams 'left-over' in containers, vessels or items of equipment which have not been properly cleaned and dried.
- Ingredient materials left in containers which are then reused without proper cleaning, or powders which have been spilt (for example, in a dispensing operation).
- 'The uncontrolled release of dust, gases, vapours, sprays or organisms from materials and products in process' (the UK Orange Guide to GMP (Sharp, 1983)).

This type of contamination tends to be called 'cross-contamination'. It may also be caused by the dust on the clothes and shoes of people who have been using or weighing bulk chemical substances (see Part Three: Personnel).

Since many of the chemical/biological substances used in modern medicinal products can have very powerful effects in and on the body, even in very small amounts, the potential hazards of this sort of contamination hardly need emphasising. It would seem obvious that the dangers will vary widely with the nature of the contaminant, and that indeed is largely true. The most dangerous will be highly potent substances that are taken in low doses; things like steroid hormones, cytotoxic substances, and sensitising agents, such as certain antibiotics. But problems can be caused by other, apparently less potent substances.

The well-known Association of the British Pharmaceutical Industry (ABPI) training film/video *You'll Soon Feel Better* shows, as an example of the hazards of cross-contamination, the manufacture of a batch of an over-the-counter analgesic tablet which is unevenly contaminated (that is, only part of the batch has the contaminant) with digoxin, with serious, life-threatening consequences. This happened because the equipment used to mix/granulate the powders from which the digoxin tablets were compressed had not been properly cleaned before it was used for the analgesic. This left a slug of digoxin-mix to fall (late in the process) into the analgesic mix, where it was only partially blended-in. It was thus missed in the laboratory tests made on the sample taken for assay.

Now assume that the analgesic tablet was aspirin. The 'standard' aspirin tablet contains 300 mg per tablet, with a usual dose of 1 to 3 tablets every 4–6 hours as necessary. The maximum dose is 4 g per day. Digoxin is a powerful, prescription-only heart stimulant. It generally comes in tablets of 62.5, 125, or 250 *micro*grams of digoxin. Daily dose varies according to circumstance, but 125 to 250 *micro*grams is common. A very big difference, therefore, between the dosage, potency and severity of action of the two active drug substances. So there is no argument. Even the smallest traces of something like digoxin in aspirin tablets are dangerous, and must be avoided. But what about the reverse situation – for example, small traces of aspirin in digoxin tablets? There are many medicinal substances which, although they are well tolerated and safe in normal doses when take by most people, can cause severe reactions in a sensitive minority. The classic case is penicillin and similar antibiotics. For the majority of patients there is no problem, but in some they can cause serious reactions. In general, the safest thing is to assume that somebody, somewhere, could react to traces of these 'non-living active' contaminants. Moderate doses of aspirin, taken as recommended do not cause harm to most people. In a few it causes marked sensitivity reactions. As the UK Orange Guide (Sharp, 1983) put it:

> 5.1   The presence in a medicinal product of any chemical or micro-biological contaminant, of such a nature and in such a quantity as may have the potential to affect adversely the health of any patient or impair the therapeutic activity of the product is unacceptable. Particular attention should be paid to the problem of cross contamination, since even if it is of a nature and at a level unlikely to affect health directly, it may be indicative of unsatisfactory manufacturing practices.

In practice, many regulatory authorities take a distinctly strict view of cross-contamination. (There is no question about micro-organisms in products that are required to be sterile. They are clearly and absolutely not permitted.) Various suggestions have been made about quantitatively specifying acceptable levels of cross-contamination, based upon the potency, or activity, of the contaminant, for example: 'No more than 1/1000th of minimum daily dose of X (the contaminant) in maximum daily dose of Y (the contaminated product)'. However, there is no universal agreement on this point. Some cynics have argued that acceptable levels vary in accordance with the sensitivity of the analytical methods available to detect them, and that as analytical chemical technology advances, and methods become ever more sensitive, so do the levels considered to be acceptable get lower. Nevertheless, the dangers of this 'active contamination' are fairly obvious. Perhaps not quite so obvious is the significance of inert non-living contamination.

Inert non-living contamination

The concern here is with particles, fibres, flakes, dusts, and the like, which do not have any specific chemical or biological activity in or on the body. Contamination by the inert excipients (or 'fillers') that are used in some medicinal products could be regarded as 'inert cross-contamination'. Other commonly used terms (particularly in the USA) are 'particulate contamination', 'particulate matter' or just 'particulates'. 'Particles', 'particulate matter', 'particulate contamination' and 'particulates' all mean the same thing – little bits floating about in the air or in liquids, or deposited on surfaces, or in products.

The list of such particles is almost endless, and includes:

- Atmospheric and house dust.
- Fine soil.
- Sand.
- Ash.
- Smoke.
- Dandruff.
- Skin flakes.
- Pollen.
- Fibres (from natural and artificial textiles, or from paper).
- Flaking paint.
- Powdering plaster or masonry.
- Metal particles from moving machine-parts or from drilled or ground metals.
- Rubber or composition particles from belt-drives in machines.
- Inert powders from other products.

There has been much discussion and argument over the dangers (or otherwise) of fine particles contaminating medicinal products, particularly those which are injected or inserted into the body. Clearly, it is important to avoid hard particles in eye drops, and it is well known that excessive inhalation of a wide range of dusts causes serious lung problems. Particles in products intended for application to body surfaces can abrade the skin and give rise to infections.

The dangers of inert particles in products taken by mouth will vary with the nature and level of the contamination, but even small amounts of relatively harmless materials can spoil the look of tablets, or liquids that are meant to be clear.

Surprisingly, some workers have argued that the *injection* of inert particles is not as dangerous as it may at first seem. Others have claimed that there *are* hazards, and that injected particles can block small blood-vessels, or pass to the lungs and block the fine bronchial tubes, or lodge in the liver and cause damage, and so on. So, in spite of some of the arguments, it is generally considered necessary to control the level of particles in injections (and other sterile products), and the pharmacopoeias specify the levels that are permitted for particles in certain injections and other sterile products. This in turn means controlling the numbers of particles in the rooms (in the air and on surfaces) in which such products are made.

There is another very good reason for keeping down contamination by inert particles. It is that most airborne bacteria and other micro-organisms do not merely float around in the air on their own. They are usually attached to particles. So, if the level of particles in general is controlled, a step has been made towards controlling the level of micro-organisms.

One form of possible contamination so far not mentioned is oil, grease and other lubricating materials. At best it can spoil the look of products. At worst it can be toxic and/or harbour micro-organisms.

Pyrogens

Although it is non-living, this form of contamination is produced by living organisms which may be present, for example, in water or in a solution. It may also be present on the surfaces of containers, vessels, instruments, devices and other materials that have been in contact with liquids which contained organisms, or which have been left wet so that micro-organisms could develop. These bacteria-produced contaminants are the pyrogens. (Another expression which means *more-or-less* the same thing is 'bacterial endotoxins'.) Pyrogens are poly-liposaccharides produced from the outer cell walls of certain Gram-negative bacteria. When injected or otherwise inserted into patients they can cause a rapid rise in body temperature (hence 'pyro-gen' – 'giving rise to heat'), with chill, shivering, vasoconstriction, pupillary dilation, respiratory depression and an increase in blood pressure. There may also be pains in joints and back, headache and nausea. In seriously ill patients, the effects of pyrogens can be very dangerous. Since most sterilisation processes do not necessarily remove or destroy pyrogens, it is very important to guard against the development and growth of micro-organisms, and the concomitant formation of pyrogens. The sterilisation process alone cannot (usually) be relied on to ensure that the product is both sterile *and* free from pyrogens. Very careful control over the entire manufacturing cycle is essential, to ensure that pyrogen-producing organisms are excluded, or at least kept to a minimum, throughout the process.

Summary

To sum-up on types of contamination:

1. There are two main types of contamination: living and non-living.
2. By 'living (or 'viable') contamination' is generally meant micro-organisms. That is, bacteria, moulds, yeasts and viruses.
3. There are many millions of millions of these micro-organisms. They can reproduce themselves and spread very rapidly.
4. Some micro-organisms are very dangerous to people. Others are quite harmless or even useful, in some circumstances. *All of them must be kept away, or removed, from sterile products* and they must be kept under control when making *all* types of medicinal products.
5. Non-living contamination, whether it is an active chemical substance, or just inactive dust, powder or fibres, must also be kept tightly under control.
6. Living micro-organisms can produce dangerous pyrogens. These must not be allowed to develop in, or on, products intended for injection.

Sources of contamination

Contamination by active chemical substances can be caused by dust and powder, spilt or released during processing, which is 'floating' in the air, or which has settled on surfaces, or in vessels or equipment. It can also arise from residues ('leftovers') in or on containers, vessels and equipment which have been used for other products or materials, and which have not subsequently been properly cleaned. Other possible sources include traces of materials which have been used for cleaning and disinfection.

There are many possible sources of what we called inert non-living contamination (or 'particulate contamination'), for example:

- *Buildings* – unsealed stone-work, brick, mortar, plaster, flaking paint, etc; sawdust, brick chippings, metal filings generated during repair, maintenance, installation and restructuring.
- *Raw materials* – ingredients which might not be highly active in themselves can nevertheless be a big source of highly undesirable particles.
- *Equipment* – dirty equipment, moving machine parts, and belt drives; and the materials used to lubricate equipment.
- *'The general environment'* – dust, dirt, soil, sand, smoke, ash, etc.
- *Containers, packages, paper, cardboard* – fibrous contamination.

Filtered air-supplies to the rooms in which products are manufactured, although intended to reduce particulate contamination, can have the reverse effect if the filters are damaged, or if the system is not properly maintained. Air extraction systems, if badly designed, installed and maintained can in fact be a *source* of contamination by withdrawing it from one location, only to blow it all over another.

There is thus a very wide range of possible sources of contamination. A further major source is *people and their clothing*.

By the use of rooms with a special filtered air supply quite a high level of control over particles can be achieved. Put people in a room, and it is a different story.

The human animal sheds thousands of millions of dead skin cells and fragments, per day. This amounts, it has been claimed, to a total weight of somewhere between 5–15 g per day per person (ASPI, 1972). The more we move, and the more vigorously that we move, the greater the shedding becomes. We shed three or four times more particles when we move about than when we are at rest. Depending on the type of cloth, we also disperse large numbers of fibres from our clothing. This amount also increases as we move about.

Personnel moving from one location to another can carry powders, dusts, fibres (and micro-organisms) about with them as they go – on their bodies, clothes and shoes.

The human male sheds something like 1000 bacteria-carrying particles per minute. People are, indeed, a major source of both living and non-living contamination.

Sources of micro-organisms

To the question 'Where do micro-organisms come from?' the simple answer is that, like all other organisms (including people), they don't just 'happen'.

They come from 'parent' micro-organisms. The big difference is, of course, that in favourable conditions they multiply so much more rapidly than, for example, we do.

Micro-organisms are almost everywhere. Some have managed to flourish in strong acids, some in hot springs and some in certain disinfectants. They are found, by the millions, in or on:

- *The environment around us.* That is, in the air (indoors and out), on the ground, in the soil, on walls, floors and surfaces generally – almost everywhere.
- *Water.* They exist in the water from the tap, in rivers, seas, and lakes; in puddles, on wet surfaces and wet floors; in damp surfaces of containers and equipment that has not been properly dried. In general, bacteria will be found in all forms of water, whether it is in large quantities or just light surface films, except water that has been specially sterilised and sealed-in against any recontamination.
- *Raw materials* used for making products.
- *Containers and closures* used for packaging products.

All these are sources of contamination that something can be done about. It is not always easy, but it is possible. One source of contamination, and it is a major one, is rather more difficult to deal with. It is, as we have said, people. In spite of increasing automation, it is still necessary to involve people in the manufacture of medicinal products, and people generally object to being sterilised (in the microbiological sense), treated with strong disinfectants, or eliminated altogether (see Part Three: Personnel).

Control of contamination

The control of contamination is a major issue in the design, construction and layout of a manufacturing facility, and indeed in QA/GMP as a whole. Much depends on people and the way they behave, and on the protective clothing they are wearing. (Note: the reference to 'protective' here is to clothing worn to protect products and materials from contamination by people.) Other important control measures are the application of well planned and proven cleaning and disinfection procedures. Crucial factors are also the design, structure, surface finishes and layout of factories, the design, installation and maintenance of equipment, and the design, installation, efficiency and maintenance of factory services such as ventilation, heating, lighting and water supply. Proper factory/equipment design and layout can also reduce the risk of what can perhaps be regarded as extreme cases of contamination – the complete mix-up of one product with another, of one in-gredient with another, or of one packaging material (especially pre-printed materials) with another. That is the reason for this diversion into the question of contamination. An understanding of the problems is crucial to an appreciation of the quality-influencing aspects of buildings and equipment.

Relevant paragraphs from the EC GMP Guide (EC, 1992), as reproduced in the *MCA's Rules and Guidance for Pharmaceutical Manufacturers and Distributors* (MCA, 1997) under 'Premises and Equipment', read:

Production area

3.6   In order to minimise the risk of a serious medical hazard due to cross-contamination, dedicated and self contained facilities must be available for the production of particular medicinal products, such as highly sensitizing materials (e.g. penicillins) or biological preparations (e.g. from live micro-organisms). The production of certain additional products, such as certain antibiotics, certain hormones, certain cytotoxics, certain highly active drugs and non-medicinal products should not be conducted in the same facilities. For those products, in exceptional cases, the principle of campaign working in the same facilities can be accepted provided that specific precautions are taken, and the necessary validations are made. The manufacture of technical poisons, such as pesticides and herbicides, should not be allowed in premises used for the manufacture of medicinal products.

3.7   Premises should preferably be laid-out in such a way as to allow production to take place in areas connected in a logical order, corresponding to the sequence of operations . . .

3.8   The adequacy of the working and in-process storage space should permit the orderly and logical positioning of equipment and materials so as to minimise the risk of confusion between different medicinal products or their components, to avoid cross-contamination and to minimise the risk of omission or wrong application of any of the manufacturing or control steps.

3.14   In cases where dust is generated (e.g. during sampling, weighing, mixing and processing operations, packaging of dry products) specific provisions should be taken to avoid cross-contamination and facilitate cleaning.

3.15   Premises for the packaging of medicinal products should be specifically designed and laid out so as to avoid mix-ups or cross-contamination.

The subsection on 'Prevention of Cross-contamination in Production' reads:

5.18   Contamination of a starting material or of a product by another material must be avoided. This risk of accidental cross-contamination arises from uncontrolled release of dust, gases, vapours, sprays or organisms from materials and products in process, from residues on equipment and from operators' clothing. The significance of this risk varies with the type of contaminant and of product being contaminated. Among the most hazardous contaminants are highly sensitising materials, biological preparations containing living organisms, certain hormones, cytotoxics and other highly active materials. Products in which contamination is likely to be most significant are those administered by injection, those given in large doses and/or over a long time.

5.19   Cross-contamination should be avoided by appropriate technical or organisational measures, for example:

    (a)   production in segregated areas (required for products such as penicillins, live vaccines, live bacterial preparations and some other biologicals), or by campaign (separation in time) followed by appropriate cleaning;

(b)   providing appropriate air-locks and air extraction;

(c)   minimising the risk of contamination caused by recirculation or re-entry of untreated, or insufficiently treated, air;

(d)   keeping protective clothing inside areas where products with special risk of cross-contamination are processed;

(e)   using cleaning and decontamination procedures of known effectiveness, as ineffective cleaning of equipment is a common source of cross-contamination;

(f)   using 'closed systems' of production;

(g)   testing for residues and use of cleaning status labels on equipment.

5.20   Measures to prevent cross-contamination and their effectiveness should be checked periodically according to set procedures.

References

ASPI (1972). *Hygiene Recommendations*. Stockholm: Association of the Swedish Pharmaceutical Industry.

EC (1992). *The Rules Governing Medicinal Products in the European Community, Vol. IV: Good Manufacturing Practice for Medicinal Products*. Luxembourg: Commission of the European Communities. Available from The Office for Official Publications of the European Communities, Luxembourg. Also available from The Stationery Office (HMSO), London, and The EC Information Service, Washington, USA. Also stated *verbatim* with guidance on the detailed interpretation of these rules in MCA, 1997. (Referred to as the EC GMP Guide.)

MCA (1997). *Rules and Guidance for Pharmaceutical Manufacturers and Distributors*. London: Medicines Control Agency. Available from The Stationery Office (HMSO), London.

Sharp J, ed. (1983). *Guide to Good Pharmaceutical Manufacturing Practice*, 3rd edn. London: HMSO. Also stated *verbatim* with guidance on the detailed interpretation of these rules in MCA, 1997. (Referred to as the UK Orange Guide.)

US FDA (1990). *Code of Federal Regulations, Vol. 21, Ch. 1, Part 210*, Current good manufacturing practice in manufacturing, processing, packaging or holding of drugs, general; *CFR Vol. 21, Ch. 1, Part 211*, Current good manufacturing practice for finished pharmaceuticals; *CFR Vol. 21, Ch. 1, Part 820*, Good manufacturing practice for medical devices (revised 1995). Washington: US Food & Drug Administration. (Collectively referred to as the US CGMPs.)

9

Premises: location, design, structure, layout, services and cleaning

I thought the best thing to do was to settle up these little local difficulties
Harold Macmillan, British Prime Minister, 1958

Many established manufacturing facilities are situated where they are for historical, and long-forgotten reasons. Sites for new factories have been selected for many different, and not always the best, reasons. That the executive vice-president likes the look of the local golf course ought not to be a major influence.

Location

Factors truly relevant to the siting of pharmaceutical manufacture are:

1. Is the site suitable for the erection of a building of the size, shape and height proposed? Will the existing terrain allow the insertion of foundations which will support such a structure?
2. Is the site of sufficient area to accommodate not only the building, but also access roads, parking areas, hard standing for delivery and despatch vehicles and, one hopes, a certain amount of pleasing external landscaping and planting?
3. Do national and local regulations permit a building of the size, type and shape proposed?
4. What are the risks of water damage, flooding, pollution, pest/vermin infestation, or contamination and/or objectionable odours from other nearby activities? What control will the manufacturer have (e.g. via the local authority) over any possible future development of such activities?
5. Will it be possible to attract suitable staff?
6. Will local and personal transport allow convenient staff-access to the site?
7. The convenience and economics of getting materials to the site, and distributing products from it.

8. The logistics and geographical relationships between the site and any other company-owned facilities, its subsidiaries, warehousing and distribution agents, wholesale and retail outlets.
9. Availability of services – water, power, electricity, fuel oil, telecommunications, waste and effluent disposal.
10. Potential for future expansion.

Other relevant factors might include altitude (at high altitudes physical characteristics, e.g. boiling point of some materials, are altered), climate (extremes of temperature can affect products and materials, as may excessive rain/flooding, snow or fog – or at least they may necessitate more extensive ventilation and temperature control systems), prevailing wind (risk of airborne pollution), local noise, and tax incentives/development grants (possible more money available for a higher standard of plant and equipment).

All these considerations, albeit that some may seem to be more of an economic/commercial nature, do indeed bear upon product quality, directly or indirectly. Some are obvious. What if the local terrain, building regulations, and area available do not permit the construction of the quality preserving/enhancing aspects of the building (with all the flows, segregation, grouping, servicing, etc. that has been conceptually planned)? It is no good constructing a factory in an area where the required numbers, and quality, of workers cannot be recruited. Crucial consideration must be given to the availability of staff capable of grasping and responding to the special disciplines, and indeed the culture, appropriate to the manufacture of pharmaceuticals and other healthcare products. Even noise can affect quality, at least indirectly, by affecting the powers of concentration of operators on the matter in hand. Anything that causes chaos and confusion (late arrival of ingredients and packaging materials, 'panic production', over-stocked stores, trying to expand or re-layout buildings that resist it) can result in error, mix-up and contamination.

Site security

Protection of the site against intrusion, theft and vandalism is not just an economic, but is also an important quality, issue. Break-ins, for whatever purpose, can result in mix-ups and contamination, which may escape immediate detection. All but the smallest facilities should, ideally, be surrounded by a secure perimeter fence. Access to the site (staff, contractors, visitors) must be strictly by authorised persons only, using some form of personal identification badges.

Structure and finishes

There are many ways to build factories. The most widely adopted approach is based on a steel or reinforced concrete frame with fill-in external walls of brick, building block, coated steel panels or combinations of these. Such structures provide a degree of flexibility in arranging internal non-load bearing walls, which can be constructed from structural blocks rendered, made smooth and finished with a hard drying, smooth impervious surface finish, or from prefabricated partition panels of various types. Internal wall surfaces (and indeed all surfaces in processing areas) should be impervious, non-porous, non-shedding and be free of cracks, dirt retaining holes and flaking paint. They should be washable and able to resist repeated applications of cleaning and disinfecting agents. Internally there should be no recesses that cannot be cleaned, and a minimum of projecting ledges, shelves, fixtures, fittings and the like.

Services pipework/ducting/conduit should be installed so as not to create uncleanable dust-traps – preferably within walls or above ceiling voids. If pipework, etc. must pass through walls, it should be thoroughly sealed-in on both sides.

In certain highly critical processing areas (e.g. sterile production), walls need to be smoothly coved to floors and ceilings.

An economic approach which has been successfully adopted for small-scale manufacture has been to purchase, or lease, a standard factory or warehouse unit of sound construction and construct the manufacturing rooms inside it, from rendered blocks or partitioning.

Floors should be even-surfaced, free from cracks and allow for ready cleaning and removal of any spillages. They should conform to the requirements similar to those indicated for walls above. They need also to be tough. Expansion joints should be flush-sealed with a suitably resilient compound.

Where drains or drainage gullies are installed they should be easily cleanable (and clean) and trapped to prevent reflux. Floors should fall to drains, not vice versa, although there still seems to be an extraordinary number of drain installers who seem convinced that, left to its own devices, a liquid will flow uphill.

Overhead ducts, pipes and roof joists should be avoided. A common approach is to employ suspended or false ceilings, with the void above the ceiling being used for pipework and services. Ceiling panels or tiles should be close fitting and sealed or clamped together at joints. The entire ceiling should have a smooth impervious surface, easy to keep clean. Acoustic tiles are generally inappropriate in processing areas, except perhaps where product is not exposed.

Lighting should be fitted flush, or suspended from the ceiling in such a manner that the fittings may be kept clean.

Doors and window-frames should all have a smooth, hard, impervious finish, and should close tightly. Window and door-frames should be fitted flush, at least on sides facing inwards to processing areas. (That is, for example, a door/window between a transit corridor and a processing room may need only to be flush fitted (no window ledges etc.) on the processing side. A door/window fitted between two processing rooms should be flush fitted both sides.)

Any windows from production areas to the exterior should be tightly sealed and not normally openable.

Doors, except emergency exits, should not open directly from production areas to the outside world. Any such emergency exit doors should be kept shut and sealed, and designed as to be openable only when emergency demands.

Despite the space-saving advantages, sliding doors should be avoided because of the difficulty of maintaining the sliding gear in a clean condition.

Basic design and layout

As already stated, fundamental to good pharmaceutical factory design are the concepts of:

- Segregation of different types of operation.
- Grouping together of related types of activity or product.
- Smooth, mainly unidirectional, flows of materials (starting, packaging and in-process), intermediates and products, with minimal crossing over of work flows, or back-tracking. Similar considerations apply also to personnel flows.

In any but the simplest facility, it is perhaps not possible to achieve ideal segregation, grouping and flow, but the objective is clear. It is, essentially, to avoid mix-up and contamination and additionally to create and maintain an orderly, efficient working environment in which supervision, rapid appraisal of just what is going on, and communication are all facilitated. In addition to the quality aspects, it is hardly necessary to add that there are of course the economic benefits of more efficient production and higher productivity. The current trend among the larger multi-product companies to 'rationalise' manufacturing sites to single product types (e.g. tablets and capsules, or liquids only) is doubtless driven by quality as well as economic considerations.

The immediate surrounds of the building should be such that they may be, and are, maintained in a clean, tidy and orderly condition. Around the entire perimeter there should be a width of concrete, tarmacadam or similar material, which should fall to drains and prevent water seepage into the building. All outside walls should be sealed to prevent entry of dust, damp and insects through cracks and gaps, as should all cutouts for windows, piping and duct work. All external loading and unloading points should be provided with protection from the weather.

The building, and the site as a whole, should be secure, with access restricted to authorised personnel at authorised times only. This, too, has quality as well as economic implications. Intruders, even if their intent is no more than petty pilfering (and it could be worse), could be the cause of contamination and mix-up. The access of vermin, birds, insects and pests should also be prevented.

The general external appearance ought not be neglected. It might be argued that aesthetics have nothing to do with product quality, but a good, clean, attractive external (and internal) appearance does help to encourage desirable operator attitudes.

Layout concepts

A very basic block design showing a simple single-storey linear flow layout is given in Figure 9.1. Another popular layout is the horizontal U-flow, as shown in simplified form in Figure 9.2.

A rough schematic drawing of a partially two-storey factory building – based upon an existent and successfully operating facility that meets, in three dimensions, the requirement for smooth, mainly unidirectional, flows – is shown in Figure 9.3.

The western side of the building is largely a high-rise stores area. Starting and packaging materials are received, at ground level, towards the north-western corner of the building. Following quarantine, testing and release the goods are held as pallet loads, on racking. As required, released starting materials are lifted to the dispensary (on upper floor only) by high-reach fork-lift truck (FLT). Dispensed materials are delivered to the appropriate manufacturing room via the upper corridor. Bulk manufactured products are delivered to the packaging area via the corridor (bulk liquid products are piped). Finished pack products are lifted down to the stores from the southern end of the corridor from specially constructed bays. As required, finished products are dispatched from a goods outwards bay, at ground level at the southern end of the store.

It is not difficult to picture a number of variations on just these three simple patterns alone. In practice *total* realisation of the ideal layout is rarely found. Nature of the site, local conditions, availability and placement of services all tend to dictate modifications, and as business and product range change and develop, and premises expand, supplementary flows (or subsidiary production loops) tend to be grafted on to the original pattern. Nevertheless the aim should always be to remain as close to the ideal as possible.

With the current general trend among larger companies to rationalise away from multi-product sites and towards factories producing just a single product type, the achievement of ideal factory layouts is probably becoming somewhat easier.

Internal building requirements vary according to the nature of the operations carried out or type of product produced within the various departments, sections or rooms. Not surprisingly, there are special requirements for the design, finishes, layout and environmental control of premises for the manufacture of sterile products. These are matters which will be considered later.

Plant services, systems and utilities

A factory, built and finished as designed, still requires various other inputs, in addition to people, equipment and materials, before the manufacture of

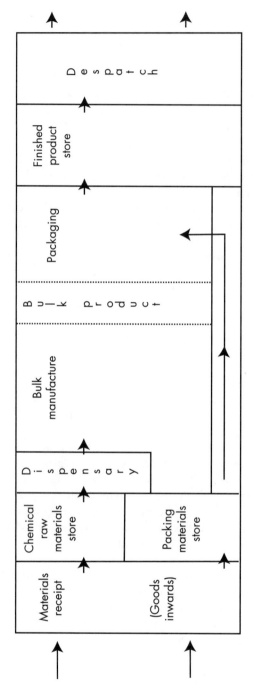

Figure 9.1 Simple single-storey linear flow pattern for pharmaceutical manufacturing. Sampling, quarantine and release stages not shown. Not to scale.

128

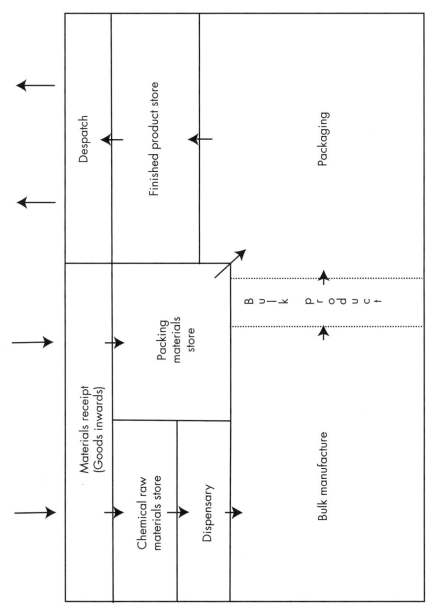

Figure 9.2 Simple horizontal U-flow pattern for pharmaceutical manufacturing. Sampling, quarantine and release stages not shown. Not to scale.

129

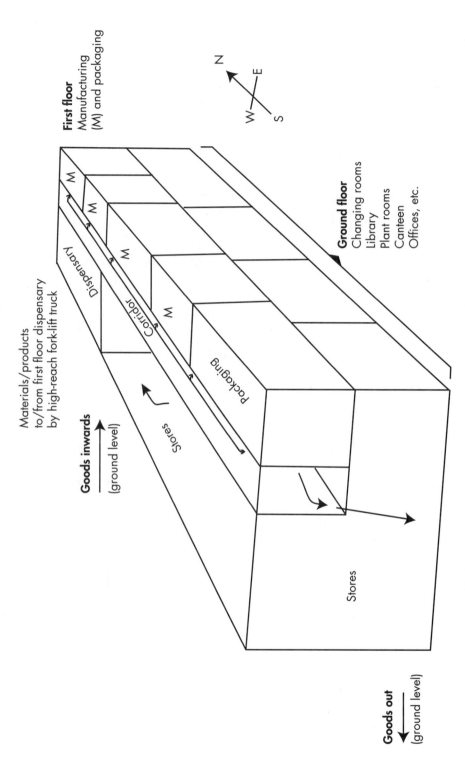

Figure 9.3 Two-floor design for pharmaceutical manufacturing. Sampling, quarantine and release stages not shown. Not to scale.

products can begin. These can be referred to, collectively as 'plant services, systems and utilities'.

First and foremost, air must be provided for those working in the factory to breathe. That air will need to be at a comfortable temperature so that the workers' innate enthusiasm for work will remain unimpaired. Providing ventilation by simply opening the windows and doors will just not do. Some form of forced, conditioned air supply is required, and this in turn has further implications for the control of potential airborne contamination.

Attention must also be given to the other needs of the factory and the people in it. Water is needed – for drinking and washing, as well as to clean, to rinse, to produce steam and as a major ingredient.

Services are needed to permit equipment to function, as are systems for dust control and collection, and systems for the disposal of waste and effluent. Cooling systems may also be required.

So, under the general heading of 'plant services, systems and utilities', manufacturing requirements include the following:

- Heating, ventilation and air conditioning (HVAC)
- Lighting
- Water (of various grades)
- Steam
- Compressed air
- Various other gases
- Vacuum
- Electricity
- Cooling systems
- Dust control/collection systems
- Effluent and waste disposal systems/drainage
- Bulk solvent, and other bulk liquid supply systems
- Lubrication services.

To this list may be added the provision of cloakroom, toilet, canteen and communication systems.

It would be a mistake to think that these things are all 'just plant engineering' issues. All have strong quality implications. If these services are not adequately provided, and operating satisfactorily, then the quality of the product will suffer, either directly or indirectly, and as a further consequence, patients may also suffer as a result of failure of product quality. Furthermore if some of these services are inadequately provided, factory personnel may suffer (from discomfort or inconvenience, or worse) and if they suffer, so will product quality.

Heating, ventilation and air-conditioning (HVAC)

'Natural' ventilation (via doors and windows) is not acceptable because of the risk of product contamination from the outside world (particulate matter, dust, dirt, micro-organisms, insects, etc.). Control of humidity is also important for a number of products, particularly effervescent products. Non-effervescent tablets, gelatin capsules, and tablet coatings, packages and packaging materials, and various other medicinal and similar products can also be adversely affected by humidity, which can also encourage microbial growth.

Windows from production areas to the outside world should thus normally remain shut, and preferably not be openable. External doors should be air-locked, or only openable in an emergency. Therefore some form of forced, conditioned, usually filtered air supply is required. The nature and quality of that air supply will depend on the nature of the process being performed and the products produced in the area concerned. Perhaps the most critical requirements are for the manufacture of sterile products (see later).

Air systems can, therefore, have a positive effect on product quality if they are properly designed, installed, operated and maintained. If not, they can have an adverse effect – on the product and on operators.

Care must be taken to ensure that an air supply system is doing what it is supposed to do. That is, supplying air of a higher quality than the outside environmental air at an appropriate temperature and level of humidity. The purpose is immediately defeated if the system is drawing air from a source which contains contaminants of a nature and at a level which the conditioning and filtration systems are not adequate to deal with. Siting of the air intake is therefore critical.

Maintenance of the system to ensure it continues to operate to designed standards is also critical. Damaged/holed trunking can cause more contamination than no system at all, by drawing in contaminated air/dust from service voids, lagging material, etc. by venturi effects. Air filters should be functioning to the standard required and as specified. If they are damaged they too can become a source of contamination. As they become blocked and their efficiency decreases, they need to be changed. The system should be designed, and the changing operation carried out, so that changing filters does not have the effect of merely spreading around all the dust that has been collected on the filter over a period of time.

Air supply trunking must be installed, preferably in 'voids' or above false ceilings, but in any event where it does not create uncleanable surfaces or recesses. It is essential that HVAC systems are subject to a formalised programme of planned preventative maintenance (PPM). This will need close liaison between the manufacturing and maintenance departments to ensure that production does not continue in ignorance of a 'down' HVAC system.

Lighting

Lighting levels should be adequate to permit operators to do their work properly, accurately and attentively. Too little light may cause operators to miss things they should be noticing, or to work without the necessary precision. It will cause eye-strain and fatigue, which in turn can have indirect adverse effects on product quality. Too bright a light, producing glare and dazzle, can also be fatiguing and have similar ill effects on quality.

Although daylight is preferable from a number of aspects, it needs to be noted that a number of pharmaceutical products and materials are affected by UV light. The design and layout of a modern pharmaceutical factory also usually makes artificial lighting inevitable. It should be installed so as not to create uncleanable dust traps, e.g. preferably flush-fitted to the ceiling, or with smooth easily accessible and cleanable surfaces.

Water

Water is, generally, by far the biggest single usage item in pharmaceutical and similar manufacturing. A number of applications, types, or grades, of water may be distinguished. It is used:

- As an *ingredient* (many products consist mainly of water).
- As an *in-process material* at some stage in the manufacture of a product, but which does not appear in the final product, for example, water used in granulating and coating solutions in tablet manufacture, although little of it remains in the end product – except, of course, any non-volatile impurities, or even micro-organisms it may have contained.
- For drinking.
- For washing (people, floors, walls, equipment, containers).
- For rinsing.
- For cooling.
- As a source of steam.

Basic considerations, all of which have significant product-quality implications are:

- The quality of the feed water to the plant.
- The uses to which the water will be put.
- The quality standards to which the waters used for different purposes must comply.
- The pretreatment and treatment methods which must be applied to ensure water used for various purposes complies with the appropriate standard.
- The design and installation of water treatment and installation systems.
- The control and monitoring of the output quality.

Put simply, the nature and extent of the water treatment will depend on the quality of what is available as source water, and on what is needed as the end product of the treatment process.

Water may be obtained from a number of sources. Water from wells or bore-holes, given suitable treatment, has been used to manufacture pharmaceuticals. In many countries, the most usual source is normal mains water of potable (drinkable) quality.

For pharmaceutical purposes, it may be considered that there are four basic types of water:

- Potable (mains) water.
- Purified water.
- Water for injections.
- Other (ancillary) water.

Potable water

Potable water is water that is fit and safe to drink – that is, the stuff that comes from the mains and out of the taps.

As far as it is possible to ascertain, no monograph on potable water appears in any pharmacopoeia. Some pharmacopoeias refer to it in terms such as 'Suitable water freshly drawn from the public supply . . .' and 'palatable and safe to drink . . .', but no monograph. An international standard was published by WHO in 1971, and an EC guideline in 1978 set standards for appearance, pH, limits for toxic substances and microbial contamination, and so on, but the precise definition of quality standards for water tends to vary with location.

To produce potable water, the primary source material (from rivers, lakes, wells, etc.) needs some form of treatment (flocculation, settling, filtration, chlorination . . .). Potable water can contain a range of dissolved organic and inorganic substances, suspended colloidal matter, and relatively low levels of micro-organisms. Although it has been suggested that potable water can be used as an ingredient in the manufacture of some non-sterile pharmaceutical products (creams, ointments and tablet granulations have been mentioned), informed opinion holds that potable water should only be used for drinking, personal washing, and also for the initial washing and rinsing of equipment and containers, provided (in the case of surfaces in contact with product) this is followed by rinsing with either purified water or water for injections, as appropriate and relevant.

Although it may seem strange that water which is fit to drink is not fit to be used as an ingredient of pharmaceutical products, this is indeed generally considered to be so. Tap water (or 'mains water') usually (dependent on location and ultimate source) contains small but not insignificant quantities of dissolved, and possibly suspended impurities. Some of these, although harmless to normal fit people when swallowed, can cause harm to those who are ill and weak and/or when administered by other routes than by mouth. They can also adversely affect formulations, for example by causing precipitation, or through ionic solutes disturbing the delicate balance of some emulsions. Potable water will also contain at least some level of (ever-multiplying) micro-organisms. These can cause infection in patients and/or break down formulations.

Particular care is necessary when potable water (and indeed any water) is held in a storage tank, where microbial growth could be prolific.

Purified water

Purified water is potable water which has been treated to conform with defined official standards. Specifically, in Britain and the EU generally, it is water which complies with the monograph on *aqua purificata* of the European Pharmacopoeia. A similar monograph appears in the British Pharmacopoeia (BP), and there is one in the United States Pharmacopoeia (USP). These monographs set down tests and limits for *chemical* purity, based on specific limit tests, and more general techniques such as electrical conductivity and residue on evaporation, but do not specify allowable microbial levels.

It is usual, however for manufacturers to define their own in-house limits, with a limit of not more than 100 organisms per mL being common. Commonly adopted 'warning limits' vary from 10 to 50 organisms per mL. Often the complete absence of particular types, or groups, of organisms (e.g. coliform, pseudomonas) is specified.

Purified water is produced from potable water by distillation, ion-exchange, reverse osmosis or other suitable means.

It is used for 'general' manufacturing purposes, that is, generally as an ingredient of non-sterile products but certainly NOT of injectable products. Also it is used as a final rinse for washing of containers and other primary packaging components, and in final rinses when cleaning equipment – in both cases when these are intended to be used only for non-sterile products.

Water for injections

It is necessary to draw an important distinction between water for injections which is in bulk (e.g. in a bulk holding tank and/or circulating in a ring-main distribution system) and water for injections which has been sterilised and is in fact sterile.

Various pharmacopoeias make this distinction in various ways. The BP defines water for injections as distilled water which is free from pyrogens and which is obtained by distilling potable water or purified water from a neutral glass, quartz or suitable metal still fitted with an efficient device for preventing the entrainment of droplets. It adds that the apparatus must be correctly maintained to ensure the production of pyrogen-free water and that 'the first portion of the distillate is discarded and the remainder collected and stored in conditions designed to prevent the growth of microorganisms and to avoid any other contamination.' Water for injections is required to comply with the requirements for purified water, with further limit tests, including that for pyrogens (or 'bacterial endotoxins').

Having thus generally defined water for injections, the BP then defines 'water for injections in bulk', in effect, as water which is used in the preparation of bulk solutions intended ultimately for injection (and which will be sterilised at a later stage in the process) and 'sterilised water for injections'. This is specifically defined as water for injections which has been filled and sealed into 'suitable containers' and then sterilised by *heating in an autoclave.* Thus, this definition is specifically directed at the water in sealed ampoules or vials which is used to dissolve or suspend sterile powders immediately prior to injection. However, it is of course possible to have bulk sterile water for injections.

Note that the BP requires that water for injections should be produced by distillation. Some other countries permit the use of reverse osmosis. The USP also distinguishes between 'water for injection', 'sterile water for injection', 'sterile water for irrigation' and 'bacteriostatic water for irrigation'.

Water for injections (not necessarily sterilised if the product is later to be sterilised, but most certainly sterilised, and *sterile*, if it is not) is used for the manufacture of injections, ophthalmic products and other sterile products intended for critical clinical applications. Here we encounter a matter of fundamental importance, and although it will be encountered again when we turn later to consider Sterile Production in more detail (see Part Six), it is so important that it is well worth stressing now: *It must **never** be thought that what happens (microbiologically speaking) before a product is sterilised is of no great importance. Careful control over contamination levels 'all along the line' is vital, so as to present the lowest possible challenge to whatever the chosen sterilisation process* – and, of course, to prevent the development of pyrogens. Having sterilised a product or material, very careful steps must be taken to prevent recontamination.

Thus, although 'water for injections in bulk' is not required to be sterile, this does not mean that it can contain an abundance of organisms, and it is usual for manufacturers to set their own in-house limits. Opinions tend to vary on what these should be, but not more than 500 cfu (colony forming units) per litre, with not more than 100 cfu/litre as a 'warning limit' and a complete absence of specified organisms (e.g. coliforms), is commonly suggested.

Water for injections (bulk quality) is also used for the final rinse of equipment and containers to be used for the manufacture of sterile products.

Other water

This includes water used for cooling and as boiler feed for the production of steam.

Cooling water used for cooling equipment does not have any defined standard. Nor does it need any, provided that it is retained within a sealed system and does not come into contact with product or the production environment. It has been suggested that it is prudent to add chemicals to such water in order to minimise microbial growth. However, in the accidental event of contact with product or environment, it would need to be recognised that, while the microbial risk may have been reduced, the chemical contamination risk has been increased.

The water used, following the sterilisation cycle, in some types of autoclaves to cool the sterilised load is a different matter altogether. It should be sterilised water for injections quality, to protect against the potentially hazardous consequences of water (or residues from it) remaining on the load, or, say, entering a vial through a faulty seal, or a crack.

The quality of water used to feed boilers is, from a pharmaceutical point of view, of no importance – *provided* there will be no contact (direct or indirect) between the steam produced by the boiler and the products manufactured, or with the contact surfaces of the equipment used to manufacture them. Where the steam *will* come into contact with products, containers, medical devices or the contact surfaces of manufacturing equipment, the water used to produce it should not contain volatile additives like amines or hydrazines. If the steam is intended to be used for sterilisation (e.g. in autoclaving, live-steaming, or sterilising in place (SIP)) then it must be 'clean steam' (or pure steam), produced from deionised (or reverse osmosis) water by a well-designed clean steam generator which will yield a condensate that complies with the requirements for water for injections.

Water treatment and supply systems

The EC GMP Guide Annex on Sterile Products (and the statement is relevant to water used for other purposes) states (paragraph 35):

> Water treatment and distribution plants should be designed, constructed and maintained so as to ensure the reliable production of water of an appropriate quality. They should not be operated beyond their designed capacity. Water for injection should be produced, stored, and distributed in a manner which prevents microbial growth, for example by constant circulation at a temperature above 70°C.

Many would argue that the temperature at which the water should be held and circulated should be not less than 80°C.

To conclude this important digression on water: it is not merely a question of the correct selection, installation and maintenance of the major items of equipment (e.g. stills, deionisers); it is a matter of viewing the whole water production, supply and distribution process as an integrated system, and controlling it and monitoring it to ensure the consistent supply of water of the required quality (or qualities). This requires consideration of the source water arriving at the plant, its nature and quality, and what sort of settling, coarse filtration, scavenging or other pretreatment it may require; through to the deionisation equipment, its installation, monitoring, maintenance and regeneration; on to the still itself, its installation control and monitoring, via any holding vessel (with provision for elevated temperature storage, and with vent valves protected by hydrophobic bacteria-retentive filters) and the recirculation system; to final delivery to production areas.

The overall concept should be that of what has been termed a 'sanitary design' – a system which aims at minimising microbial growth, at minimising chemical and particulate contamination arising from the system itself, and which permits cleaning and sterilisation in place. Except in the very smallest systems, where water is taken direct from the still as required, water should be distributed to the required production outlets via holding tank(s) and a recirculating loop, in all of which the water (at 80°C) is maintained in constant turbulent motion. Tanks and pipework should be constructed of 316 stainless steel with internal surfaces (including all welds) highly polished to prevent mini-pockets of stagnant water where organisms can flourish. The following sources of contamination should be avoided, or kept to a minimum:

- Excessive length of pipe runs.
- Too many valves.
- Non-sanitary valves and joints.
- Threaded joints.
- 'Dead-legs'.
- Undrainable loops and bends.
- Unprotected vents.
- Pumps.
- Tanks.

It is no use installing a system which works well just for the first week or so. It needs to be monitored and maintained to ensure that it continues to work well. Here there is a vital need for close cooperation between microbiological quality control which will perform the microbiological monitoring, and the engineers who will need to service and maintain the system to ensure it remains capable of supplying the quality of water required. Care needs to be taken to ensure that in the very act of sampling for microbiological testing the system is not contaminated.

Steam

Possible uses of steam include:

- General factory heating.
- Production process heating (steam-jacketed vessels, heating coils).
- Steam cleaning.
- Sterilisation (autoclaving, 'live-steaming' of vessels and pipes, steralising in place).

Where steam is not associated with product manufacture, and does not come into contact with product or manufacturing materials (or with surfaces that will contact product or materials) then, pharmaceutically speaking, the quality of that steam is not particularly relevant. Where there is any such contact (and the steam is not used for sterilisation, or directly associated with sterile products or materials) then the steam should be of such a quality that, when condensed, the water thus produced would comply with the requirements for purified water. When used as the sterilising medium (e.g. in autoclaves, SIP systems) the steam should be 'clean steam'; that is, steam which when condensed will form water-for-injections quality water.

Gases/compressed air

Various gases may be used for a variety of purposes, e.g. inert gases used as a protective blanket or to displace air in an ampoule head-space; as propellants in aerosol manufacture; as sterilants (e.g. ethylene oxide); as a source of flame in glass ampoule sealing.

Any gas which may come into contact with a product (or product contact surfaces), or is used in the manufacture of a product, must be treated as if it were a raw material, and must therefore be subject to standard quality control procedures to ensure that it conforms to predetermined quality standards. A number of gases are used in laboratory test procedures. If these are not of the required/specified quality, then the reliability of the test results may suffer.

Gases supplied in cylinders should be properly colour coded (BS 1319), and additionally identified as to lot or cylinder number. Cylinders should be stored under cover, without exposure to extremes of temperature, and in such conditions that their markings remain clearly visible. Pressure gauges should be regularly checked and calibrated. Gas pipelines, from cylinders or from bulk gas storage, should be clearly marked as to contents. It should not be possible to switch pipelines and connections and thus to supply the wrong gas. Dedicated, pin-indexed valves and connections, as used in hospital gas supply lines, should be employed where possible.

Gases (including compressed air) may need to be filtered when supplied to production areas generally. Gases (including compressed air) when supplied to manufacturing areas for sterile products (and other controlled environments) will certainly need to be filtered (as close to the point of use as possible) to ensure that it conforms to the particulate and microbial standards for the area.

Electricity

Although there is no need to dwell on the importance of electricity supplies to any modern manufacturing facility, a few matters of critical importance to pharmaceutical manufacturing are worthy of emphasis.

Continuity of electricity supply is essential for a number of systems or processes (air supply/extraction, particularly for sterile manufacture; fermentation plants; incubators) and thus back-up systems should be available in the event of mains failure. Ideally, there should be automatic changeover and reset from mains to emergency generator supply. Just what the needs and priorities are for emergency back-up should be a matter of discussion and agreement between the production, engineering and quality functions. The actions to be taken on mains failure should be agreed and set down as a standard operating procedure (SOP), with out-of-hours contact telephone numbers of relevant key personnel (Engineering, Production, Security).

Certain equipment (computers, microprocessor control systems, some analytical instruments) may need voltage stabilisation in order to operate reliably.

Solvents and other bulk liquids supplies

Large manufacturing organisations may well receive a number of liquid materials in bulk (solvents, sugar syrup, 'liquid glucose', glycerin, etc.), which are pumped from the supplier's delivery tanker to storage tanks. Often it is not a practical proposition to keep the tanker waiting in the yard while full quality testing is carried out, and the material may thus be provisionally accepted and pumped to storage on the basis of passing, perhaps, just one or two tests (including a specific identity test), with full testing to follow later. It is therefore important that (if and as necessary) storage tanks, pipework and valve systems are installed so that liquids held pending full test cannot be used before formal release by Quality Control. Bulk liquid storage and pipework systems should be installed and maintained so as to prevent, as far as is humanly possible, mix-up, cross-contamination and inadvertent switching of pipelines. All pipes should be marked clearly to identify their contents, and the direction of flow should be indicated.

Lubricants and lubrication

To say that moving parts need lubrication is to state the obvious. What should be just as obvious, but does not always seem to be so, is that there is a world of difference between the lubrication of a piece of equipment which is used to fabricate machine parts, and one which is used to manufacture pharmaceuticals. Industrial lubricants should not be allowed to come into contact with starting materials, products or product containers. Care needs to be taken to avoid hazarding product quality through contamination from leaking seals, lubricant drips and the like. Gland packing materials should be inert and non-reactive and wherever possible, food-grade lubricants should be used. All those concerned with lubrication should be aware that pharmaceutical manufacture is a different world – lubricants are potentially serious contaminants.

Waste disposal and drainage

Careful control of waste material and its disposal is important for a number of reasons. If reject or scrap product and/or material is allowed to accumulate in an uncontrolled fashion it can represent a cross-contamination hazard. If it is a vehicle of microbial growth, then it could also become a viable contamination hazard.

Clearly, product scrap and waste can also become an environmental and public toxic hazard and must therefore be disposed of in accordance with all national and local legal requirements. Chemical/solvent wastes may require agreement with the local authority as to their disposal, and any necessary pretreatment. Emitted gases and vapours may also need treatment, not only to avoid environmental pollution but also to prevent product contamination.

Similar care and control is necessary over the disposal of scrap/

rejected/discarded packaging materials. All waste printed packaging materials (printed containers, tubes, labels, cartons, leaflets – the lot) must be kept under secure control and then destroyed, under close supervision, as soon as possible, to prevent unauthorised (either inadvertent or deliberate) re-use.

Drains (internal and external) should be sufficient in size, number and location to do the job intended. They should not be, or allowed to become, vehicles of contamination. They should have trapped gullies, with air breaks as necessary to prevent back siphonage. Internally, open drainage channels should be avoided if possible. If they are necessary, they should be shallow to facilitate cleaning and disinfection. There should be written cleaning and disinfection procedures for internal drains. These procedures should be strictly adhered to.

In the critical areas of sterile products manufacturing areas, drains should not be installed.

At the beginning of this chapter, mention was made of the provision of cloakroom, toilet, canteen and communication facilities. All these have product-quality implications. If operators are not comfortable (e.g. hungry, thirsty, need to use the toilet) their work will suffer, and so will product quality. They should not eat or drink in production areas, and they need to be properly dressed in the correct standard protective clothing. They need to observe hygienic personal practices. Supervisory staff, at least, will need to be able to communicate with each other over distances. Hence the significance to quality of the provision of good standard cloakrooms, toilets (**not** opening direct to production areas), canteens and communication systems. The good, or alternatively bad, effects on operators' morale, motivation and attitude can be considerable. No management can reasonably expect operators to respect the ideals of high quality standards when they provide them only with ugly, wretched and inadequate canteens and dark dismal and dirty cloakrooms and toilets.

Cleaning and disinfection

Cleaning is quite simply the removal of dust, dirt, debris and residues. The more difficult question to answer is 'How clean is clean?' and inevitably the answer is 'It all depends'. One normally expects domestic dwelling places, kitchens for example, to be clean. It is generally expected, with good reason, that areas used for the manufacture of medicinal and other healthcare products should be cleaner than merely 'domestically clean'. How *much* cleaner will depend on the nature of the product being manufactured, its intended route or method of administration, and the potential hazards of any contamination of the product. It is thus reasonable to suggest that the highest conceivable level of cleanliness is required for the manufacture of sterile products intended for injection. On the other hand, a significantly lower level may well be acceptable for, say, the manufacture of foot-dusting powders.

The 'dust, dirt, debris and residues' can arise from a number of sources:

- Air-borne dust, dirt and particles.
- Particles, fibres, hairs and exudates shed by humans.
- Spillages and breakages.
- Particles from friction in machines.
- Oil and grease from lubricated moving parts.
- Residues from previous products.
- And just plain dirt – it is one of the fundamental laws of the universe that things which are not regularly cleaned get dirty.

For obvious reasons, areas, surfaces and equipment in and on which products are made must be kept clean. Dirt, and the microbes which it can harbour, must not get into or onto products. But there is another good reason for regularly and scrupulously cleaning away this dirt.

Floors, walls, ceilings and work surfaces often need to be disinfected. Disinfectants can be inactivated by dirt. Dirt (particularly oily or greasy films, and protein-like matter) can also protect micro-organisms against the action of disinfectants. So, before disinfection, it is important first to clean surfaces.

Where gross amounts of dirt are present, it may be first necessary to remove most of it by scrubbing. Then surfaces may be cleaned by the application of a cleaning agent, followed by rinsing. In most normal circumstances all that is needed for the cleaning of floors, walls, and work surfaces is clean water with the addition of detergent, followed by a clean water rinse. The quality of the water used will depend on the nature of the operations carried out on, or near, the surfaces in question. Obviously, it must be microbiologically clean, and it may be appropriate (for example, in sterile product manufacture) for at least the final rinse water to be of high quality 'water for injection' standard.

Manufacturing tanks, pipelines and associated equipment need also to be cleaned and rinsed after use, and before any sterilisation that may be necessary. This may be done by simple manual methods, or by clean in place (CIP). Here cleaning is accomplished by automatically pumping cleaning agents, and rinsing liquids, under pressure, around the entire system without necessarily dismantling it (see Chapter 10: Equipment).

Disinfection

A disinfectant is a chemical substance or combination of substances which, when applied to surfaces, will kill micro-organisms, with the exception of some bacterial spores. Disinfection is not the same as sterilisation which is the destruction or removal of all micro-organisms, and indeed of all organisms generally – when something is sterilised, if it is done properly, all living organisms are destroyed, or removed. A disinfectant is something which cannot quite achieve that. It is not possible to be certain that, by use of chemical solutions alone, *all* living organisms will be destroyed, particularly bacterial spores.

However, usually the aim with walls, floors, ceilings and work surfaces is not necessarily that they should be rendered sterile, but that they should be as clean as possible, with any microbiological contamination kept to a minimum.

Other words which mean more-or-less the same as 'disinfectant' are 'germicide', 'bactericide' and 'biocide'. There is a possibility of confusion here, because these words mean different things to different people. It is generally best to stick to the term 'disinfectant'. Another word, 'antiseptic', means a milder substance which can, for example be used on skin surfaces and wounds to control or prevent infection without harming the patient. Even so, some people confuse antiseptics with disinfectants. Another term 'sanitise' has been used in so many different senses (e.g. after the bombing at the Atlanta Olympic Games, the local police chief declared, on international TV, that the area was now safe as it had been 'sanitised') that it is virtually devoid of meaning, and therefore its use in any scientific/technological context should be abandoned.

Types of disinfectants

A wide range of substances are used as disinfectants. They may be single substances, like alcohol or phenols, and there are a number of commercially available mixtures. It is usually best not to make 'DIY' mixtures. It could be dangerous, and some disinfectants can neutralise each other's activity.

Disinfecting agents vary in the range of their activity and in the concentrations at which they are effective. All have their own special advantages, and also disadvantages. For example, alcohols are inflammable, phenols and chlorine compounds can be dangerous and corrosive, iodine compounds can stain some surfaces, and so on (see Table 9.1).

Disinfectants should always be used in accordance with instructions, and at the right dilution (instructions as given either in the supplier's literature, or in company procedures). Dilutions of disinfectants should not be stored unless they are sterilised. Otherwise, dilutions should be made up freshly each time they are needed since some micro-organisms can grow quite successfully in dilute disinfectants.

Another, traditional, method of disinfecting clean rooms is by fumigating or 'gassing', usually with formaldehyde gas, although this can present problems due to the unpleasant, choking and toxic nature of the gas.

Rotation of disinfectants

Many manufacturers use different disinfectants over a period of time, on an alternating, or rotating, basis. The reasoning behind this is to prevent the development of disinfectant-resistant strains of micro-organisms. Although there have been some arguments about whether or not it has this effect, alternation of disinfectants remains a recommendation of a number of experts, and it may be a worthwhile practice.

Table 9.1 Disinfectants for premises – types and applications

Substance	Suitable concentration	Effect on bacteria	Effect on spores	Effect on vegetative fungi	Advantages	Disadvantages
Ethanol	70%	Good	Fair	Fair	• Quick acting • Evaporates rapidly, leaving no residues	• Limited range of effects • Flammable
Phenols	0.5–3%	Excellent	Good	Excellent	• Broad range of effects • May be combined with surfactants	• Corrosive on some surfaces (including skin!)
Formaldehyde		Excellent	Good	Good	• Broad range of effects • Used for 'gassing'	• Premises not accessible during treatment • Can be corrosive • Short- and long-term human toxicity problems
Isopropanol	70–90%	Good	Good	Good	• Quick acting • Evaporates leaving no residues	• Not the most effective
Iodine and iodophors	75–150 ppm	Excellent	Good	Excellent	• Quick acting • Effective in low concentrations	• Can be corrosive • Stain some surfaces
Chlorine compounds (hypochlorite, chloramine, etc.)	1–4%	Excellent	Good	Excellent	• Broad range of effects	• Corrosive
Quaternary ammonium compounds	1–5%	Good	Fair	Fair	• Some cleaning effect • Odourless	• Limited effect • Inactivated by soap detergents

Cleaning and disinfection in processing areas

Routine cleaning and disinfection in clean rooms and other processing areas should be regularly carried out in accordance with an established programme, following a standard written procedure. That is, cleaning and disinfection is not something to be done when it 'seems like a good idea', or only when time permits.

Written programmes and procedures will, naturally, vary in detail from manufacturer to manufacturer, and in accordance with the type of product being manufactured. Some important general points on cleaning and disinfection of rooms, areas and surfaces may be set out as follows:

1. There should be an approved written programme and procedure which must always be followed exactly.
2. It is necessary to *clean* thoroughly first, before disinfecting.
3. It is important to ensure that the cleaning and disinfecting process does not, in fact, create more contamination.
4. All cleaning and disinfecting agents and materials should themselves be clean and not shed fibres or particles.
5. Cleaning implements and wiping cloths, having been applied to a surface should not be re-wetted by direct return to the container of cleaning or disinfecting agent, but first rinsed (and squeezed out) in a second bucket of clean water.
6. Non-shedding materials should be used for wiping surfaces, and dry, dust-creating brushes should not be used. If it is necessary to remove significant quantities of powdery materials, then wet or vacuum methods are preferable.
7. All cleaning and disinfection of a room should start at the part of the room furthest from the entrance, otherwise there is a danger of the cleaner 'painting himself/herself into a corner', and having to cross the cleaned area in order to get out.
8. When cleaning walls and other vertical surfaces, work should always start at the top and work down – again to avoid recontamination of parts already cleaned/disinfected.
9. It is vital that the right cleaning and disinfecting agents are used, in the right dilutions, as directed in the company's written procedure. Remember, dilutions of disinfectants should be made up fresh, in clean containers. They should not be stored for later use unless they are sterilised.
10. All cleaning equipment and implements must themselves be thoroughly cleaned after use, and stored in a clean, dry condition.
11. All spilled materials (liquids or powders, or breakages) should be cleaned up in a way which will minimise the possibility of creating further contamination. Again, dry brushing should be avoided and wet and/or vacuum methods employed. If there is a risk of microbial contamination the cleaned-up area or surface should then be disinfected. Any spilled material which represents a microbiological hazard should be placed in a container, immersed in disinfectant, covered, and removed from the room.

10

Equipment

With shabby equipment always deteriorating in the general mess of imprecision of feeling

T S Eliot, *East Coker* from *Four Quartets*, 1944

Pharmaceutical manufacturing equipment should be capable (and, more than that, be *demonstrably* capable) of producing products, materials and intermediates which are those intended, and which conform to the required/ specified quality characteristics. In other words, not only should products be 'fit for their intended purpose', so should the equipment used to produce them.

Equipment requirements

The equipment must be designed and built so that it is possible (and relatively *easily* possible) to clean it thoroughly. Surfaces which come into contact with product should have smooth polished finishes, with no nooks and crannies, difficult corners, uneven joints, 'dead-legs', projections and rough welds to harbour contamination and/or make cleaning difficult. Equipment must also be capable of withstanding repeated, thorough cleaning. Traces of previous product, at levels which might be acceptable in other industries, are totally unacceptable in the manufacture of medicines. It may also be necessary for equipment to be sterilised before use. It then becomes important that it is capable of withstanding the sterilisation treatment – for example, the stress of steam at elevated temperature, under pressure. The questions of CIP (clean in place) and SIP (variously used to mean 'sterilise in place' or 'steam in place') are covered later in this chapter.

Lubrication of moving parts should be so designed and performed that the product cannot be contaminated by the lubricant – or by, for example, metal particles from parts which have not been properly lubricated.

Materials used for equipment

As far as the properties of the materials of construction of the equipment are concerned, there are two major concerns.

1. The possibility of contamination, or degradation, of the product by the material from which the equipment is constructed.
2. The action of the product or material in process on the material from which the equipment is constructed.

Contamination of product can arise from shedding or leaching of contaminants from the equipment into the product, or from reaction between the product and the material of the equipment. Product could otherwise be degraded by this sort of interaction, or by absorption or adsorption of components of the product onto, or into, the equipment.

Corrosive action of product on the equipment can damage that equipment, and in turn lead to further product contamination or degradation.

It is worth remembering that there are two aspects of the potential release of product contaminants by equipment: they could be toxic to patients, even in very small amounts, and they could cause product decomposition. As an example of the latter – penicillin can be inactivated by trace heavy metals. This is not the place for a detailed discussion of the properties of the materials of construction of pharmaceutical plant and equipment, but it is worth noting that each case must be considered on it merits. For example, although stainless steel is widely, and generally successfully, used, there are a few examples of liquid solution products where the active ingredient can be degraded by contact with stainless steel mixing and storage vessels. In some cases, specialised plastic vessels have been found to be the best alternative. This illustrates the crucial importance of selecting equipment fabricated from materials appropriate to the product(s) to be manufactured.

Fixed equipment should be installed, piped-in and supplied with services in a manner which creates a minimum of recesses, corners or areas which are difficult to get at for cleaning. The pipework mazes beloved of some fitters should be avoided. Where pipework/ducting passes through walls/partitions, it should be sealed in, on both sides.

Good manufacturing practice for pharmaceutical equipment

A digest of statements on equipment which appear in the official GMP guides is as follows:

Pharmaceutical equipment should be designed and located to suit the processes and products for which it is to be used. It should have been shown to be capable of carrying out the processes for which it is used (that is, it should be properly commissioned, or 'qualified' – see later), and of being operated to the necessary hygienic standards. It should be maintained so as to be fit to perform its functions and it should be easily and conveniently cleanable, both inside and out. Parts which come into contact with materials being processed should be minimally reactive or absorptive with respect to those materials and there should be no hazard to a product through leaking seals, lubricant drips, and the like, or through inappropriate modifications or adaptations. It should be kept and stored in a clean condition and checked for cleanliness before each use. Washing and cleaning equipment should not itself become a vehicle for contamination. All measuring, weighing, recording and control equipment should be serviced and calibrated at defined intervals, according to an established procedure. Fixed pipework should be labelled as to contents, with an indication (where applicable) of the direction of flow. Defective equipment should be removed from manufacturing areas, or clearly labelled as defective.

Within the last 25 years there has been a most significant trend away from machines 'borrowed' from other industries (such as bakery, confectionery or dairy) and from machines adapted or designed for pharmaceutical use with scant regard to GMP principles. The trend has been towards equipment designed and built specifically for pharmaceutical use. To this end some particular trends have been:

1.   Towards more precision in control and adjustment.
2.   Towards closed systems of manufacture.
3.   Towards more efficient, more automatic control, monitoring and recording.
4.   Towards multi-sequential purpose-built machinery, which performs a series of operations *in situ* (e.g. mixer/drier/granulators).
5.   Towards built-in local environmental and contamination control.
6.   Towards easy and readily confirmable cleanability.

Many of these trends are epitomised by the evolution of the hard gelatin capsule filling machine. For many years it seemed to be readily accepted that the only way to fill capsules was by using the early semi-automatic double ring-plate machines with manually actuated powder hoppers. Those machines were:

- Noisy.
- Prodigiously dust generating.
- Requiring of constant attention (one operator per machine).
- Very demanding of operator skill and judgement.
- Much affected by physical nature of powder.
- Liable to produce wide-ranging fills.
- Slow (say <10 000 per hour)
- Unpleasant for operators.

By contrast, modern advanced capsule filling machines are:

- Relatively quiet in operation.

- Enclosed with dust extraction.
- Once set up, in need of little attention (one operator per several machines).
- Precise, and fitted with automated weight check and adjustment.
- Not so affected by powder nature and density.
- Fast (150 000 or more per hour).
- Pleasant to work with.

There are, of course, other examples of this type of evolution, and equipment manufacturers have become increasingly attentive to the special needs of the pharmaceutical and related industries.

Cleaning of equipment

Between batches (or 'campaigns') all manufacturing equipment and vessels must be thoroughly cleaned, and (as necessary) disinfected or sterilised.

There should be written procedures for doing this, which must be followed exactly. Each different piece of equipment has its own particular areas where there is a risk, given the right conditions, of microbial growth.

The best modern equipment is usually designed and built to reduce these risks as far as possible. It needs to:

- Be easy to dismantle and clean.
- Have internal surfaces which are smooth, continuous, with no pits or rough, unpolished welds.
- Have no 'dead-legs', or water or dirt-traps.

It may be necessary to strip (or partially strip) equipment down before cleaning it. A written standard procedure should always be followed. With mobile equipment there is the advantage that it can be removed from the manufacturing room for cleaning in a wash bay.

Once equipment has been cleaned and disinfected or sterilised, steps should be taken to ensure that it cannot become recontaminated. Care must also be taken to ensure (by labelling and/or segregation) that there is no possibility of mix-up between items which have been cleaned and disinfected or sterilised and those which have not.

Clean in place (CIP) and sterilise in place (SIP)

The traditional way of cleaning between batches or products was (and to a significant extent, still is) to do it by hand. Attention must be given to the internal contact surfaces of equipment, mixing vessels, storage vessels and any associated pipework. This requires the opening up of vessels, dismantling and stripping down, with subsequent re-assembly. The efficacy of cleaning by simple manual methods will be crucially influenced by the zeal (or lack of it) of the human cleaner. It will also result in long down times and thus poor plant utilisation. It also introduces the potential hazard of recontamination of internal surfaces when the equipment is re-assembled. Well designed clean in place (CIP) systems provide an answer to these problems – but the crucial phrase is 'well designed'. For the manu-facture of products intended to be sterile (or microbiologically clean or with a 'low count'), the concept is extended to 'sterilise in place' (SIP). It needs always to be remembered that, before sterilisation (or disinfection) it is first necessary to *clean*. If traces of product, or other material, remain on surfaces through ineffective cleaning, these can build up, protecting organisms from the sterilising agent (e.g. steam) and thus prevent proper sterilisation.

There are a number of advantages of CIP/SIP, especially if (as it should be for maximum efficiency and efficacy) the process is automated. These include:

- Reduction in equipment down-time/increased plant utilisation.
- Reduction in labour costs.
- Elimination of the variability of the human factor, and thus a more consistent and reproducible process.
- Elimination of the recontamination hazard on reassembly.

The major disadvantage is the higher initial cost of plant purchase and instal-lation.

Clean in place (CIP)

Effectiveness of cleaning is a function of a number of factors, including time; temperature; rate of turbulent flow of the cleaning solutions(s); the concentration (and activity in relation to the soiling material to be removed) of chemical cleaning agents in the cleaning solution; and the surface finish (smoothness or roughness) of the surfaces to be cleaned. All these factors interact. For example, all other things being equal, it will take a longer time to clean completely a relatively rough internal surface as compared to a high-polished smooth one. Higher temperatures will need lower times and flow rates, and so on. Cleaning solutions commonly employed contain caustic agents and detergents, and it must be remem-bered that, before cleaning is complete, it is necessary to ensure removal of the cleaning agents themselves. That is, there must be a rinsing stage, using (for aqueous products) water of a quality appropriate to, and com-patible with, the product(s) to be manufactured in the equipment.

To attempt to 'bolt-on' CIP/SIP systems to existing plant and equip-ment is to court disaster. The process, and the system, must be designed and built in from the very start; that is, at the process development, or scale-up stage. The plant needs also to be designed and built so as to be able to with-stand (and *safely* withstand) the temperatures involved.

By the very nature of a CIP process it is not possible to take a look to see if the equipment is clean. Indeed, to do so would defeat the whole object of the exercise. This makes validation of the CIP cleaning process especially important.

Cleaning validation

It is increasingly being considered that it is not sufficient merely to apply *ad hoc* cleaning methods, and then *assume* that things (particularly equipment, manufacturing and holding vessels and the like) are clean just because they look clean, and as we have noted, in a CIP process it is just not possible to see if the internal surfaces of the equipment 'look clean'. It is necessary to employ fully documented, *validated*, cleaning procedures. That means cleaning procedures for which there is documented experimental evidence that they do, in fact, achieve the level of cleanliness which is both intended and appropriate in the given circumstances. Validation of cleaning processes is discussed in Chapter 23.

Sterilise in place (SIP)

'Sterilise in place' is the term applied to a process of sterilising the internal product-contact surfaces of a complete system of manufacturing, including holding tanks and associated pipework (transfer lines, filling lines, etc.) while that system is assembled and in place, without having to take the system apart, separately sterilise the various elements of the system, and then reassemble it aseptically.

The sterilising agent employed is steam at sterilising temperature, and it thus necessary to design the system, from the outset, so that it is able to withstand the temperatures and pressures required. As with CIP, 'bolt-on' SIP is not a practical proposition. Nor is it a safe one.

Removal of air, and condensate, is crucial to ensuring that saturated steam, at the required temperature, for the required time, makes contact with all internal surfaces of the equipment. Evacuation is not usually possible, and air must be removed by properly designed and positioned bleed valves. In most systems, there will be significant amounts of condensate, which must be removed by drainage points placed in all horizontal and low parts of the system. Wherever possible, pipework should be angled so as to assist drainage. The process can be controlled automatically so as to maintain sterilising conditions throughout. At the completion of the sterilising phase, air or nitrogen is introduced through a bacteria-retentive filter, and the system purged of any residual steam or condensate. A flow of pressurised gas is then maintained to dry the system, which should then be kept under positive sterile air (or nitrogen) pressure, to maintain internal sterility before the system is used. The efficacy of any SIP system must be demonstrated by appropriate process validation (see Chapters 22 and 23).

Calibration

A number of items of equipment used in manufacturing are themselves measuring devices (e.g. balances, scales, volumetric measures, metered valves) or have measuring devices associated with them (from quite complex pressure gauges, strain gauges and load cells, to the more humble dipsticks and sight glasses). All need to be calibrated, and maintained in a state of calibration.

Confusion sometimes exists between the two terms 'metrology' and 'calibration'. Metrology is the science or study of measurement. It is not unusual, particularly in companies with US affiliations, to hear of 'Metrology Departments'. These perhaps might be more properly termed 'Calibration Departments', for they usually are concerned with just one aspect of metrology – calibration.

In the EC GMP Guide (EC, 1992), calibration is defined thus:

> *Calibration:* the set of operations which establish, under specified conditions, the relationship between values indicated by a measuring instrument or measuring system, or values represented by a material measure, and the corresponding known values of a reference standard.

This definition is only partially satisfactory, although linguistic purists might argue that that is, indeed, what calibration *is*, and that nothing more is needed. However, it gives no indication of *purpose*, or of what is the next step once the relationship has been established. For that reason, the following (from the US National Standards Laboratory) is to be preferred:

> *Calibration:* The comparison of a measurement system or device of unknown accuracy to another measurement system or device with a known accuracy to detect, correlate, report or eliminate by adjustment, any variation from the required performance limits of the unverified system.

There is no doubt that calibration involves a comparison of the unknown (or uncertain) with the known, and it is usually taken that the next step is to make any correction or adjustment that this comparison has shown to be necessary.

International standards

We measure many things; for example, time, linear dimensions (length/distance), area, volume/capacity, mass/weight, temperature, heat, pressure, velocity, electrical values (current, voltage, resistance). Some of these are fundamental measures (e.g. time, linear dimensions, mass), others are derived from them (area, volume, velocity). The units used have been established in various ways, and some 'absolute standards' have changed over the passage of years:

- A *metre*, for example, was originally defined as 1/10 000 000th of the length of the polar quadrant through Paris. The definition has changed

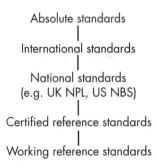

Absolute standards
|
International standards
|
National standards
(e.g. UK NPL, US NBS)
|
Certified reference standards
|
Working reference standards

Figure 10.1   Hierarchy of standards for calibration.

a number of times since, and the current definition (since 1983) is the distance travelled by light, in a vacuum, in 1/299 792 258th of a second.

- A *second* was originally 1/86 400th of a mean solar day. It is now defined as the duration of 9 192 631 770 cycles of the radiation associated with a specified transition of the caesium atom.
- A *kilogram* is more simply defined as the mass of a platinum/iridium cylinder held at Sèvres, near Paris.

In ordinary routine work it is hardly necessary (or practicable) to refer each time to the ultimate, or absolute standard for any measurement, and it is usual to make the necessary comparison with something lower in the league table, but which has in turn been reliably calibrated and certified against a higher standard. This introduces the concept of a 'hierarchy of standards' (as seen in Fig. 10.1).

Laboratories, calibration departments, technicians and the like will tend to have available reference standards (e.g. weights) or devices (e.g. thermometers), which have been certified (for example by the UK National Physical Laboratory or the US National Bureau of Standards) and from which their own internal working standards are derived or against which they are compared.

Terminology

The terminology of calibration tends to be akin to that used in analytical validation (see Chapter 17). Thus, in the context of calibration/metrology:

- *Accuracy* is the closeness of an observed or measured value to the true, or a reference, value (closeness to the truth).
- *Precision* is the closeness of agreement between different measurements of the same value, in a series of measurements, using the same measuring device (closeness to each other or 'togetherness').
- *Range* is the interval over which a device or system will operate with suitable accuracy and precision.
- *Sensitivity* is the degree to which the device or system can detect small differences in a measured value.

Official statements on good calibration practice

The EC GMP Guide (under 'Premises and equipment') quotes the following:

> 3.40 Balances and measuring equipment of an appropriate range and pre-
> cision should be available for production and control operations.
>
> 3.41 Measuring, weighing, recording and control equipment should be cali-
> brated and checked at defined intervals by appropriate methods. Ade-
> quate records of such tests should be maintained.

The US CGMPs (US FDA, 1990), in Section 211.160 (b) (4), state that
laboratory controls shall include:

> (4) The calibration of instruments, apparatus, gauges, and recording devices
> at suitable intervals in accordance with an established written program
> containing specific directions, schedules, limits for accuracy and pre-
> cision, and provision for remedial action in the event that accuracy and/or
> precision limits are not met. Instruments, apparatus, gauges and record-
> ing devices not meeting established specifications shall not be used.

Since the quality of a product will depend so much on the quality (i.e. fitness
for purpose) of the measuring devices used in its manufacture and testing,
it is important that the calibration of all measuring and testing equipment
(whether it be intended for manufacturing, or laboratory use) should not be
conducted on a whim, or only when a device is clearly not functioning. It
should be *managed* as a well-controlled operation, run according to pre-
planned programmes and schedules, with written, approved procedures for
the calibration of each type of instrument or device, and with records maintained of calibrations carried out. Whatever the format of the documentation system employed, it should clearly signal when next an instrument or
device is due for calibration.

Good calibration practice summarised

The main steps to good calibration practice may be set out as follows:

1. Carefully review all manufacturing and control processes, to deter-
    mine and record all the measurements which need to be made, and to
    define the accuracy and precision required when making them. On this
    basis, select and obtain the necessary test/measuring equipment
    accordingly, or discard and replace any test equipment found to be
    unsuitable, or inadequate for the purpose.
2. Mark, or by some other means (e.g. by reference in documents/records
    to plant or model numbers) identify all measuring equipment to ensure
    it is calibrated at defined intervals against certified reference standards.
3. Prepare and implement written calibration procedures, programmes,
    schedules and records, which will ensure that measuring devices are
    indeed calibrated, as intended, at the prescribed time intervals. The
    careful determination of the intervals between routine calibrations of
    a given instrument or device is critical to the success, or otherwise, of
    a calibration programme. It should not be a general, overall figure,

applicable to all instruments, which just seems like a good idea. Each time interval should be carefully selected for each device, after consideration of:

— Type of measuring device.
— How crucial is the accuracy and precision of the device in relation to quality, and hence consumer safety.
— Degree of accuracy and precision required.
— Device manufacturer's recommendations.
— Extent of use.
— Stress placed upon device in use.
— Any tendency of device to display drift.
— Previous history, and records, of device in use.
— Environmental conditions.

4. Keep calibration records, detailing what calibrations have been carried out, when and by whom. Regularly review these records to ensure that the required calibrations are, in fact, being carried out at the specified intervals.
5. Ensure visibility of calibration status. That is, label the equipment with an indication of when last calibrated, and when next is due, or record this information in an immediately accessible document or record book.
6. Ensure the calibration status of any measuring device or instrument before it is used.
7. Carry out documented retrospective assessments of the validity of previous measurements/tests whenever a piece of measuring or test equipment is found to be out of calibration. (It is irresponsible to fail to consider the potential effects of false previous results when a measuring device is found to be reading incorrectly, and to act accordingly, no matter what might be the economic consequences.)
8. Ensure that measuring equipment is handled and stored so that its accuracy and general fitness for use is not hazarded.
9. Protect the equipment, and any associated software, against unauthorised adjustments which would invalidate its setting.
10. Ensure that calibrations, inspections, tests and measurements are carried out under suitable environmental conditions, and that reference standards are very carefully protected against damage or deterioration. (Instances have been observed where the pristine condition of a company's set of standard balance weights was maintained by a vigorous weekly application of brass polish, and another that identified its set of standard weights each with a dab of red paint.)

The most important requirement is the need to ensure that calibration work is carried out by trained, experienced personnel who really know what they are doing, and the importance of what they are doing. It is also important that there is a formally assigned, accountable responsibility for calibration.

If calibration work is carried out under external contract, it should be subject to a formal written contract, clearly defining the nature and extent of the work required, and the content and format of the resultant test report(s).

Machine maintenance

All machinery is subject to the deleterious effects of wear, dirt, stress and corrosion, acting individually or in combination one with another. To mini-mise these adverse effects, and the inevitable consequent decline in machine performance, efficiency and useful life, and (most importantly) in product quality, it is vital to take appropriate preventative measures. Thus, a com-prehensive written maintenance programme should be prepared, for each piece of mechanical production equipment, setting out each and every required maintenance activity in detail. It should include statements of the frequency with which each activity should be performed, in terms of real time (e.g. daily, weekly, monthly, yearly) or machine time (e.g. number of hours machine running time). The frequency and time base should be clearly defined in the written programme(s) for each maintenance procedure to be carried out on each machine. Machine maintenance should be carried out on a planned preventative, not on an emergency curative, basis. In the manu-facture of pharmaceuticals the adage, useful perhaps on a domestic basis, 'if it ain't bust, don't fix it' is definitely not applicable.

Formal maintenance records, which can be readily related to the overall maintenance programme, should be compiled as each maintenance operation is performed. These records should be held on file, in order to ensure, and to make it possible to demonstrate, that all required maintenance operations are indeed carried out as and when required by the programme.

Hazards to be avoided

Matters generally to be considered in order to combat the deleterious effects mentioned above include, but are not necessarily limited to:

1.   Dirt (e.g. dust, grit and other abrasive particulate matter) can be a major cause of loss of machine efficiency and useful machine life, especially when mixed with moisture, oil or grease. Maintenance pro-grammes should ensure that machine surfaces are kept in an appro-priately clean condition. Build-up of dirt can be minimised by ensuring that surfaces (except of course those which require lubrication) are free of oil, grease and moisture.
2.   Wear between moving parts in contact is inevitable. The extent of wear and the rate at which it occurs can be minimised by the application, at a specified frequency, of the correct, defined lubricants. It should be noted that over-lubrication can be almost as damaging as insufficient lubrication. Moving parts should be inspected for wear at regular, defined, intervals. Failure to monitor wear can lead to machine failure, and possible serious damage.

3.   Regular inspections for corrosion should be made, looking for signs such as discoloration, chemical deposition, and flaking or 'bubbling' surface finishes. Inspection should not be limited to the machine itself, but should cover brackets, supports and ancillary equipment. If corrosion is discovered, immediate steps should be taken to treat it, to discover the cause(s) and to prevent recurrence.

4.   All machinery should have been constructed and installed so as to tolerate the strains to which it will be subjected when used for its intended purpose, over its expected operational lifespan. It should not, however, be assumed that faults will never occur through stress and/or fatigue. Regular inspections should be made to detect any signs of this (e.g. stress cracks) on all parts of the machine under any stress.

Other more specific points which need to be covered in the maintenance programme include (but are not necessarily limited to) checking and confirming the correct operation of (as relevant):

• Electric motors and pumps.
• Automatic valves and switches.
• Any other automatic systems.
• Steam traps in SIP systems.
• Thermocouples and resistance temperature detectors (RTDs).
• Alarm systems, both visible and audible.

The written maintenance programme should also cover any special maintenance specified or recommended by the manufacturer of any given piece of machinery.

Equipment and maintenance change records

Formal change control procedures and documentation should be in place that will ensure that no significant engineering changes or modifications to machines can take place without prior authorisation, nor without full assessment of any potential effects on product quality.

Unless maintenance programmes, maintenance records and change control procedures, are developed and implemented (to ensure that manufacturing equipment and attendant instruments and control devices remain in the same qualified and maintained state as they were during any validation studies conducted using that equipment) then any assurance hopefully derived from those validation studies could well be negated.

Ancillary equipment

Requirements for equipment design, specification, qualification, calibration and maintenance apply equally to equipment, installations or services which are ancillary, subsidiary, or provide support to, manufacturing equipment; that is, to things such as electrical power supplies, HVAC systems, steam generators (both clean and 'plant' steam, to ensure that the steam produced does indeed comply with the required specification), air compressors (to ensure, for example, the supply of appropriate quality, oil-free, compressed air), heat exchangers, chillers, water purification and supply systems, CIP and SIP systems, and to all measuring, indicating, controlling, together with monitoring and recording instrumentation associated with these various items of equipment, systems and services.

References

EC (1992). *The Rules Governing Medicinal Products in the European Community, Vol. IV: Good Manufacturing Practice for Medicinal Products.* Luxembourg: Commission of the European Communities. Available from The Office for Official Publications of the European Communities, Luxembourg. Also available from The Stationery Office (HMSO), London, and the EC Information Service, Washington, USA. (Referred to as the EC GMP Guide.)

US FDA (1990). *Code of Federal Regulations, Vol. 21, Ch. 1, Part 210,* Current good manufacturing practice in manufacturing, processing, packaging or holding of drugs, general; *CFR Vol. 21, Ch. 1, Part 211,* Current good manufacturing practice for finished pharmaceuticals; *CFR Vol. 21, Ch. 1, Part 820,* Good manufacturing practice for medical devices (revised 1995). Washington: US Food & Drug Administration. (Collectively referred to as the US CGMPs.)

Part Three

Personnel

11

Personnel management

The quality of a product ultimately depends on the quality of those producing it

Sir Dereck Dunlop (1971)

References to the 'four Ms' (men, materials, machinery and methods) or to the 'four P's' (personnel, premises, plant and procedures) as the essential elements in any quality-orientated industrial enterprise are commonplace, and such generalisations do at least serve to focus attention on basic requirements. There can be no doubt that of these elements, it is the people that are the most important in the assurance of quality. This is true of all levels within an organisation, from company president or managing director to the most junior employee. It may well be possible (if not altogether desirable) for high-quality, well-trained, dedicated personnel to compensate for some lack or deficiency in the other elements. Nothing, not even the finest premises, equipment, materials or procedures can compensate for the quality hazard represented by low standard, ill-trained or badly motivated staff. In a manner matched in only a few other industries (e.g. food), questions of personal hygiene also assume significantly more than a mere social acceptability significance.

Certainly, most GMP guidelines place early and emphatic emphasis on people, and their management, organisation and training. It is worth stressing that good staff, well trained, managed and motivated will work more effectively and more productively, that is, there are *quantity* as well as *quality* benefits.

Organisational structure

Many and varied statements have been made about the objectives, or purpose of any commercial business. The elements are, generally, that a business exists to deliver goods or services for which there is a demand (or for which a demand can be created), and thus to make a profit.

Although some of the products with which we are concerned may be manufactured without any specific aim or desire to yield a profit the vast majority (in terms of type, product or number of units) are manufactured in situations where profit is a prime motive. To some this represents an ethical dilemma, and they have seen the profit motive as inimical, as representing an opposing force, to the special dedication to quality required in the production of medicines. Others can see no reason for considering the making of a profit from the manufacture of pharmaceuticals as in any way different from profiting from the manufacture and provision of other basic human needs, such as food, shelter and clothing. Discussion of the ethics of capitalist society is somewhat outside the scope of this book, as indeed is the thought-provoking question of creating the demand mentioned above for, say, a medicinal product. Whatever one's stance on these politico-philosophical issues, it needs to be noted that even if ethical considerations do not provide a sufficiently powerful impetus, it would still be a foolhardy manufacturer who did not allocate sufficient resources to the prevention of the production of poor quality or defective products, since if he does not do so he will run a risk of damaging or killing (quite literally) his market, losing his profit, and ultimately (for one reason or another) going out of business altogether. Ethical imperatives are thus reinforced, rather than opposed, by practical and regulatory considerations, and as the UK Orange Guide (Sharp, 1983) states:

> ... assurance that products will be of a quality appropriate to their intended use ... requires the involvement and commitment of all concerned, at all stages

The EC GMP Guide (EC, 1992) somewhat clumsily apes this with '... requires the participation and commitment by staff in many different departments and at all levels within the company ...' This spirit of involvement, this commitment, must first reside at top management level and thence diffuse throughout the organisation as a whole.

The 'Qualified Person'

In establishing an organisational structure for the manufacture and quality assurance of medicinal and similar products, the most generally accepted view is that there should be two separate persons, each with overall responsibility for production OR for quality control, neither of whom is responsible to the other. This organisational concept is explicitly stated, or is implicit, in a number of 'official' GMP publications, including the US CGMPs. In some European countries the concept is traditionally overlaid or replaced by a statutory requirement that there shall be a single person designated as a 'Responsible Person', 'Qualified Person', 'Responsible Pharmacist' or some such similar title. A requirement that each manufacturer shall have available the services of at least one 'Qualified Person' (in a special, defined sense) has now become embodied in European Community, and thus UK, law.

The requirement for a manufacturer of medicinal products to have the services of at least one 'Qualified Person' was established in European law, in Directive 75/319/EEC. This will be covered a little more fully later in this chapter. For the present, it just needs to be noted that the term 'Qualified Person' has a specialised, defined, meaning: it does not simply mean a person who is qualified. A Qualified Person (QP) functions specifically in relation to the release of product to the market, and the matters which a QP needs to consider before releasing a batch of product have already been outlined in Chapter 4.

The production and quality control functions

The World Health Organisation, in its GMP guidelines, also indicates the need for the supervision of quality control by an appropriate expert, reporting directly to top management and independent of other departments.

Since the implementation of the UK Medicines Act (1968), pharmaceutical manufacturers in the UK have been required, when making application for a Manufacturer's Licence, to name separate persons (with their qualifications) as responsible, respectively, for production and for quality control. These persons, who should be managerially independent one from the other, are also named on the Manufacturer's Licence.

Reference to European Directive 91/356/EEC, will reveal (under 'Quality control') that:

> This department shall be placed under the authority of a person having the required qualifications [what those qualifications are and by whom they are required are not stated] and shall be independent of the other departments.

The independence of the production manager or department is not specifically stated in the directive, but is no doubt to be assumed. Certainly the point is made in the EC GMP Guide, which includes the following (under 'Key personnel'):

> 2.3 Key Personnel include the head of Production, the head of Quality Control, and if at least one of these persons is not responsible for the duties described in Article 22 of Directive 75/319/EEC, the Qualified Person(s) designated for the purpose. Normally key posts should be occupied by full-time personnel. The heads of Production and Quality Control must be independent from each other . . .

There is something distinctly odd about this statement. As the perceptive reader will have noticed, whilst the 'heads of Production and Quality Control must [note **must**] be independent from each other' it is implicit in the paragraph quoted that it is permissible for the Head of Production to be the Qualified Person responsible for certifying that a batch of product is of 'fit' quality, prior to its release for sale. That is, it would appear (in European terms) to be acceptable for a Production Manager to make the final quality decisions on his own products. This would seem to be both a contradiction and a paradox, and it is a problem to which it is not possible to offer an answer.

The PIC (see Chapter 3, Annex II) 'Basic Standards of GMP' (1987) (which are now harmonised with, i.e. virtually the same as, the EC GMP Guide) require both separate Production and QC Managers, *and* an authorised or responsible person to release product. This person may or may not be one or other of the two managers.

Defining roles and responsibilities

Despite the potential for confusion introduced by the EC 'Qualified Person' concept, the need (and the general acceptance of the need) for separately defined and managed responsibilities for production and for QC is widely established. Surprisingly, the USA appears to stand somewhat alone in not *explicitly* requiring, in its current good manufacturing practice regulations, a specific separation of QC and production management structures, although independent management of the production and quality control functions is standard US practice. The UK GMP Guide (Sharp, 1983) is emphatic regarding separation and independence in the management of QC and production.

Aside from any statutory requirements, the separation of quality control from production has on occasions been challenged by some quality experts on the grounds that it removes from production personnel the healthy sense of responsibility for product quality that they so very rightly should have. This is largely to miss the point, and to misunderstand the special nature of medicines manufacture and of good *pharmaceutical* manufacturing practice.

The more generally accepted view is that it is sound sense that the person ultimately responsible for quality control should be freed from the need to consider, or be influenced by, questions of *quantity* of production, meeting production schedules, sales estimates, etc., all of which are quite properly the province of a production manager. The quality control manager should thus be able to make decisions regarding quality standards and procedures, and to approve or reject materials and products entirely unbiased by such pressures. This is by no means to say that the production manager and his staff do not have a responsibility for implementing quality policies and procedures which, remember, 'requires the involvement and commitment of all concerned' and for quality assurance. Perhaps the misguided challenge to this view arises from differing conceptions of the precise meanings of the terms 'quality control' and 'quality assurance', which, as already discussed, have indeed been the subject of considerable confusion. If 'quality control' is defined as being concerned with sampling, specification and testing and with release/reject systems and decisions; and if 'quality assurance' means all activities and systems concerned with the attainment of the appropriate product quality, then this sort of objection to the managerial separation of production and quality control very largely disappears. That is, it does if it is understood that attainment of the required quality is everyone's responsibility, even though some specific quality responsibilities may be assigned more especially to the quality control manager, and others to the production manager.

While there is fairly general agreement about the way many of the differing responsibilities for quality control and production should be allocated, there are in practice some differences in detailed approach. In addition, there are certain functions which can be, and indeed are, seen as being joint responsibilities of both production and quality control. It is essential that these various responsibilities are defined and understood, and this point was well made in the UK Orange Guide:

> The way in which the various key responsibilities which can influence product quality are distributed may vary with different manufacturers. These responsibilities should be clearly defined and allocated.

The EC GMP Guide deals with the separate and joint responsibilities of production and QC managers as follows:

2.5   The head of the Production Department generally has the following responsibilities:

    i.   to ensure that products are produced and stored according to the appropriate documentation;

    ii.   to approve the instructions relating to production operations and to ensure their strict implementation;

    iii.   to ensure that the production records are evaluated and signed . . . before they are sent to the Quality Control Department;

    iv.   to check the maintenance of his department, premises and equipment;

    v.   to ensure the appropriate validations are done;

    vi.   to ensure that the required initial and continuing training of his department personnel is carried out.

2.6   The head of the Quality Control Department generally has the following responsibilities:

    i.   to approve or reject, as he sees fit, starting materials, packaging materials, and intermediate, bulk and finished products;

    ii.   to evaluate batch records;

    iii.   to ensure all necessary testing is carried out;

    iv.   to approve specifications, sampling instructions, test methods and other Quality Control procedures;

    v.   to approve and monitor the contract analysts;

    vii.   to ensure that the appropriate validations are done;

    viii.   to ensure that the required initial and continuing training of his department personnel is carried out . . .

(Other duties of the Quality Control Department are summarised in Chapter 6; that is, in the EC GMP Guide chapter on Quality Control.)

2.7   The heads of Production and Quality Control generally have some shared, or jointly exercised, responsibilities relating to quality. These may include . . .

    —   the authorisation of written procedures and other documents, including amendments;

    —   the monitoring and control of the manufacturing environment;

- — plant hygiene;
- — process validation;
- — training;
- — the approval and monitoring of suppliers of materials;
- — the approval and monitoring of contract manufacturers;
- — the designation and monitoring of storage conditions for materials and products;
- — the retention of records;
- — the monitoring of compliance with the requirements of Good Manufacturing Practice;
- — the inspection, investigation, and taking of samples, in order to monitor factors which may affect product quality.

The reader may have noticed in the above a degree of inconsistency in ascribing to the 'head of Quality Control' the responsibility for approving or rejecting (*inter alia*) finished products. As already noted, this is the responsibility of a/the Qualified Person, who may *or may not* be the Head of Quality Control.

The UK Orange Guide deals with the same general issues rather more succinctly:

> The person responsible for Quality Control should have the authority to establish, verify and implement all Quality Control Procedures. He should have the authority, independent of Production, to approve materials and products, and to reject as he sees fit starting materials, packaging materials and intermediate, bulk and finished products which do not comply with the relevant specification, or which were not manufactured in accordance with the approved methods and under the prescribed conditions. (His authority in relation to packaging materials may be limited to those which may influence product quality and identity.)
>
> The Production Manager, in addition to his responsibilities for production areas, equipment, operations and records; for the management of production personnel, and for the manufacture of products in accordance with the appropriate Master Formula and Method, will have other responsibilities bearing on quality which he should share, or exercise jointly, with the person responsible for Quality Control.
>
> These shared or joint responsibilities may include monitoring and control of the manufacturing environment; plant hygiene; process capability studies; training of personnel; approval of suppliers of materials and of contract acceptors; protection of products and materials against spoilage and deterioration; retention of records. It is important that both direct and shared responsibilities are understood by those concerned.

Job descriptions

The way in which the technical management of different manufacturing companies is structured can (and does) vary considerably on points of detail. It is essential that all concerned are fully aware of both their functional and reporting responsibilities, by means of organisation charts and written job descriptions, and that is a European legal requirement under Directive 91/356/EEC.

Although organisation charts are a requirement of European law, they make good business and quality sense in all types of manufacturing enterprise, anywhere in the world. Everyone should surely be clearly aware of who reports to them, and who is their manager – a simple and obvious truth that has escaped the notice of a number of companies in the past. The need for job descriptions, as well as being legally required for all managerial and supervisory staff is another equally simple and obvious truth. A job description should, state as minimum:

- To whom the person reports.
- The main purpose and objectives of the job.
- Tasks, and responsibilities expressed in resources (human and inanimate), technical and financial terms.

An illustrative example of a job description for a Production Manager is given in the Annex to this chapter. Note particularly that the description carries a reference number, date, and date for review. It also should be signed and dated by the job holder, and by their immediate superior. This is to ensure that there can be no doubt on any side as to just what are the boundaries and the responsibilities of the job.

The question arises of the level in the organisation down to which formal job descriptions should be prepared. Here the EC GMP Directive, 91/356/EEC, may be taken as giving sound advice as well as laying down the law. It requires that 'job descriptions should be available for all managerial and supervisory staff'. It could be argued that, at operator level, the applicable (say) batch manufacturing instructions plus the relevant standard operating procedures fill the place of job descriptions. Certainly, operators should be trained in the understanding and application of these instructions and procedures. It also makes sound quality sense to maintain records of this training, signed by the operator to confirm that they have received and understood the training given. As with job descriptions, this should not be seen as a policing exercise. The object is to ensure that there is no doubt, on any side, as to just precisely what the job is about, and to avoid the sort of situation observed by the author, a number of years ago at the major site of a large pharmaceutical manufacturer. In the dispensing area it was noted that scant concern was given to accuracy in the weighing of ingredients (usually an excess of the formula amount was provided). When questioned about this, one of the dispensers commented that it did not matter, because 'all the weights were checked again, before use, in the production area'. In the production areas it was conspicuously noticeable that there were no such second checks, because, it was said 'there is no need – all the materials have already been carefully weighed up in the dispensary'. This one small incident reveals a lack of training, a lack of communication, and a dismal failure of management.

To return to organisation charts (or 'organograms'): although the formal drawing-up of organisational structures is essential to the clear understanding of responsibilities and reporting relationships, it is important that it is also realised that in the pursuit of quality, such divisions are not to be regarded as watertight compartments. It would, for example be difficult to see how there could be true assurance of quality in an organisation where there was failure to communicate between the production manager and the QC manager. Perhaps the starkest example of the dire consequences of communication failure were the deaths of patients following the intravenous infusion of contaminated fluids at Devonport Hospital in 1972 (Clothier, 1972). (This was not the only problem. The whole wretched affair is a text-book of BAD manufacturing practice. For full details, see the report of the Clothier committee of enquiry into this incident.)

This need for cooperation between various functional units, however, goes wider and deeper. The setting up of the master formula and processing method for a new product (or an established product to be made by a modified method) must surely be a cooperative effort between Production, QC *and* Research and Development. There can also be a significant impact on quality by Engineering and perhaps not so obviously, Marketing. Some of these 'wider implications' we have already discussed (Chapter 6). For the moment let it just be stressed that the personnel, recruitment and training policies of a company are crucial to the attainment of quality.

The Expert and the Qualified Person

Amongst the many things introduced by various EC Directives are two virtually new professional titles, 'the Expert' and 'the Qualified Person'. Although their functions are entirely different, one from the other, it is convenient to consider them together and to draw a distinction which, in some minds, tends to be blurred.

The Expert

The concept of 'the Expert', and the requirement for 'Expert Reports', written by 'Experts' on defined parts of the data submitted in support of a application for a Marketing Authorisation, (as a sort of professional second opinion) was introduced into EC law by Directive 75/319/EEC.

There are three different sorts of Expert in this context – in medicine (or 'clinical aspects'), in 'pharmaco-toxicology' and what the text of the original directive refers to as an *Expert Analyst*. However, in later non-statutory guidelines, and as reflected in the way that this piece of European legislation has been implemented, the Expert Analyst has been transmuted, for reasons difficult to explain, into an 'Expert in Chemistry and Pharmacy'.

Applications for Marketing Authorisations from an EU member state need to be supported by an Expert Report on each of these aspects of the submission, each written by a person acceptable as an Expert in the relevant field.

It needs to be appreciated that a person who is an expert (small 'e') in a particular field is not necessarily an Expert (capital 'E') in EC terms. For example, in the area of chemistry and pharmacy (or strictly, chemical analysis), pharmacists are regarded *ex officio* as 'Experts', whereas the expert status of non-pharmacists is not accepted without justification, and in some member states not at all. Thus, in EC terms, a chemist is not necessarily considered to be an expert in chemistry.

To write an acceptable Expert Report on the pharmacological/toxicological aspects of an application, a formal qualification in toxicology and/or pharmacology, or other relevant discipline, and 'sufficient practical experience' are required. To be an Expert in clinical aspects 'a formal qualification in medicine, with relevant practical experience' is necessary.

The Qualified Person

The Expert Reports are specifically related to Marketing Authorisations. In relation to the ongoing processes of manufacture, another new European concept has emerged, that of the 'Qualified Person'.

Two important essentials which it is necessary to grasp are:

1. The Expert and the Qualified Person are not the same thing, although it **is** possible to be both.
2. A person who is qualified, even in a relevant discipline, is not necessarily a Qualified Person.

Furthermore, it needs to be noted that whereas the role of the Expert is in the area of applications for authorisation to market individual products (Marketing Authorisations; cf. UK Product Licences and the US NDAs), that is he/she is concerned with aspects of quality of design, the Qualified Person functions in the area of the ongoing processes of quality of manufacture.

Every EC company manufacturing pharmaceuticals, and/or importing pharmaceuticals from outside the Community must have at least one Qualified Person. The QP's functions are simple to describe.

In the case of manufacture, the QP is legally required to:

> Secure that each batch of product has been manufactured and checked in compliance with the law in the member state . . . and in accordance with the Marketing Authorisation [and he/she must certify to that effect] . . . in a register or equivalent document.

In this context, an appropriately signed batch manufacturing record (for example) is considered to be an 'equivalent document'.

What is the difference, it may well be asked, as compared with the release of product by a QC Manager, or QC Unit, independent of Production, as is the practice in the USA and UK, and which is a legal requirement under both the UK Medicines Act, and (as one reads them) the US CGMPs?

The concept derives from the traditional setup in some European countries, notably France and Belgium, where it was a legal requirement for a manufacturer to appoint a 'Responsible Pharmacist', who could be in charge of both Production *and* QC, or not necessarily a full-time employee at all. In the EC Directive, the Responsible Pharmacist was converted to the 'Qualified Person', and now in the UK there is this somewhat strange legalistic graft of a traditional Gallic approach on to the pre-existent requirement for separate QC and Production Managers.

A UK Manufacturers Licence has to name, as it always has since the implementation of the UK Medicines Act, a Production Manager and a QC Manager. But now, in addition, one or more Qualified Persons have also to be named, who may or may not be the same person(s) as the QC Manager or the Production Manager.

Under 'grandfather' transitional provisions (now virtually expired) it was relatively easy for anyone already in post to be accepted as a QP. Under the Permanent Provisions, the requirements in terms of education, professional/academic qualifications, knowledge and experience are somewhat more rigorous.

Requirements

The EC requirements (EC Directive 75/3129 of 1975) for a QP include:

FORMAL QUALIFICATION . . . after recognised course of Study . . . bearing at least upon

— Applied physics
— Microbiology
— Organic chemistry
— Pharmacology
— Inorganic chemistry
— Pharmaceutical technology
— Pharmaceutical chemistry
— Pharmacognosy
— General and applied biochemistry (medical)
— Physiology

The requirements in terms of *practical experience*, must be 2 years or 1 year or 6 months (depending on the nature of the 'formal qualification').

In the UK, the Health Ministers have delegated to the relevant professional bodies (The Royal Society of Chemistry, The Royal Pharmaceutical Society, and The Institute of Biology) the responsibility for maintaining and publishing registers (now, in fact, a single joint register) of those considered, in terms of all the criteria, acceptable as Qualified Persons. Whilst the MCA has the last say on the acceptability of an applicant to be named on a Licence, it is not normal for them to reject a person who is listed in the joint professional register.

Whilst in origin the concept may have been foreign to UK traditions, it has to be said that the overall effect is beneficial in helping to promote a high level of all-round expertise in the industry. In the UK it has all been taken very seriously The three professional bodies have produced a joint statement on knowledge and experience requirements. Colleges also run

3-year postgraduate courses for aspirant QPs. It is believed that the intention is that there should be a reciprocity of Qualified Person status across the EC, but that has yet to be tested, and it could be that some member states will not be inclined to accept that any person other than a pharmacist could be a Qualified Person.

One other function of the QP has still to be mentioned. In the case of the importation of pharmaceutical products, into the EC from a non-EC source, the QP must also ensure that each imported batch undergoes a complete re-analysis in the importing state, even if certificates of analysis of confirmed reliability are available, and he must certify in writing to that effect. (In some specific cases a waiver may be permitted.) No such requirement for re-analysis applies to export/import between EU member states.

As already noted, the three professional bodies have jointly issued a Code of Practice for Qualified Persons, as an appendix to their joint Register of Qualified Persons – Section 5 of which delineates the 'routine duties of a Qualified Person', particularly in relation to the matters to be considered before a batch of product is released for sale or supply (see Chapter 4). This statement of the routine duties of a QP will be noted with profit, not only by actual and aspiring QPs, but also by all who are interested and concerned about the factors which need to be considered in the determination of the quality (fitness) of medicinal and similar products. Its contrast with the 'all tests meet specification so it must be OK for release' philosophy which pervaded but a few decades ago is both salutary and marked.

Management and motivation

The manufacture of quality products cannot be expected from a mismanaged, poorly motivated workforce. Mismanagement may occur at all levels, from the top (e.g. Chairman, Chief Executive) to first-line supervision (charge-hand, foreman). Mismanagement from the top is wider-ranging, deeper-reaching and more insidious in its ill effects. First-line mismanagement may have more immediate, and more immediately noticeable, but usually more readily curable, effects. A not entirely inappropriate analogy may be drawn with a chronic, as compared with an acute, disease state.

Self-responsible, motivated, activity is more efficient than commanded activity. Other things being equal, well motivated staff will produce more goods, with a greater assurance of the quality of those goods, than will poorly motivated staff. Conversely, in the special context of medicines manufacture, poorly motivated staff can represent a hazard both to themselves, to the public, and to company profits.

Job satisfaction

Motivation and engendering of high morale in healthcare workers should be a relatively easy task. Indeed it is difficult to understand why in any pharmaceutical manufacturing operation there should be ill-motivated workers. Work of any type, far from being just a curse and a punishment to man for his sins can be itself a motivator. By and large people *want* to work. Work defines a person's status. It places them in society. It provides a major source of social interaction. A person is very much what they do. We all tend to ask of a new acquaintance 'What do you do?'

It has been argued by some management theoreticians that pay and conditions are the less important, even insignificant, motivational factors. It is, however, difficult to see how a feeling that one is being paid less than one's worth (or less than others who are doing comparable jobs), or how a sense that the working environment and facilities are of a standard lower than the job requires, could be other than *de*-motivating factors. In any event, while remuneration is a matter of company policy, legislation and basic GMP requirements should guarantee that generally, apart from a few 'dirty jobs', the working environment will be more congenial than many. Even 'dirty jobs' are acceptable when it is realised that the 'dirt' is an inevitable part of the job – coal miners do not usually complain about coal. It is when the working environment is seen to be more dirty or unpleasant than it need be, that it becomes demotivating. A source of low morale which needs to be noted, and which can arise in the most modern, clean, air-conditioned, window-less, immaculately finished, pharmaceutical factory, is the sense of isolation, segregation, and lack of contact with others and with the outside world, which can arise in such circumstances.

In addition to the basic need to work, and the social satisfactions gained from working (plus the *possibly* debatable contributions of rewards and conditions), the other main motivating factors may be summarised as *sense of purpose, sense of pride* and *sense of belonging*.

The stimulation of such senses in the worker should be particularly easy in the healthcare industry. Medicines serve a recognised, significant social purpose. Workers will easily understand this, and should readily take a pride in that purpose. From induction training onwards, they should be encouraged to see that they have a role to play, however marginal, in achiev-ing the socially useful purpose of supplying products to cure, alleviate or prevent illness. They should be made to feel that they belong to a team (top management to most junior shop-floor worker) the aim of which is to achieve that purpose. The most important word is 'communication', not just of facts but also of ideals, attitudes and objectives. Motivation and main-tenance of morale must be easier in the pharmaceutical industry than in most others. There is such a good peg to hang it all on.

Where morale and motivation are low, the blame must be laid squarely at the door of senior management. That said, the road to moti-vation and communication is *not* via 'quality' posters bearing slick slogans of the type 'Object '98 – Total Quality Attainment' or '1999 – Quality Commitment Year' or 'Our Objective – World Class Quality'. Such trite statements are rarely understood by the workers, achieve no purpose and can, and do, become objects of derision. More will be achieved in terms of motivation, and two-way communication, by a more 'visible' senior management prepared to take the trouble to walk around the factory, to see what is really going on and also *to be seen*. It is important however, to avoid giving the impression that such a walk-round is just a high-level policing exercise, and also for managers to be prepared to listen sympathetically, and to comment amiably.

Recruitment

Clearly, senior, supervisory or managerial staff in production and quality control must have the education, experience and professional or technical qualifications appropriate to the jobs they perform. In many countries this is mandatory, and not just a 'guideline' recommendation. A vital point which can be overlooked is that they should also have the *ability* to do the job. Specifically they should have the ability to *manage*. In assessing a prospective senior employee's admirable 'paper' qualifications and his proven technical ability, it is perhaps a little too easy to forget that a major part of his prospective role will be to *manage* – to lead, to direct and to motivate those people reporting to him. Top management should bear in mind that while the possession of outstanding technical ability and exemplary professional qualifications by no means excludes the ability to manage, neither does it guarantee that ability.

In all but the very smallest organisations, junior unqualified staff (production operators and maintenance men; cleaning, stores and service personnel) and their first line supervision, form the vast bulk of the workforce. It is these people and the way they are trained, directed and motivated that form perhaps the key element in the assurance of product quality. By far the largest proportion of reported defective medicinal products are the result of simple human error or human misunderstanding, and not of failure at a level of high technology. Advanced qualifications are not normally required at, for example, basic operator level. Nevertheless such personnel must, at minimum, have the education and intelligence to read and fully understand written instructions, and carry them out. They must also be able to respond effectively to the very special challenges of medicine manufacture, and to understand the nature and purpose of good manufacturing practice. They must also have innately good standards of personal hygiene. Management needs therefore to be in a position to exercise some degree of selectivity in the recruitment of such staff. It follows that it should tailor its policy regarding monetary and other rewards, conditions of employment, and prospects of advancement, accordingly. It should also aim at creating a working environment in which staff turnover is reduced to a minimum, since it is difficult, if not impossible to maintain a well-trained and motivated workforce where there is rapid staff turnover. The pharmaceutical/healthcare industry is not really a job for those who are 'just passing through' nor is it an industry where a policy of 'paying peanuts and getting monkeys' makes any sort of sense at all.

References

Clothier C M (1972). Report of the committee appointed to inquire into the circumstances, including the production, which led to the use of contaminated infusion fluids in the Devonport Section of Plymouth General Hospital, July 1972. London: HMSO.

EC (1992). *The Rules Governing Medicinal Products in the European Community, Vol. IV: Good Manufacturing Practice for Medicinal Products.* Luxembourg: Commission of the European Communities. Available from The Office for Official Publications of the European Communities, Luxembourg. Also available from The Stationery Office (HMSO), London, and the EC Information Service, Washington, USA. (Referred to as the EC GMP Guide.)

Sharp J, ed. (1983). *Guide to Good Pharmaceutical Manufacturing Practice,* 3rd edn. London: HMSO. (Referred to as the UK Orange Guide.)

Annex

Example of a job description

Form 11.1 may be used as a basis for job descriptions.

Ref. No. MMJD/123

Date prepared......
Review Date.........

JOB DESCRIPTION – PRODUCTION MANAGER
Milleniapharm Manufacturing Co. Ltd.
Megatown, Anycounty.

Reports to: Technical Director

Principal Objectives: To ensure that staff, equipment, services and all other relevant resources are available and capable of functioning in accordance with defined standards, in order that product can be supplied to the market, in the quantity, of the quality, and at the time required (in accordance with production plans and schedules), and at a cost consistent with overall budgetary requirements.

General responsibilities:
1. To assess, and ensure availability, of the human and equipment resources, necessary to fulfil production planned to meet forecasted sales.

2. To ensure, through optimum utilisation of those resources, that products are in fact manufactured in accordance with that plan, and are thus available to serve the forecasted sales.

3. To propose capital investments necessary, to comply with 1. and 2. above.

4. To ensure that all manufacturing operations are performed in accordance with Good Manufacturing Practice, including:
   a. Ensuring, in collaboration with the Training Manager, that all staff under his/her command are properly trained to perform their tasks and undertake their responsibilities.
   b. Ensuring, in collaboration with the Engineering and Maintenance Manager that all premises, plant and equipment in his/her area of responsibility are maintained in a serviceable condition, in accordance with planned maintenance schedules.

Specific responsibilities:

1. General Management:

a. To define, with the agreement of the Technical Director, the organisational structure and staffing of the Production group of departments.
b. To direct, control and motivate the six production departments under his command (Liquids, Creams and Ointments; Tablets Capsules and Powders; Sterile Products (I); Sterile Products (II), Aerosols, Packaging).

Form 11.1 continues over

c. To agree annual objectives of those who report directly to him/her, and to monitor the attainment of those objectives.

d. To delegate responsibilities to those reporting to him/her, as necessary and appropriate.

e. To ensure that information (on company policy and developments, regulatory matters, technological developments and the like) is disseminated, as appropriate, throughout his/her organisation.

f. To work with the Quality Control Department on the setting-up, revision and maintenance of Batch Manufacturing and Packaging Instructions, Standard Operating Procedures and other written production procedures. To ensure that current practices are in accordance with the written procedures, and also that the written procedures reflect current practice.

g. To assist management in defining staff policy and in keeping staff records.

h. To ensure the implementation of Health and Safety and other legal requirements.

i. To take part in staff recruitment, and oversee the career development of his/her staff.

2. Technical:

a. To keep abreast of all relevant technological developments, and advise on, and oversee, the implementation of these new technologies.

b. To remain aware of all relevant regulatory developments, and ensure implementation as appropriate.

c. To work closely with the Research and Development, Marketing and Regulatory Affairs Departments, in the scale-up and launch of new, or modified, products.

3. Financial

a. To produce annual budgetary estimates of expected departmental expenditure.

b. To ensure departmental costs remain within approved budget limits.

c. To monitor and control departmental cost-effectiveness.

Functional interrelationships

According to circumstances, close cooperative liaison with Quality Control, Training, Engineering/Maintenance, R&D and Regulatory Affairs Departments will be necessary.

Signed..............................   Signed.............................
   (Production Manager)   (Technical Director)
     Date...................   Date...................

12

Training

People who have been trained by example that high production is more important than extreme care are going to make mistakes
Edmond Fry, former senior official, US FDA (c. 1985)

It is virtually an article of faith that sound training of staff, at all levels, is of pre-eminent importance in the assurance and maintenance of quality. Official guidelines and regulations respectively recommend and require it. Regulatory inspectors aim to enforce the requirement. Yet it is sadly true that training, even in some of the most distinguished and richly endowed manufacturers, is often something that is indifferently, even poorly, done, and regarded as an irritant to which only occasional, makeshift, resource needs to be allocated. The purpose of this chapter is to suggest ways in which training can be approached with the seriousness of purpose that it needs and deserves.

The need for training in QA and GMP

The necessity for training arises whenever there is any deficiency in the knowledge, understanding, attitudes and specific skills possessed by a person as compared with the knowledge, understanding, attitudes and specific skills required for the successful performance of any task assigned to that person. The new recruit, or a person newly transferred to a department, is almost certain to display a deficiency in one or more of these areas, and is thus a prime candidate for training.

This need for training can, and does, emerge at all levels in an organisation from senior management to most junior employee. The balance of skills training in relation to general/orientation training will vary between different jobs and different levels, both as to nature and extent. A new employee may have already acquired the basic skills required, from previous employment, but still needs to learn how to exercise those skills in the new working environment, and to demonstrate this to any new employers. The person will still need to be made familiar with that new environment, and with company background, traditions, attitudes and policies. Crucially a new employee will need training in GMP, or require any previous GMP training reinforced. In no other industry can the need for sound training be more obviously apparent, yet it is sadly true that, across the industry as a whole, there has been a wide spectrum of personnel policies and training approaches, from well organised, efficient enthusiasm to lip-serving, indifferent inadequacy.

The concept of sound training implies a formal, systematic approach. Merely 'sitting with Nellie' on grounds that this constitutes 'on-the-job training' is just not good enough. Nor does viewing a video or tape/slide show (and there are precious few good examples of these) constitute anything approaching adequate training. There is no objection to the use of videos, tape/slides etc. *per se*. But to use such things in isolation, and not just for illustrative and reinforcement purposes within the context of a well-planned interactive training presentation, is to make no more than a feeble pretence at training. No better are the 'training' sessions, where the 'instructor' merely stands up, and reads in inexpressive parrot-fashion style from someone else's prepared text. Indeed, this sort of thing is probably worse than no training at all. The trainees are not fooled (never underestimate the intelligence of the ordinary operator), and the whole exercise becomes the object of demotivating derision.

Who needs training?

In general terms, training needs to be directed at three categories of employee:

1.   Employees new to the company or division.
2.   Existing employees – when the nature or content of their job changes.
3.   Existing employees whose performance at a particular task declines below required standards.

Basic training should also be reinforced from time to time by ongoing training programmes designed to ensure that employee performance, skills, knowledge and attitudes remain up to standard. That is, the aim should be to ensure that point 3 above does not arise. As in so many other things, prevention is better than cure.

Costs and benefits of training

Training of manufacturing staff takes up time and costs money. It is not outrageous, and is indeed relatively conservative to suggest, that somewhere between 2% and 5% of overall available man-hours need to be absorbed by training. The precise amount of time will depend upon the size and complexity of the manufacturing operation and upon (a) how far behind a company is in meeting its training obligations, and (b) the extent to which a company is recruiting new staff and/or expanding into new products/technologies. A company manufacturing and packaging, say, just one simple liquid product will need to spend a relatively small percentage of its time on training. In the context of more complex manufacture, in a company with a long-standing, well-established, sound and effective training programme, with a relatively stable workforce, and which is not significantly expanding into new manufacturing areas, the time needed for training will be at the lower end of the scale. On the other hand, in a company which has historically allocated inadequate resource to training, which has an unstable workforce, but which is also expanding its range of activities, the time required for training will be at the upper end of the range. As training programmes bed down, and become increasingly effective, the overall time required will reduce.

It needs to be clearly understood that training is costly. In addition to the cost of providing the training resource (trainers, in-house or consultants, training facilities and equipment, documentation) there is the unproductive time spent by the trainees. There are, however, benefits. Although these may be difficult to quantify, as has been observed, good staff, well trained and motivated, will work more effectively and productively. They will make fewer of the sort of mistakes which result in rejects, scrap and rework, and consequent production delays. The majority of product recalls are the result of 'human error'. Reduce the potential for error by good training, and the possibility of encountering a recall situation correspondingly diminishes. Any company which has experienced the overall expense of a full-scale recall, with the consequent loss of consumer confidence, and the possibility of regulatory action will acknowledge that the benefits of training outweigh its cost.

In any event, it is a statutory requirement in the European Union, and failure to comply will give a manufacturer further grief. The European Directives on GMP (91/356/EEC and 91/412/EEC) state (Chapter II, Article 70):

> 4.   Personnel shall receive initial and continuing training including the theory and application of the concept of quality assurance and good manufacturing practice.

The US CGMPs (US FDA, 1990) require that:

> 211.25 (a)   Each person engaged in the manufacture, processing, packing, holding of a drug product shall have education, training and experience . . . to enable that person to perform the assigned functions. . . . Training shall be in the particular operations that the employee performs and in current good manufacturing practice.

Here, therefore, is another example of regulatory requirements reinforcing something which is, inherently, a 'good thing'.

The major training elements

The fields in which training needs to be given may be considered as forming three basic training elements:

1. Introductory, background ('induction' or 'orientation') training for new employees.
2. GMP training, including training in hygienic practices.
3. Specific skills training.

None of these elements should be neglected.

Background training

All new employees in any job, in any industry, need to acquire a certain basic knowledge of the company in which they will work; its pay, personnel and promotion policies; its physical layout (they need to find their way about); its supervisory and management structure, and so on. In the pharmaceutical industry it is also important that employees are aware of the ethical, social and legal significance of the company's activities. The task of impressing upon employees the importance of the end product, and of the *quality* of the end product, should be relatively easy, since 'treatment by medicine' is a great 'human interest' subject – if the popularity of television doctor/hospital/nurse drama series is anything to go by. Every opportunity should be taken to stress that the company is making medicines for patients. Not only is it a powerful factor in employee motivation, it is indisputable that people learn quicker and better, and function more effectively, when they can relate what they are learning and what they are doing to a wider context. The employee in the pharmaceutical industry needs to be able to relate his job not only the work of the factory as a whole, but also to the social – *the human* – significance of what his company is doing. This is not just high-minded ethics. It is also, like so much of QA/GMP, good hard-headed business sense.

GMP training

GMP training is necessary for all production and quality control workers, and also for any other personnel whose duties take them into production or control areas, or in any way bear upon the nature and quality of a company's products.

To provide a context, to stimulate interest, and to supply motivation, this training should be related to the general background of the history and use of medicines and their role in society, briefly and simply explained.

The following is a brief checklist of topics which should be considered:

○ Brief history of medicine: the 'therapeutic revolution'.

○ Background of the healthcare industry and the company's place in it.

○ Benefits/risks of modern medicines.

○ Cost of medicines: R&D.

○ The need for GMP.

○ Quality assurance and quality control.

○   Pharmaceutical dosage-forms and packs.

○   Company product lines.

○   Problems of faulty batches and recall.

○   The need/reasons for documentation, records and written procedures.

○   The company's documentation system – and the importance of abiding by it.

○   Cleanliness, hygiene and simple microbiology.

○   Personal hygiene.

○   Plant and equipment cleaning methods and schedules.

○   Nature and problems of micro-organisms.

○   Microbial and cross-contamination.

○   Clothing.

○   Effects of legislation/regulation/inspection.

○   The overall company manufacturing and control cycle.

(See Annex I to this chapter for more details.)

The emphasis placed on different topics may need to vary in different organisations. Always the main motivating thrust should be that the reason for being 'GMP minded' is for the sake of the sick patient who needs the products. A secondary motive can be that if the company produces significantly defective goods it will rapidly cease to be able to pay employees. Whilst staff must obviously have an understanding of relevant statutory and regulatory matters, and of the need to abide by the law, an approach based solely on 'We have a quality system, and we follow GMP, and we do it this way because the man from the Health Department says so, and if we do not we will be in trouble', is likely to have a much lower motivating force.

Skills training

A wide range of skills, and of types of skills, is required. Some jobs are simple, routine and repetitive. Others may require a considerable level of expertise, concentration and judgement. It is neither possible nor appropriate to dwell here in detail on training in all possible specific skills. Suffice it to say that skills (e.g. operating a machine, servicing equipment) cannot be satisfactorily acquired in the classroom. This is pre-eminently a case for showing, for demonstrating, and for hands-on practice.

The learning process

It may be useful to discuss briefly both the learning process, and the main points to be considered by anyone (i.e. a trainer or instructor attempting to

impart knowledge, or aid the acquisition of skills) aiming effectively to acti-
vate that process.

In any consideration of approaches to training, there are two essential
factors which need constantly to be borne in mind.

These are that people learn quicker, more thoroughly, and are better
able to use the knowledge or skill acquired if:

* The specific skill or knowledge is placed in a wider or more general
  context, so the trainee is aware of 'how it all fits', and is not expected
  to acquire information as isolated, disconnected scraps.
* The reason WHY something is done, or required, is explained (and
  understood), as well as what is to be done and how to do it.

Reception

The first stage in any learning process is the *reception* of new information.
This information is initially received via the senses, and thence transmitted to
the brain. All senses can or may be involved: sight, hearing, touch, smell, taste,
plus that muscular sense of movement and balance, which has sometimes
been considered to be a sixth sense and given the somewhat clumsy title of
'kinaesthesis'. Of these various senses, it is generally accepted that sight provides the strongest stimulus to the learning process. It is also true that the
simultaneous stimulation of more than one sense has a powerful reinforcing
action. Thus, trainees will learn quicker, better and more retentively if they
are not merely *told*, but also *shown*, and, in practical skills training, allowed
to touch and try out ('get the feel') for themselves. Even in more theoretical,
non-skills, training, the learning process is facilitated if a verbal presentation
is reinforced by pictures, slides, diagrams, charts, and concrete examples.

The stimulation of the senses of smell and taste generally have a more
limited application in the industrial training process, although they can
assume considerable importance in the food and perfumery businesses. On
the whole, however, the use of the sense of taste in the manufacture of pharmaceuticals is probably something to be discouraged.

Perception

A distinction may be drawn between the mere *reception* of sensory stimuli,
and their useful and effective *perception* in the brain. There can be few people
who have not sat musing, or dozing, with half an eye on the television screen.
In such circumstances, clearly some stimulus is being applied to both eye and
ear, albeit that the level of organised *perception* by the higher sensory centres
may indeed be very low. A number of factors, such as fatigue, can affect levels
of perception (and, indeed, reception). Trainees who are so fatigued that they
fall asleep are unlikely to receive any relevant sensory stimuli, and thus will
fall at the first hurdle. Perception affecting factors include:

* Inherent interest (or otherwise) of the subject, and/or its manner of
  presentation.

- Health/fatigue of trainees.
- General physical condition of trainees (hunger and over-repletion both inhibiting the learning process, as does the need to attend to other natural functions).
- Environmental conditions in the training room – heating, lighting and ventilation.
- Presence or absence of distractions.
- Trainee familiarity, or perhaps over-familiarity, with the subject.
- Motivation and the will, or desire, to learn.

Cognitive learning leading to validation

We cannot learn without sensory stimuli, but the mere reception and perception of such stimuli does not constitute learning. The brain must be able to organise, evaluate and make judgements on the perceived sense-data, relate them to other relevant, previously learned information and 'file them away' in memory for later retrieval. This has been termed the *cognitive* or *assimilation* phase of learning.

The final, clinching, phase in the learning process has been termed the *effector* phase, although perhaps in our present context the smarter (not to say 'cooler') term might be the *validation* phase. This is where trainees, either verbally (by the spoken or written word), by practical demonstration or both, reveal or attempt to put into practice what they have learned. This phase serves both to monitor progress and most powerfully to reinforce the overall learning process. This overall four-phase process is shown diagrammatically in Figure 12.1.

It could be argued, with some justice, that this classification into four phases is an artificial division of what is an essentially continuous process. But most human divisions and classifications of data are artificial. We find it easier to understand and learn when information is presented in discrete but related packets. Hence classification, as in the physical, chemical and natural sciences. This applies to learning about learning. Hence classification.

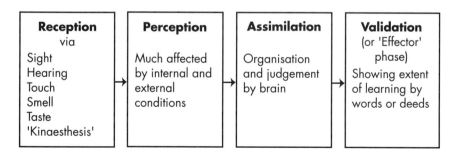

Figure 12.1   The phases of learning.

Further factors influencing the overall learning process

In addition to the factors already mentioned, which bear particularly on the reception/perception phases of learning, others which influence the learning process include:

1. *Length and frequency of training sessions.* Although it varies from person to person, there is a limit to the amount of new information with which the brain can cope (that is, receive, perceive, assimilate and use) at any one time. Just as muscles need time for recovery following physical effort, so brains need time to recover after hard learning effort. Shorter, periodic learning sessions are better than occasional long ones.

2. *Planned, structured training.* Training which proceeds in accordance with a preconceived, well thought-out and structured training programme is more effective than unplanned, casual *ad hoc* training. This does not mean that a training plan should be so inflexible as to allow no scope for adjustments to meet individual needs, different persons' ability to absorb knowledge, or to concentrate over different periods of time.

3. *Sequence.* Information which is presented in a logical sequence is far more readily and effectively absorbed than information which is random. This applies both to the sequence within a given learning session, and also to the logical sequence from one session to another.

4. *Feedback.* People learn better if they are made aware how well (or how badly) they are doing. This is, of course, a two-way benefit. The instructor needs to be in touch with how well his or her message is getting across, in order that suitable adjustments in content, style and presentation can be made. For a trainee to know that they are progressing satisfactorily is both motivating and reinforcing. The revelation of if and where they are going wrong will enable further assistance to be given, and suitable corrections to be made. Over-emphasis, at too great a frequency should, however, not be placed on failure. This will only serve to demotivate trainees.

5. *Vividness of original reception/perception.* Mere exposition in a dull and lifeless manner inhibits learning and fails to impress the memory. Interesting learning sessions, presented by instructors who are able to project enthusiasm and some degree of 'character', and who can both communicate and also encourage active trainee involvement (as distinct from just sitting and listening), all backed-up by memorable visual images and/or direct hands-on contact with any relevant hardware, stimulate learning and fix things in the memory.

6. *Repetition.* That repetition is a major factor in the learning process is well known and acknowledged – practise makes perfect. It needs also to be noted that over-repetition is counter-productive, and that it is just as easy to learn bad habits by repetition as it is good habits. One should not practise one's mistakes.

7. *Frame of reference.* Learning is faster and more effective, and retention is better, if the learner can relate new knowledge or skill to that already

possessed. People do not all learn with the same facility, or at the same rate. There is considerable variation in the ability of different people to absorb and retain new information, although skills once acquired tend to be retained more readily than factual information. (Does anyone ever completely forget how to swim, or ride a bicycle?)

Training – approach and technique

The above excursion into the learning process has been taken in order to provide a basis for a discussion of the way training should be organised, approached and presented.

As a preliminary, we may isolate some key factors which influence the effectiveness of training:

1.   Training should not be haphazard, 'as and when'. It should be conducted in accordance with a planned structured programme, with records maintained of the training given, and assessments made of trainee progress. Training records should be kept in two forms:

    (a)   A record of the training received by each individual employee.
    (b)   A tabular record, where the names of employees are listed and the training modules are ticked off as they are received (see Forms 12.1 and 12.2).

2.   Training is not a 'one-off' business. All training should be reassessed from time to time, and augmented and reinforced as necessary.
3.   Understanding and retention of information are greatly assisted by:

    (a)   An understanding of *context* – of 'how it all fits in'.
    (b)   An understanding of the Why's as well as the What's and How's.

4.   Training presentations should be made as interesting and as attractive as possible, with the engagement of as many of the trainees' senses (particularly sight) as possible. In other words, do not just talk, *show*.

Thinking through a training session

When contemplating/giving a specific training session, or a series of inter-linked sessions, trainers need to pay attention, before the event, to:

• Defining in their own mind what the *objective(s)* of the training is/are.
• The *preparation* for the training.

During the training session itself, although probably guided by preparations made in advance, trainers will need to consider:

• How they are *transmitting* the prepared material, in order to best achieve the desired objective(s).

MEGAPHARM Co.

Personal Training Record

Name ....   Date joined company ....

Job Title:

1. ....

2. ....

3. ....

Training Received (Module ref. and Title)	**Date**

Name	GI/1	GI/2	GMP/1	GMP/2	GMP/3	GMP/4	GMP/5	GMP/6	STT/1	STT/2	STT/3	STT/4	STT/5	STT/6	STT/7

- How the transmitted information is being *received/perceived* and *assimilated* by the trainees.

A more detailed consideration of some of these basic training elements from the trainer's point of view is given below.

Objective(s)

Before attempting to train, the trainer must have an absolutely clear understanding of the objective(s) of the training which is to be given. This applies whether the session is of the more formal training-room type, or is less formal 'on-the-job'. That is, the training should proceed in accordance with a preconceived, carefully considered training programme. It should be intended and designed to impart a definite amount of specified knowledge, understanding or skill, with both trainer and trainee having a clear appreciation of how the specific session relates to the latter's overall training needs. This does not mean that a training schedule should be a rigid, inflexible, dehumanised affair. But it also means that merely leaving it to Nellie (or Fred) to 'show the new girl (or chap) around to give them an idea of what to do' is just not good enough.

Careful mental framing of objectives will provide a salutary concentration of the trainer's mind on the job in hand, and provide a measure for the later determination of how well those objectives have been achieved.

Preparation

Sound preparation is obviously essential. The trainer's own training, knowledge and skills (both job-skills and skill as a trainer) form the bedrock of the preparation. In addition a trainer should take the trouble to prepare properly for each session. The effort required for this preparation will vary widely according to circumstances. It could be extensive where, for example the trainer is starting from scratch, on the basis only of his own store of knowledge of the subject. Then it will be necessary to collect thoughts, organise and concentrate knowledge, plan a logical sequence for the presentation, prepare speaking notes (or at least jot down headings to maintain the proposed presentation properly sequenced and on track), prepare or obtain visual aids, and so on.

On the other hand, where the basic preparation of a training module has already been done (either by the trainer or by someone else) and the trainer is well used to giving the particular presentation, the effort required in preparation may well be considerably less. It may involve little more than a consideration of the numbers and abilities of the trainees, with an appropriate mental adjustment in accordance with that consideration, and a check that all necessary materials, training aids, demonstration equipment and suchlike will be available at the right time and in the right place.

At the very least, any person about to impart any knowledge, or teach any skill, should keep very firmly in mind that although this may be the fiftieth time for them, it may well be the first time for the trainees. Every attempt should be made to keep the approach fresh, and the way to do that is *not* merely to stand up and read a previously prepared text. Even if such a text is available, it should serve only as a basis for the trainer's own presentation, in his/her own individual style. Just to read out someone else's text is to court disaster. Trainees are rarely fooled, and may treat the whole exercise with cynical contempt. However experienced the trainer is in relation to the topic in hand, it makes good sense to review notes, consider sequence, to think if an updating of information is required and to consider if there are any topical examples (good or bad) which might usefully be cited. With practice, a trainer will become more and more able to function without constant reference to notes. Broad general headings, however, should keep things in sequence, and help to ensure that what should be dealt with is, indeed, covered. One of the spin-off benefits of slides, or overhead transparencies, is that they also serve as sequence-headings for the trainer. Provided, that is, that the trainer carefully checks in advance that they are all in the correct order. Many a potentially good presentation has been ruined by slides or overheads which have got out of order either during, or since, they were last used. The effect on the hapless trainer's composure can be dire.

Training-room facilities

Having considered the trainer's mental preparation, the mention of slides and overheads leads naturally to a consideration of the hardware preparation. Here is a checklist of possible requirements in the training room:

○ Room available at time required?

○ Adequate capacity?

○ Sufficient seating (if required)?

○ Tables, or other surfaces, available (if trainees will be required to write, take notes, answer question papers, consult documents)?

○ Writing implements available, or trainees told to bring them?

○ Overhead projector available? Does it work? Spare bulb?

○ Transparencies prepared? Undamaged? In correct order?

○ 35 mm projector available? Does it work? Spare bulb?

○ Remote control? Trainer familiar with remote control? If no remote control, who will operate projector?

○ Chalkboard or flip chart?

○ Chalks or felt pens?

○ Videos?

○ Video player and screen? Do they work? Trainer knows how to start (and stop)?

○ Demonstration material (equipment, samples, documents, etc.) – available as and when needed?

Careful pre-planning to ensure that all these aspects have been considered in advance can be crucial to the success, or otherwise, of training. Non-avail-ability, or failure to function, of these physical components of training can lead to distracting pauses in a training session, and perhaps worse can so discompose a trainer as to turn a professional presentation into a display of apparent bumbling amateurism. A little time spent in attention to these things in advance will be amply repaid.

Transmission

The way the training message is received depends to a significant extent on the personal qualities of the trainer, for example:

- *The trainer's knowledge.* The trainer's own knowledge of the subject and/or ability in the skill concerned are self-evidently significant factors. A trainer who does not know a subject is clearly in no posi-tion to teach others about it. Most important is the recognition by the trainees that the trainer speaks or demonstrates with authority. Respect for that authority will stimulate attention, and hence learning. If that respect is not granted, attention will wander.
- *Appearance.* A bespoke three-piece suit, or upper-set garden party ensemble, is not necessarily required for an instructor in good prac-tices in the manufacture of say tablets, but a scruffy overall and an unkempt appearance should be avoided. A smart, well-groomed appearance inspires confidence and helps to command attention.
- *Voice, manner and approach.* It is difficult to train successfully if the voice is dull, monotonous or very quiet. Such things *may* be improved by practise, but very quietly spoken persons can, realistically, only be expected to train groups of no more than two or three people, if they are able to do it at all. A trainer's manner should be outgoing, firm but friendly, aimed at establishing contact, and putting trainees at their ease. Trainers should, however, be themselves and not attempt to act a part. There is nothing wrong with laughter. Indeed a little humour can be a positive aid to learning. It can ease any tension and make the learning memorable. It should not, however, be overdone.

Encouraging feedback and discouraging resentment

Feedback from the trainees should be encouraged and obtained:

- Can they see/hear properly?
- Are they comfortable, not too hot or too cold?
- Do they understand?
- Have they any questions?

Every effort should be made to turn a one-way lecture into a live (and lively) two-way event.

On no account should a slow learner be ridiculed, even lightly. It does that person, or the trainer no good, and it can provoke resentment in the other trainees. Difficulties should be treated sympathetically and sarcasm avoided.

Securing the best attention

In addition to the personal qualities and approach of the trainer, other factors which affect the transmission (and the reception/perception) of information include:

- *The training environment.* The questions which need to be asked are: Is it neither too hot, nor too cold? Is it well ventilated? Can all the trainees see and hear? Far too many training sessions are ruined by a dark, hot and stuffy training environment, where the general tendency is to doze. The keen trainer will check on the comfort of the trainees, and on whether or not they can see and hear properly as the session proceeds. A little advance attention to these factors will pay dividends.

- *Presence or absence of distractions.* Random sights and noises can distract the attention of trainees. Given the choice, there are usually many other things that a trainee would rather be hearing, seeing, doing or handling. Efforts should be made by the trainer to ensure, as far as possible, concentration on the matter in hand. What can be done will be, to an extent, dictated by the place available for training. Some things can only be taught and practised on the factory floor, where inevitably there will be distractions. Yet in even a well-appointed, dedicated, training room there may well be distractions. It is a strange but nevertheless very real aspect of human behaviour that what is going on outside the window, or materials left over from, or intended for, other training sessions (e.g. diagrams, charts, writing on flip-charts/blackboards, etc.) always seem more interesting than the matter under discussion. Such distractions should be removed, as far and as quickly as possible – and that includes pictures, diagrams, writing on flip-charts and so on that the trainer has used earlier in a session. Anything that is no longer immediately relevant should be removed or erased. It is a false economy to attempt to cram as much as possible on one sheet of a flip chart. Use one side to explain one point, and turn over. External distractions, such as persons passing by windows, may be more difficult to control. Use of some form of blind may be helpful.

- *Quality and impact of visual aids.* As already discussed, visual images both reinforce and facilitate the reception and assimilation phases of learning. This statement should perhaps be modified by saying that *relevant* visual images, properly used, can have this effect. No doubt stimulated by the oft-repeated, and generally accepted, advice to illustrate and emphasise by the use of slides and the like, some trainers tend to over-do the visual aids, to an extent that training sessions become more like picture shows. Visual images could be regarded as rather like the jam on the bread. They certainly help the bread to go down, and assist in its assimilation, but a trainer should not offer all jam, and too little of the sold bread of training.

Visual aids

The visual aid materials in common use have their advantages and pitfalls.

The blackboard (or whiteboard) and chalk (or erasable pen)

Points to be aware of:

- Yellow chalk usually shows up better on black than white.
- Write, or draw in sufficient size to be clearly visible to all.
- Right-handed trainers should have the board on their left (as they face their audience). This way they will obscure less of the board as they write or draw.
- The temptation to talk to a board or screen, rather than the audience, needs to be fiercely resisted.
- The board should be cleared as soon as the trainer has finished with what is on it. To leave old material can distract trainees from the new topic to which the trainer has turned.

Flip charts (or other pads of large white paper sheets)

Points to consider:

- A common fault is too small a drawing or writing. It must all be bold and simple.
- As above, material which is finished with should be removed from view.
- Trainers should ensure, in advance, that sufficient felt pens (which are not exhausted or dried out) are available.
- Again, the temptation to talk to the chart, rather than the audience, needs to be fiercely resisted.

35 mm slides and overhead transparencies (OHTs)

These have become perhaps the most commonly used form of visual aid. Opinions differ as to which of the two forms is to be preferred. One can only say that the great advantage of the use of an overhead projector and 'transparencies' or 'acetates' is that it gives the speaker greater and more immediate control of things. Given that the trainer has taken the trouble, in advance, to assemble the OHTs in the right order, with a sheet of white paper between each, then little should go wrong.

If a 35 mm projector, without a remote control, is used the trainer has to rely on a projectionist to show the right slide at the right time. Even with a remote control, operated by the speaker, there is always the problem of mechanical (or electrical) failure of the projector, or jamming of slides.

A remote control, hand-held by the speaker, although it eliminates divided control, does not diminish the potential for such problems. And it adds the problem, which all too frequently surfaces, of the trainer in full flight, pressing the 'backwards' instead of the 'forwards' button, and then panicking and taking some embarrassing time to get back on track. Reversed, or inverted 35 mm slides are more difficult to correct (and can result in spilled slides) than overheads. It is also much more difficult to refer back to previously displayed images with 35 mm slides.

There are a number of failings common to the use of both 35 mm slides and overheads:

- Projected words, rather than pictures or diagrams, are of debatable value.
- Words that cannot be read, or images that cannot be clearly seen and interpreted are a positive, distracting menace. (The all too commonly heard 'I don't know if you can all read/see this' should be taken as an abject admission of failure. If it cannot be clearly seen and interpreted, then it should not be shown.)
- The ever-increasing availability of computer graphics and clip-art packages has led to the blossoming of irrelevant images on slides and overheads. Some trainers, and other presenters, seem to be obsessed with the thought that any image is better than no image at all. They are very wrong. No matter how charming, arresting or amusing the image, if it is not relevant, then it is a distraction.
- All too often slides and overheads are too wordy, too complex, or too crowded. All these faults should be avoided, and things made simple, bold, relevant and direct.
- Once a slide or overhead has made its point it should be removed, or it will become a distraction. Again this is probably easier with over-heads. If a break is intended in the showing of a series of 35 mm slides, then a blank should be inserted and/or the projector switched off.
- Another commonly encountered failing is where a speaker displays a relatively complex and detailed slide, and says words to the effect '. . . this is all clearly illustrated by this slide' and then goes on, without explanation, to talk about something entirely different. The slide will neither teach nor illuminate, nor will the trainees be giving full attention to the new topic.

The technique of pointing, and the use of pointers, needs to be considered:

- When pointing at a board (or a screen, or a flip-chart) the trainer should point with the hand which is on the same side as the board, so as to remain facing the audience.
- If a pointer is used, it should not be allowed to wander around the

board (or screen). It should be pointed directly at the item to be stressed, held motionless for a sufficient time for the point to sink in, and then taken away. Laser pointers are a particular problem for all but the steadiest of hands. For those with the slightest inclination to wobble, some additional support should be found. A little red spot, dashing about, can be very distracting.

- A pointer should be used only as a pointer, not as a walking stick, a swagger stick, a conductor's baton, or as a device to tap out interesting rhythms on the floor or table.

Handout material

Longer-term retention of information will be greatly assisted if trainees are encouraged to make a few notes and/or are handed out some form of printed material, written and presented in a readily absorbable and attractive fashion, to take away and read at leisure. This can take the form of material prepared in-house.

Trainers' checklist

To conclude this review of training, the following is a summary/checklist for actual and potential trainers.

○ Know your subject. It is usually necessary to know rather more than the bare bones of the topic to be presented, in order to be able to deal with questions. A trainer lacking in knowledge of his subject will not be able to fool all his audiences all of the time.

○ Be absolutely clear about what your objectives are.

○ Try to approach each session as something new, no matter how many times you have spoken on the subject.

○ Check the availability of the training room, and on the heating, lighting, ventilation and sound/noise level.

○ Make sure that all required equipment, materials, handouts, slides etc. are readily to hand. Check that the equipment works. (Spare bulb for projector? Felt pens? Chalks?)

○ Look smart and sound bright.

○ Speak up, and check up on how your message is being received.

○ Avoid/eliminate distractions.

○ Establish contact with the audience. Be friendly, but do not let the session become just a genial chat.

○ Use humour (if it works for you) but be careful not to over-do it, or cause embarrassment.

○ Encourage trainee participation (questions, discussions, workshops). Training should be a two-way, not just a one-way exercise.

○ Have sympathy for those in difficulties. *Never* ridicule.

○ Present the subject in a logical, pre-planned sequence.

○ Place the subject in its wider context.

○ Explain the Why's as well as the What's and How's.

○ Avoid distracting mannerisms (tapping, shuffling and the like).

○ Engage as many senses as possible – especially sight, but remember to remove slides, drawings, etc. as soon as they have made their point.

○ Don't carry on for too long. Several short sessions, with breaks for mental recovery, are better than one long one.

○ Look at your audience (not at screens, boards or notes), but do not stare at anyone in particular.

○ Hammer home important points by repetition and summary, but do not bore by overdoing it.

○ Do not 'act'. Be yourself, but your best self.

Selection and training of trainers

The easy options are to employ consultants to present on-site training courses or to send trainees to external courses/seminars/symposia. The former tend to be expensive; the latter very expensive. They both can be of variable quality and utility. It is essential to establish, before engaging consultants or electing to send trainees on external courses, the credentials of those who will be presenting the training. When considering the use of a consultancy body to present on-site training, it is essential to agree, and to tightly specify, in advance a programme of topics to be covered, and in what degree of depth. If this is not done beforehand, it is both pointless and too late to complain after the event that the required topics were not covered, that subjects not required were presented, or that the level was pitched too high or too low for the trainees. All this should be agreed, in writing, in advance, as should the price structure.

All this is not to say that training given by persons from outside the company is of no value. On the contrary, outside experts and specialists can present a more profound or wider view. When it comes to training in quality assurance, GMP or regulatory matters, for example, they can ensure that the requirements in such areas are seen by the trainees, not as company quirks but as important issues of wider application and relevance. However, any large company is well advised to provide much of its training needs from its own internal resources. This is not just a question of economics. This way the company has full control over the training provided, its content, and when and where. It is salutary for trainees to feel that colleagues, or more senior personnel, have the knowledge, skill and ability to teach them what they need to know. To permanently opt out and use external people could be seen as an admission of failure or inadequacy. To opt in, it will be necessary, in addition to devising training programmes and syllabuses, to select and train trainers.

Training trainers

To throw people in at the deep end, just because they know (or are believed to know) about a subject, without any consideration of their actual or potential ability to teach that subject is just not good enough. A prime consideration is willingness, interest and enthusiasm to be a trainer. No person who is unwilling should be forced into the job. This is very definitely a case where one volunteer is worth infinitely more than 10 pressed men.

At this stage it is worth setting down some basic concepts:

- It is a mistake to think of training as something which is easy to do. It is not. To be a good trainer is hard work, although it can be very rewarding, and useful for personal development, particularly in terms of confidence-building.
- Some people are naturally brilliant trainers, public speakers and the like. On the other hand, there are a few who, no matter how they try, will never make it as trainers. Between these two extremes there is the great mass who, with a little effort and practice, and with appropriate practice and encouragement can become more than adequate at it.
- Potential trainers who are nervous at the thought of standing up and speaking to a group of people need to be assured that everyone has 'nerves', even experienced speakers and particularly at the start of a presentation. With a little practice, trainers learn to control, or cope with those 'nerves', and far from letting it all spoil their presentation, they can in fact energise themselves on the adrenaline flow.

Any organisation intending to set up a training scheme based on its own corps of internal trainers, having determined what are its training needs, and at least roughed-out training programme(s) and basic syllabuses, should then identify potential trainers. The first criterion is the obvious one that a trainer should know his or her subject. Other judgements will have to be based on personal attributes and qualities. Can the person under consideration be expected to be able to explain and teach that subject in a clear, confident and interesting manner? Those who seem to be suitable should then be approached and asked if they are interested in taking on a training role in addition to their normal function. Acting as a trainer should be made to appear as attractive as possible, and a little encouragement given, but absolutely no pressure should be applied to force anyone to do anything they do not want to do. It may be possible to offer financial incentives, but in any event the job of trainer must be presented as a positive move, leading to greater job satisfaction and personal development, and certainly not as some additional chore that the company regrets having to ask anyone to take on. An alternative is to announce generally the establishment (or re-establishment) of a training scheme, and call for volunteer trainers. Any company which, through either approach, fails to recruit an adequate body of potential trainers must ask itself what is wrong with its motivational and personnel policies and practices. In any company where there is a good, well motivated sense of belonging, and where there is a healthy relationship between management and labour, there should be no great problem in finding a sufficient number of people ready and willing to be trained as trainers.

An approach which has been found to work well on a number of occasions is first to call a meeting of all those selected, and/or who have volunteered. At this meeting the proposed training programme should be outlined, and the basic principles and techniques of training, as discussed earlier in this chapter, should be explained. It would be useful to distribute handouts of the major points. The trainee trainers should then be allocated topics (with a summary of the points to be covered) upon which they are requested to develop a training module – outline script, slides/overheads or other visual aids, complete with any other demonstration material. It is generally better to allocate any given topic to more than one person, say to two or three, so that they can assist each other in the preparation. All should then be asked to return in, say 2 months' time, in order to present to the other members of the group, the training module which they have prepared. In the interim, each member of the group should be asked to prepare a short talk on any subject they care to select (e.g. hobbies, interests) to be given to the rest of the group in say, 2–4 weeks' time. This is essentially a confidence-building exercise, and it needs careful management to prevent it becoming the reverse. While it is serious in its intention, attempts should be made to make it fun rather than an ordeal. At the end of each talk, the course leader should call for *constructive* comments from the other trainee trainers on the content, interest and presentation of the talk, and then give his/her own views. Every effort should be made to be encouraging. Depending on the number of trainee trainers it may be necessary to spread this phase over more than 1 day.

The real crunch comes when the newly prepared modules are presented. This, too, may extend over more than 1 day. This time the comments requested, while still *constructive*, should be required to be rather more detailed and specific:

- Content – adequate coverage; factually correct?
- Interest.
- Presentation.

- Voice – clear; interesting or boring; sound level?
- Contact/interaction with audience?
- Questions/feedback/discussion.
- Any mannerisms or other distractions?
- Clarity and impact of visuals.

As before, the course leader should add his or her own comments on each presentation. Where, say, two persons have prepared a given module, they could either present half each or preferably each separately present the whole module, but on different days. This will have the added advantage of affording an opportunity to compare different approaches to the presentation of the same topic. (It is of course assumed that no presentation will consist of just a slavish reading-out of a previously prepared text. The 'script' written during the preparation of a module should be considered as neither more nor less than notes upon which speakers base their own words.)

Almost certainly, on a first time round, there will be some corrections needed for the presentation of most modules. Any presentations which are judged to be first-class presentations of exemplary material may be considered to have yielded a perfectly formed trainer, and a training module for future use. This is unlikely to apply in many cases. It will usually be necessary to repeat the process after a month or two, during which time any necessary correction and polishing can take place. After this second session it should be possible to settle on the corps of company trainers, and to eliminate, as gently and sympathetically as possible, any less-able trainers. The company will also have acquired a set of training modules for future use, and for use in the later training of further trainers.

This may seem a lengthy and time-consuming process, but it is one with which the author has been successfully involved on a number of occasions, and there is no doubt that, if well managed, it does work well.

Reference

US FDA (1990). *Code of Federal Regulations, Vol. 21, Ch. 1, Part 210*, Current good manufacturing practice in manufacturing, processing, packaging or holding of drugs, general; *CFR Vol. 21, Ch. 1, Part 211*, Current good manufacturing practice for finished pharmaceuticals; *CFR Vol. 21, Ch. 1, Part 820*, Good manufacturing practice for medical devices (revised 1995). Washington: US Food & Drug Administration. (Collectively referred to as the US CGMPs.)

Annex I

Suggested outline for a basic GMP training course

The following may be used as a basis for staff training in basic good manufacturing practice.

Structure

This suggested basic course, for pharmaceutical manufacturers, is founded on a series of BGMP (basic good manufacturing practice) modules, as follows:

- BGMP/1 – Making medicines
- BGMP/2 – The principles of GMP (A)
- BGMP/3 – The principles of GMP (B)
- BGMP/4 – Cleanliness and hygiene
- BGMP/5 – Legal aspects, etc.
- BGMP/6 – Summary session

With suitable adaptations this could be used for basic training in other types of healthcare manufacturing.

Each module is intended to provide sufficient material for one training session, of say 30–40 minutes' duration, run at the rate of one or two sessions per week. Attempts should be made to make cross-references between the sessions, rather than present them as separate entities.

The programme as a whole is designed to be suitable for presentation to employees engaged in a variety of areas, e.g. Production, Packaging, QC, Warehousing, Engineering, etc. It may well need to be supplemented by further GMP training which is more specifically relevant to their field of work.

It is assumed that, before starting this course, new employees will already have received induction training in, for example:

- Pay, and conditions of employment
- Job title and description
- Management structure
- General company familiarisation
- Health and safety

- Welfare
- Disciplinary and grievance procedures.

Approach

This course is intended to be presented to new (and as required, existing) employees, off-the-job, by means of talks/demonstrations/audio-visual displays, etc. It should be supplemented by routine on-the-job training.

Learning and understanding is facilitated when the trainee is made aware of:

- The *context* (i.e. the frame of reference).
- The Why's as well as the What's and How's.

That is why this programme starts with a brief consideration of such matters as the history of medicine, and the growth of the pharmaceutical industry and of our company. Whilst these topics need only be covered very simply, they do provide the context, and if well-presented can be highly motivating.

When presenting the various sessions, the instructor should make efforts to minimise the 'classroom/lecture' atmosphere. A too-formal approach should be avoided; use should be made wherever possible of visual aids and practical examples, and questions and open discussion should be actively encouraged.

The benefits of modern medicines (the products of our Industry) to people, to sick patients, and their need for our care should receive prime and positive emphasis. While it is obviously important to deal with statutory/regulatory requirements, these should **not** be presented as the only (or even the main) reasons for GMP. The attitude should be 'We comply with GMP because this is the right and proper way to discharge our duty to our customer-patients. Because we do this, we have no fear of failing to satisfy legal requirements. However, we should all be aware that if we do fail, we can be forced to close-down.'

Those responsible for training should be aware of a not uncommon perception (fostered by some segments of the media) of the pharmaceutical industry as something 'nasty' and even hazardous to health. Therefore, the very real benefits to health should be stressed, and terms such as 'drugs' and the 'drug industry' should be avoided, where possible, as having unpleasant connotations. Expressions such as 'medicines', 'healthcare', and the 'pharmaceutical (or healthcare) industry' should be used. (This may not be possible in the USA and other countries under the control of the US FDA, as terms such as 'drug' and 'drug product' have formal regulatory status.)

Assessment of training

The effectiveness of training should be assessed during each session by oral questions and answers, and at the end of each by a simple, largely multiple-choice, question paper. (See Annex II for suggested simple question papers to be used with this course.) In the longer term, assessment should be by observation of operator performance and adherence to systems and procedures, as noted during periodic company self-audits, etc.

Retraining

Retraining and/or refresher training should be given whenever either of the following indicate the need:

(a)   Assessment of post-training effectiveness.
(b)   Changes in company organisation, systems or technologies.

Records

These should be of two types:

1.   The personal file of each member of staff should contain a record of the training received, indicated by module reference number (see Form 12.1).
2.   Departmental training records should be maintained, indicating in tabular form the training received by each member of staff (see Form 12.2).

Module BGMP/1: Making medicines

Content

1. Brief history of medicine – 'magic/herbs/faith' to modern chemo-therapy.
2. Growth and development of the pharmaceutical industry.
3. Distinction between:

   - Active substances.
   - Dosage forms.

4. Benefits of the pharmaceutical industry to:

   - Health, and quality and quantity of life.
   - National economy, exports, work/employment.

5. The place of our company in the pharmaceutical industry:

   - Company history.
   - Company organisation.
   - Our products.
   - Use of our products.
   - Advantages of our products.

6. Sale and distribution of our products (including, in the UK, the National Health Service).
7. Conclusion: 'It is not surprising that working in such an important industry, which has such an impact on people's health and well-being, is under government regulatory control, and also subject to "good pharmaceutical manufacturing practice" (GMP) regulations or guidelines. We will be dealing with these in later sessions.'

Comments

Topics 1 and 2 should be covered only in very simple terms, in order to give an elementary background. The benefits to people, to sick patients, and their need for *our* care should be stressed.

It is useful to draw an early distinction between the manufacture of bulk chemical substances ('actives' or 'primary production') and the manufacture and packaging of dosage forms ('secondary production'). Many lay people do not quite understand this distinction.

The growth of the company, from its initial establishment to its present position should be outlined and its current national and international organisation displayed.

The company's different types of business and product should be explained. Examples of our products should be shown, and their use and particular benefits and advantages explained.

In the UK, the National Health Service is something that trainees will already know something about, and it should be mentioned as the nation's single largest purchaser of pharmaceutical products. Through this, a further connection can be made both with benefits to people, and with the Government's special interest in our industry.

Suggestions for audio/visual/demonstration material

O   Slides (35 mm) illustrating:

- Aspects of history of medicine: 'ancients'/magic/herbs to present day, including 'chemotherapeutic revolution'.
- Development of industrial pharmacy.
- Development of our company.
- Our company today (home and overseas).

O   OHTs/slides showing:

- Impact on heath/life-expectancy statistics.
- Economic statistics.

O   Also have available to show:

- Pharmacopoeias.
- GMP guidelines/regulations.
- Examples of our products.

Module BGMP/2: General principles of GMP (A)

Content

1. Brief introduction, recalling previous session.
2. Meanings of QA, GMP, QC.
3. Nature of, and reasons for, GMP.
4. Potential hazards of faulty products (incorrectly made, wrongly labelled, chemically contaminated, microbially contaminated, etc.), and the need for product-consistency embracing:

    *   Danger to patients.
    *   Failure to cure patients.
    *   Recall.
    *   Cost.
    *   Loss of company reputation.
    *   Legal action (regulatory/damages).

5. Importance of following instructions ALWAYS and EXACTLY. (Mention briefly batch manufacturing instructions/records, SOPs and the vital importance of correct labelling.)
6. Show GMP video.
7. Ask questions and seek comment on film. Discuss.

Comments

The object of this session is to set the general GMP scene. (BGMP/1 built the frame: we now begin to draw in the picture.) The detail of GMP is not required at this stage, unless the need arises from the discussion. More detail will follow in the next session.

Suggestions for audio/visual/demonstration material

○ GMP video: in the UK, the ABPI video *You'll Soon Feel Better*, remains a valuable training aid.

○ Slides/OHTs illustrating:

    *   Definitions of 'quality', GMP, QA, QC, etc., and their inter-relationships.
    *   Various major points made in the lead-up to the video.

○ Examples of:

    *   Batch manufacturing instructions.
    *   Batch packaging records.
    *   A selection of SOPs to pass round.

Module BGMP/3: The principles of GMP (B)

Content

1. Introduction: recap on reasons for GMP.
2. Re-emphasise the importance of following instructions: ALWAYS and EXACTLY.
3. The nature and purpose of documentation:

   - Master documentation.
   - Batch manufacturing and packaging documents.
   - SOPs.
   - Other written documents.

4. Records, making entries on documents, and amendment of incorrect entries.
5. Labels and labelling:

   - Label security.
   - Finished product labels.
   - In-process labels.
   - Status labels.
   - Removal/defacing of old labels.
   - Line clearance.

6. Good order, tidiness and general cleanliness.
7. What to do if you make a mistake, or do (or see) something wrong on documents/records (see 5 above) or in a practical sense.
8. 'GMP is everyone's responsibility'.

Comments

The main objective of this session should be to establish the vital importance of following procedures as laid down in the various documents described. Individual variations are not to be tolerated, even if well intentioned. Mistakes must be reported and not covered up. Records must be completed properly, clearly and legibly at the time the action is taken. The correct method of correcting false entries should be described and demonstrated. At this stage, detail on hygiene/microbiology, etc. is not required. This will follow in the next module.

Suggestions for audio/visual/demonstration material

○ OHTs/slides summarising main points of text, e.g.

   - Content of master and batch documents.
   - Reasons for maintaining records.
   - Vital things to remember about records.
   - Types of labels.

- Types of contamination.

○ Examples of:

- Various company labels (cancelled or defaced).
- Typical company documents (master, batch and SOPs).

Module BGMP/4: Cleanliness and hygiene

Content

1. Introduction to elementary microbiology:

    *   Definitions (e.g. 'microbe', 'micro-organism', 'germ', 'virus').
    *   The nature and occurrence of micro-organisms in air, in water, on skin, hair, beard and in gut, etc.
    *   Effects of micro-organisms (good and bad).
    *   Methods of controlling, removing and destroying micro-organisms:

        —   cleaning
        —   disinfection/antiseptics
        —   sterilisation – the methods available
        —   importance of controlling contamination levels at all stages.

2. People as a source of contamination.
3. Personal hygiene:

    *   What is expected and why.
    *   Effects of illness or contacts.
    *   Reporting illness, injuries, etc.
    *   Company rules and regulations.

4. Protective clothing, provision and use:

    *   General factory.
    *   Clean rooms/sterile areas.

5. Cleanliness of general working areas and equipment (including special requirements for clean/sterile areas).
6. Cleaning schedules and methods.
7. Chemical contamination. (Mentioned here to ensure that trainees are clear about the different forms of contamination.)
8. Practical session. Trainees to dab fingers, palms, etc. on sterile agar plates (for incubation). Repeat after washing with antiseptic and/or normal soap. Place hair(s) from head (or beard if available) on agar plates, for incubation.

Comments

Discussion of microbiological principles need only be at a most elementary level. The whole objective is to impress the importance of good order, cleanliness and hygiene (personal and environmental) in the prevention of all forms of contamination.

Microbiological concepts will be mentioned again in the final summary session (BGMP/6), when the incubated plates will be viewed.

(Time must be allowed for incubation – hence the insertion of the next module on Legal aspects.)

[Note on the microbiological content of Modules BGMP/4 and BGMP/6: This can be adjusted in accordance with trainee requirements. It can be pitched at a lower level for those who do not work, or who are not intended to work, on sterile products. Nevertheless, the potential hazards (to already vulnerable patients) even of microbiologically contaminated non-sterile products is a useful peg on which to hang discussions of the need for clean and hygienic practices.]

Suggestions for audio/visual/demonstration material

○   Slides of micro-organisms (microscopic) and of the effects of their growth.

○   OHTs/slides summarising main points of the text.

○   Microbiological culture plates and ancillary equipment for taking finger, hand, nose 'prints', etc.

Module BGMP/5: Legal aspects, etc.

Content

1. The national legal framework. For example, in the UK:
   - The Medicines Act 1968.
   - Product Licences.
   - Manufacturers Licences.
   - Other licences/certificates.
   - The Medicines Inspectorate, its role and mode of action.

2. International legislation/agreements/formalities:
   - EC directives.
   - WHO.
   - PIC.
   - FDA.
   - Other national authorities.

3. Recap on the concepts of good manufacturing practice and quality assurance, and discuss the genesis of the GMP guides and regulations.

Comments

The whole thrust of this session should be to move from the establishment of the legal/formal framework within which we all have to operate, towards the understanding that we comply with the requirements of GMP not just because the law, and the inspectors, say we should, but because it is *right* that we should do so; right for the health of our business, and (more important) right for the health of our patients. Specific GMP content can be adjusted according to the needs/interests of the trainees.

Suggestions for audio/visual/demonstration material

- OHTs/slides summarising main points of text.
- Copies of Medicines Act 1968, SIs, etc. (to show only).
- PIC GMP guidelines.
- EC GMP Guide for medicinal products.
- Other national and international GMP guidelines, e.g. WHO, the US CGMPs, the French BPF, etc.

Module BGMP/6: Summary session

Content

1. Examine incubated plates from practical session (BGMP/4), and discuss results.
2. Use discussion to recap the various points already made about cleanliness, hygiene and good order.
3. As appropriate, outline company policy/procedures for microbiological monitoring and control.
4. For trainees involved in sterile manufacture, describe the sterility test, and stress its severe limitations as a safeguard against contaminated products.
5. Conclude with a review of a typical company production cycle (perhaps with a 'walk-through', if feasible), and the principal documents used at each stage:

   - Ordering materials.
   - Receipt of materials.
   - Warehousing/quarantine.
   - Material sampling/testing/release (or rejection).
   - Typical bulk manufacturing operations.
   - Bulk storage.
   - Packaging.
   - Labelling.
   - Quarantine.
   - Release.
   - Finished pack storage.
   - Picking and packing
   - Dispatch.

6. Follow by a discussion, prompted by questions from the instructor, on aspects of GMP (*all* aspects, not only hygiene, etc.) relevant at each stage.
7. Final question paper.

Comments

It is not intended that the concluding review of a typical manufacturing cycle should be a lecture. As far as possible, the ideas should come from the trainees, prompted by the instructor. It would be worth considering conducting this part of the session whilst touring the relevant site areas.

It would also be worthwhile, if time permits, to arrange a further meeting to discuss the results of the question papers and to clear up any misunderstandings that these have revealed.

Suggestions for audio/visual/demonstration material

○   Incubated plates from module BGMP/4.

○   Slides of on-site areas/activities to illustrate the review of production cycle.

○   Examples/illustrations of relevant documents/records/SOPs.

Annex II

Basic GMP training course – test papers

The following are suggestions for test papers to be completed by trainees at the end of the presentation of each of the first five Basic GMP Training Modules (BGMP/1 to BGMP/5). Each session could then include a discussion on the results of the previous test, with an emphasis on areas where misunderstandings may be apparent.

The final double-length paper is one of several possible selections from the other five, to be used in a final assessment of the knowledge gained by the trainees.

It is obviously important to ensure that all the points in a question paper have been covered in the corresponding training session.

Basic GMP Test Paper – No. 1

Your Name .... Date ....

*Where you are given a choice, tick the one you think is right. Where you are asked to write an answer, a **few** words are all that is needed.*

1 For how long have people used medicines of one sort or another?

a A few years ❑
b About a hundred years ❑
c Hundreds of years ❑
d Thousands of years ❑

2 What year, approximately, marked the beginning of truly scientific medicine, using synthetic chemical medicines?

a 1760 ❑
b 1820 ❑
c 1910 ❑
d 1970 ❑

3 Who is generally considered to be the 'father of modern medicine'?

a Isaac Newton ❑
b Paul Ehrlich ❑
c Louis Pasteur ❑
d Heinrich Schütz ❑

4 Who discovered Penicillin?
a Michael Faraday ❑
b Charles Darwin ❑
c James Brown ❑
d Alexander Fleming ❑

5 Has modern medicine improved people's health and life-expectancy –

a A little ❑
b A lot ❑
c Not much ❑
d Not at all ❑

6 In Britain we both import and export medicines. Do we –

a Import more than we export ❑
b Export more than we import ❑
c Import about the same as export ❑

7 Who makes most of the medicines taken in this country?

a Doctors ❑
b Pharmacists or chemists ❑
c Pharmaceutical industry ❑
d Hospitals ❑

8 Of which group of companies are we a part?
....

9 When was our company first formed –
a .... ❑
b .... ❑
c .... ❑
d .... ❑

10 Name four of our products –
....
....
....
....

Basic GMP Test Paper – No. 2

Your Name ....   Date ....

*Where you are given a choice, tick the one you think is right. Where you are asked to write an answer, a **few** words are all that is needed.*

1   What do *we* mean by 'quality'?

   a Special excellence ❏
   b Fitness for purpose ❏
   c How good something is ❏
   d Passing specified tests ❏

2   In making medicines should we –

   a Take as much care as when making anything else ❏
   b Take less care, because the product is tested ❏
   c Take a bit more care than usual ❏
   d Take extra special care ❏

3   What does 'GMP' stand for –

   a Good management procedures ❏
   b Great making profit ❏
   c Good manufacturing practice ❏
   d Good making pharmaceuticals ❏

4   Who is responsible for the quality of medicines –

   a The top management ❏
   b The QC manager ❏
   c We all are ❏
   d The Government's Department of Health ❏

5   Written instructions and procedures should be –

   a Ignored ❏
   b Followed exactly, always ❏
   c Followed when necessary ❏
   d Changed when the product is wanted quickly ❏

6   'SOP' stands for –

   a Standard operational prescription ❏
   b Simplified operational practice ❏
   c Standard operating procedure ❏
   d Superior Olympic performance ❏

7   Testing the end product will always prevent the release of defective medicines –

   a True ❏
   b False ❏
   c It all depends ❏

8   Manufacturing Instructions say '. . .rinse the vessel with distilled water . . .'. No distilled water is available. Do you –

   a Do nothing ❏
   b Use tap water ❏
   c Report that there is no distilled water ❏
   d Not bother to rinse the vessel ❏

9   Even if a defective medicinal product is released for sale, patients will usually be able to detect that something is wrong –

   a True ❏
   b False ❏
   c Very untrue ❏

10 Which of the following is correct?
   a Usually it does not matter if you make a mistake ❏
   b All mistakes should always be reported ❏
   c If you make a mistake, 'cover up' ❏
   d Workmates' mistakes are nothing to do with you ❏

Basic GMP Test Paper – No. 3

Your Name ....   Date ....

*Where you are given a choice, tick the one you think is right. Where you are asked to write an answer, a **few** words are all that is needed.*

1   What are the TWO most serious weaknesses of end-product testing of medicines (tick two)?

   a It is expensive ❑
   b It is done on samples only ❑
   c You cannot test for everything ❑
   d It is difficult ❑

2   What is the most important reason for always following written instructions exactly?

   a Because it is the law ❑
   b Because your boss says so ❑
   c Because government inspectors insist on it ❑
   d To ensure consistent quality products ❑

3   What has been the most common cause of the recall of medicines?

   a Over-strength ❑
   b Under-strength ❑
   c Contamination ❑
   d Wrong labels ❑

4   The law says that we must keep manufacturing and testing records. Give TWO other important reasons for keeping records.
   ....
   ....

5   What should you do if you make a mistake when writing a record?
   ....
   ....

6   What are the TWO main sorts of label?
   .... labels and .... labels

7   Batch manufacturing instructions and batch packaging instructions are –

   a All bound together in a book ❑
   b Made up as we go along ❑
   c Produced by making exact copies (photocopies or computer printouts) from a carefully checked master ❑
   d Written or typed-out fresh each time ❑

8   Give THREE examples of a standard operating procedure –

   ....
   ....
   ....

9   We must avoid contaminating our products with micro-organisms ('germs'). What other sort of contamination must we prevent?

   ....

10 Pharmaceutical factories in the UK are subject to inspection by the Government's Department of Health. The people who do the inspections are called –

   a Health Inspectors ❑
   b Pharmaceutical Invigilators ❑
   c Health and Safety Executives ❑
   d Medicines Inspectors ❑

Basic GMP Test Paper – No. 4

Your Name ....   Date ....

*Where you are given a choice, tick the one you think is right. Where you are asked to write an answer, a **few** words are all that is needed.*

1   What are the THREE things micro-organisms need to grow and multiply?

    ....
    ....
    ....

2   Which statement is most correct?

    a All micro-organisms are harmful ❑
    b All micro-organisms are harmless ❑
    c Micro-organisms are not useful ❑
    d Some micro-organisms are harmless, some are harmful, and some are very harmful ❑

3   What can micro-organisms grow in?

    a Water ❑
    b A hot cup of tea. ❑
    c A cream cake ❑
    d Antiseptic solution ❑
    e All of these ❑

4   In favourable conditions (for them!) how frequently do micro-organisms reproduce?

    a Every 10 seconds ❑
    b Every 20 minutes ❑
    c Twice a week ❑
    d Every 9 months ❑

5   How long can micro-organisms live?

    a Hours ❑
    b Days ❑
    c Weeks ❑
    d Months ❑
    e Years ❑

6   Which statement is most correct?

    a Boiling will kill all micro-organisms ❑
    b Boiling will not kill micro-organisms ❑
    c Boiling will kill some, but not all micro-organisms ❑

7   How many skin cells do we shed per day?

    a About 100 ❑
    b About 1000 ❑
    c About 100 000 ❑
    d Many millions ❑

8   Where do micro-organisms live on or in us?

    a Hands ❑
    b Skin surface ❑
    c Mouth ❑
    d Gut ❑
    e All of these ❑

9   Which statement is most true?

    a Refrigeration kills micro-organisms ❑
    b Refrigeration has no value ❑
    c Refrigeration prevents micro-organisms from growing and reproducing ❑

10 What should you do if you come to work with an infection (cough, cold, 'stomach trouble', etc.), or with a cut, wound or graze?

    ....
    ....

Basic GMP Test Paper – No. 5

Your Name .... Date ....

*Where you are given a choice, tick the one you think is right. Where you are asked to write an answer, a **few** words are all that is needed.*

1 When was the Medicines Act passed?

  a 1968 ❑
  b 1723 ❑
  c 1820 ❑
  d 1987 ❑

2 Under the Medicines Act, each medicinal product is required to have a Product Licence. Each pharmaceutical factory in the UK is also required to have another sort of licence. This is called a –

  a Factory Licence ❑
  b Medicines Licence ❑
  c Pharmaceutical Licence ❑
  d Manufacturer's Licence ❑

3 The conditions and practices required for the manufacture of medicines are given in detail in the Medicines Act –

  a True ❑
  b False ❑

4 Details of what is considered good practice in the manufacture of medicines are given in –

  a The British Pharmacopoeia ❑
  b The Medical Directory ❑
  c The Guide to Good Pharmaceutical Manufacturing Practice ❑
  d The World Health Standard ❑

5 If we fall below the legally required standards –

  a It does not matter ❑
  b We will be asked to improve ❑
  c We will all be arrested ❑
  d Our licence could be taken away, and our factory closed ❑

6 Medicines Inspectors are –

  a Junior civil servants ❑
  b Experienced chemists and pharmacists ❑
  c Generally incompetent ❑
  d Always men ❑

7 In addition to visiting manufacturing sites, Medicines Inspectors also inspect –

  a Hospitals ❑
  b Wholesalers ❑
  c Overseas manufacturers ❑
  d All of these ❑

8 Which of the following have laws about making medicines?

  a USA ❑
  b EEC ❑
  c Both ❑

9 What does PIC stand for?

  a Personnel Inspectors' Conference ❑
  b Pharmaceutical Inspection Convention ❑
  c Private Investigators' Club ❑
  d Pharmaceutical Investigation Centre ❑

10 What is the most important reason for following the principles of GMP?

  a Because it's a good idea ❑
  b Because it's the law ❑
  c Because it's company policy ❑
  d To protect the safety and well-being of patients ❑

Basic GMP Test Paper – General   **page 1** (of 2)

Your Name .... Date ....

*Where you are given a choice, tick the one you think is right. Where you are asked to write an answer, a **few** words are all that is needed.*

1 What do *we* mean by 'quality'?

   a Special excellence ❏
   b Fitness for purpose ❏
   c How good something is ❏
   d Passing specified tests ❏

2 Written instructions and procedures should be –

   a Ignored ❏
   b Followed exactly, always ❏
   c Followed when necessary ❏
   d Changed when the product is wanted quickly ❏

3 Who is generally considered to be the 'father of modern medicine'?

   a Isaac Newton ❏
   b Paul Ehrlich ❏
   c Louis Pasteur ❏
   d Heinrich Schütz ❏

4 Who makes most of the medicines taken in this country?

   a Doctors ❏
   b Pharmacists or chemists ❏
   c Pharmaceutical industry ❏
   d Hospitals ❏

5 What are the TWO most serious weaknesses of end-product testing of medicines (tick two)?

   a It is expensive ❏
   b It is done on samples only ❏
   c You cannot test for everything ❏
   d It is difficult ❏

6 What is the most important reason for always following written instructions exactly?

   a Because it is the law ❏
   b Because your boss says so ❏
   c Because Government Inspectors insist on it ❏
   d To ensure consistent quality products ❏

7 What is the most common cause of the recall of medicines?

   a Over-strength ❏
   b Under-strength ❏
   c Contamination ❏
   d Wrong labels ❏

8 What are the THREE things micro-organisms need to grow and multiply?

   ....
   ....
   ....

9 How long can micro-organisms live?

   a Hours ❏
   b Days ❏
   c Weeks ❏
   d Months ❏
   e Years ❏

10 What should you do if you come to work with an infection (cough, cold, 'stomach trouble', etc.), or with a cut, wound or graze?

   ....
   ....

Basic GMP Test Paper – General   **page 2** (of 2)

Your Name ....   Date ....

11 Has modern medicine improved people's health and life-expectancy –

a A little ❑
b A lot ❑
c Not much ❑
d Not at all ❑

12 In the UK we both import and export medicines. Do we –

a Import more than we export ❑
b Export more than we import ❑
c Import about the same as export ❑

13 Who is responsible for the quality of medicines?

a The top management ❑
b The QC Manager ❑
c We all are ❑
d The Government's Department of Health ❑

14 Testing the end product will always prevent the release of defective medicines –

a True ❑
b False ❑

15 Manufacturing Instructions say '. . . rinse the vessel with distilled water . . .'. No distilled water is available. Do you –

a Do nothing ❑
b Use tap water ❑
c Report that there is no distilled water ❑
d Not bother to rinse the vessel ❑

16 Even if a defective medicinal product is released for sale, patients will usually be able to detect that something is wrong –

a True ❑
b False ❑
c Very untrue ❑

17 Under the Medicines Act, each medicinal product is required to have a Product Licence. Each pharmaceutical factory in the UK is also required to have another sort of licence. This is called a –

a Factory Licence ❑
b Medicines Licence ❑
c Pharmaceutical Licence ❑
d Manufacturer's Licence ❑

18 If we fall below the legally required standards –

a It does not matter ❑
b We will be asked to improve ❑
c We will all be arrested ❑
d Our licence could be taken away, and our factory closed ❑

19 Which of the following have laws about making medicines?

a USA ❑
b EEC ❑
c Both ❑

20 What is the most important reason for following the principles of GMP?

a Because it's a good idea ❑
b Because it's the law ❑
c Because it's company policy ❑
d To protect patients ❑

13

Personnel: hygiene and health

The denunciation of the young is a necessary part of the hygiene of older people, and greatly assists the circulation of their blood

Logan Pearsall Smith (1865–1946)

Most official guidelines or regulations on good manufacturing practice (GMP) stress the importance of personal hygiene, although in some of these publications, reference to it appears under headings such as 'sanitation', which covers cleanliness of plant and equipment as well as of people.

The need for personal hygiene

High standards of personal hygiene are clearly necessary for all involved in the manufacture of pharmaceuticals and the like. This necessity is most crucial where the product is exposed, particularly when that product is intended to be sterile. Nevertheless, high standards should be demanded and achieved at all stages, and with all types of product. The primary reasons are to control contamination of product, materials or environment by that vigorous dispenser of micro-organisms and general dirt, the 'working human being', and also to prevent cross-contamination through transfer of dust and other materials via workers' hands, etc. There is a very good secondary reason. Persons with high regard for matters of hygiene will more readily be able to adopt that special attitude of care and attention that the manufacturer of medicines requires.

Micro-organisms can abound on body surfaces, and in the nose, throat, mouth, bladder and intestines. They may be transferred by shedding from body surfaces, generally in association with inanimate particles (e.g. skin flakes), via sneezing and coughing, or by direct contact with contaminated hands. The total number of micro-organisms on the skin varies from person to person, and in accordance with their personal hygiene practices. It also varies in different parts of the skin surface. It can vary from less than one hundred organisms to several million per square centimetre of skin surface. The largest concentrations of organisms are generally to be found on the head and neck, armpits, hands, feet and beard, if worn. Saliva can contain up to 100 million organisms per millilitre, and nasal excretions up to 10 million. The number of coliform bacteria alone per gram of human faeces can be of the order of 100 million.

The human body continuously sheds inanimate particles, largely consisting of skin fragments. Dependent on skin type and level of activity (the more vigorous the activity, the greater the shedding) the rate of shedding is of the order of 5–15 g of particles every 12 hours. Skin micro-organisms are most frequently shed in association with skin particles. The extent and the hazard of micro-organism dispersal increases where there is infection, especially of skin, the respiratory system or the alimentary canal. Steps need to be taken to control these hazards to product and environment, through the observations of hygienic practices by staff, and through the provision of suitable protective factory wear. Let it not be thought that the need to guard against bacterial contamination applies only to the manufacture of products intended to be sterile, or to certain creams, emulsions, suspensions, syrups, etc. which might 'grow'. There is evidence, for example, of the adverse clinical significance of microbiologically contaminated tablet products.

Other possible objectionable effects of micro-organisms, in addition to the obvious hazards of their presence in parenterals, ophthalmic products, and products for application to wounds or broken skin include:

- Possible effects on product stability.
- 'Cracking' of emulsions.
- Effects on container/closure integrity (through fermentation and consequent evolution of gases).
- Effects on bioavailability.
- Interference with analytical testing, due to products of microbial metabolism.

Hygiene measures

The first step towards ensuring hygienic practices amongst personnel is, of course, to recruit the right sort of people in the first place. That is, people who will already observe high standards of personal hygiene. It then becomes a matter of providing training which emphasises the special risks and requirements of pharmaceutical manufacturing, and of providing the necessary facilities.

There should be a general medical examination prior to employment, the extent of which may vary according to the nature of the work to be performed by the new employee. At one end of the 'risk spectrum' is the handling of exposed sterile product, at the other the handling of already packaged products. No person with a communicable disease, or with open lesions on exposed body surfaces should engage in the manufacture of medicinal products, most certainly not where product may be exposed. Further, staff should be instructed to report any such conditions and supervisors to look out for them. Steps should be taken to encourage such reporting, and no person should suffer any loss, e.g. of remuneration, for doing so.

In this context it is interesting to note the recently reaffirmed policy of the US FDA regarding the employment of HIV-infected workers in pharmaceutical manufacturing areas (Young, 1986):

> . . . a person infected with the AIDS virus should not be restricted *a priori* from working in a pharmaceutical . . . manufacturing facility. We are not aware of any epidemiological data that suggest any increased product safety risks associated with the employment of persons with AIDS under the conditions which would exist in drug . . . manufacturing, based on the fact that all . . . evidence . . . indicates that blood-borne and sexually transmitted infections like AIDS would not be transmitted under normal conditions in the workplace.

Although there is general regulatory and industrial agreement that there should be some form of initial and ongoing medical examination of persons working in, or entering, pharmaceutical manufacturing areas, it is difficult to find any regulatory instruction or official guidance which is any more detailed or specific than a vague general suggestion that it is a good thing. In 1972 the Association of Swedish Pharmaceutical Industry (LIF) published a set of 'hygiene recommendations'. As far as the author is aware, this is the most recent attempt to present any really 'solid' advice or recommendations. What follows is largely based on that Swedish publication.

Tentative guidelines on operator hygiene and health checks

1. It needs to be understood that good bodily hygiene and a high level of general cleanliness are necessary in those working on the manufacture of pharmaceuticals and similar products.
2. Hands, including nails, should be kept clean and always be carefully washed after visits to the toilet, before meals and before work commences, or recommences after a break. There is considerable risk of infection being passed on by contaminated hands. It is therefore extremely important to maintain good hand hygiene in the manufacture of pharmaceuticals and the like. So as to reduce the risk of infection through hand contact to a minimum, the following should be required of all operators:

   - Do not touch the product, nor objects that may come in contact with the product, with unprotected hands.
   - Keep the hands well groomed with short, clean nails. Hands must be free of any lesions, wounds, cuts, boils or any other sources of infection.
   - Wrist watches, rings or other jewellery should not be worn on the job.
   - Hands should be washed before work and as often as the job requires.

- Protective gloves should be worn when working with open products and when handling objects that come in direct contact with the product. Working with gloves presupposes scrupulous care and control of the gloves themselves; any failure to do that, then the use of contaminated gloves will create a hygiene risk rather than provide protection against it. When gloves of rubber or plastic material are worn, they soon become very damp inside from sweat, which contains high levels of micro-organisms. It is therefore essential for the gloves to be tight-fitting, and not torn or punctured. Reusable gloves should be cleaned and disinfected at regular intervals, after the end of each task or as often as the job requires.

3. Persons with infectious diseases, or with open lesions on the body surfaces, should not work in production areas. Employees should be encouraged, and indeed required, to report if they are afflicted in this way. They should not suffer any financial, or other form of loss, in so doing.

4. A programme for health check-ups (see suggestions in Table 13.1) should operate for all production personnel. It should provide for regular check-ups in addition to a general medical examination prior to employment. Its scope and direction should be adapted to the risks attaching to individual jobs and products.

5. The necessity to observe good oral hygiene should be stressed. Eating, chewing gum, and the ingestion of sweets or the like should be prohibited in the working area. The risks of contamination from nose and mouth can be controlled by:

- Not talking, sneezing or coughing in the vicinity of open products.
- Wearing masks.

6. The following routine should be followed to achieve the best effects from a mask, if used:

- It should cover both nose and mouth and must not be touched while in use.
- It should be replaced as soon as risks arise that its effect has been reduced, e.g. after a certain period of use, after sneezing, or when (or before) it becomes 'soggy'.
- It should be thrown away after use in a receptacle provided for this purpose.

7. When working with dusty material it may be necessary to wear protective masks of the reusable type. Such a mask should be personally adjusted to the individual using it, and should be cleaned and disinfected after each use.

8. Good care of the hair, including regular washing and cutting, reduces the risk of contaminating the product. Wearing beards, moustaches or whiskers will require the most careful grooming if these are not to pose a hygiene risk. A hair-cover should be worn in all production work areas. It should cover all hair and be replaced at regular intervals.

9. Working clothes (i.e. special protective clothing) should be worn only within the designated work areas. The material used to make protective clothing shall be dirt repellent and have a tightness of weave which makes it an effective barrier to the passage of micro-organisms, and particles from the body to the near environment. The material must not be fibre shedding. Working clothes should be kept separate from street clothes. Overalls, alternatively trousers and jackets, are preferable to smocks. Disposable protective clothes might be preferable for certain operations.

10. The nature of the protective clothing provided should be appropriate to the nature of the work carried out, and should be donned in accordance with written changing procedures. Dirty working clothes should be handled away from the production process. Laundered clothes should be dried and stored under conditions that preclude recontamination as far as possible.

11. Special working shoes, or over-shoes should be worn. The shoes should be cleaned and disinfected at prescribed intervals and be worn only within the work area. The commonly seen plastic (they always seem to be blue) shoe covers, which readily rip, are of limited value, and are little more than a cosmetic gesture.

12. Visitors and mechanics, contractors, specialists and others who have access to and enter production areas for the performance of certain tasks, should be furnished with the same type of protective clothing as used by the personnel employed in the relevant production area.

13. From the public relations aspect, visits and plant tours probably cannot be avoided entirely. Premises with passages and corridors which permit the viewing of production from the outside are to be recommended.

Note on Table 13.1

Table 13.1 is taken from the Swedish LIF publication referred to above and offers suggestions for initial and follow-up medical checks for staff employed in different manufacturing environments. The table is based on three 'area cleanliness classes' – X, Y and Z. (This relatively arbitrary classification is not to be confused with the more precisely defined 'environmental classes' of the various published Clean Room Standards.)

In the context of Table 13.1 the 'area cleanliness classes' are:

*   Class X – Environment where only closed product-units are handled.
*   Class Y – Environment where open products are handled.
*   Class Z – Environment where aseptic work is carried out.

Although put forward as no more than a suggestion, this table may provide a useful basis for discussion, particularly in a field where, although there is general agreement that medical checks are highly desirable, there is very little in the way of positive guidance as to how they should be implemented.

Table 13.1   Suggested programme for operator health checks

	Personnel who work in area class	Visual examination	X-ray	General medical examination	Faeces specimen	Nose/throat specimen
Pre-employment check-up	X	✓ ⎫	✓	✓ ⎫	✓	
	Y	✓ ⎬(a)	✓	✓ ⎬(b)	✓	
	Z	✓ ⎭	✓	✓ ⎭	✓	✓
Regular check-ups during employment	X	Once per 2 months	Once per year			
	Y	Once per month	Once per year			
	Z	Once per month	Once per year			
After illness – infection of throat or GI tract	X			✓ ⎫		
	Y			✓ ⎬(c)	✓	
	Z			✓ ⎭	✓	✓
After visits to territories where GI infections are common	X				✓	
	Y				✓	
	Z				✓	

(a) Check for incidence of allergic complaints, sores, general condition and general hygiene.
(b) Simple check to eliminate persons clearly unfit for employment, on medical grounds.
(c) More detailed health check starting after approximately 2 months' employment.

Additional points

A few further points are worth making:

- If high standards of cleanliness and hygiene and the proper wearing of protective clothes are to be observed by operators, it is necessary for supervisors and managers to set an appropriately good example.
- If hand washing facilities are to be used, not only must they be available, they must be *conveniently* available.
- From the GMP angle, the protection of the operator and his/her 'normal' clothing is only a secondary consideration. The primary purpose of protective clothing, in this context, is the protection of the product and thus the patient.
- Protective garments are of no value if they are damaged, dirty or permitted to become themselves vehicles of contamination, or cross-contamination. Suitable changing rooms should be provided, and the protective garments should not be worn outside the controlled factory environment or in any area where they could collect or distribute potential contaminants.
- Medical checks should include sight testing, including checks for colour blindness. This is something which is often neglected and it can assume great significance in jobs where visual acuity and/or distinction of colours is important.
- The question of head wear can be difficult. In aseptic production areas there can be no question. All hair on the head and face as well as on the bodily surfaces must be completely covered. In other less critical areas the importance of head covering is both variable (in accordance with the operations carried out) and, it has to be said, debatable. There is, however, a powerful argument in favour of sound head-covering, even in areas where the product is not exposed, e.g. in the labelling of filled and sealed containers, since it helps to engender a salutary attitude amongst the workforce that they are engaged in 'medical' work and they are part of a team making medicines. However, the relatively small paper objects that one frequently sees would seem to have little direct practical or psychological value. The selection of suitable head wear and the peaceful persuasion of operators to wear it properly can call for considerable management skill. But, **all** matters concerned, directly or indirectly with the quality of pharmaceutical products call for considerable management skill.

Reference

Young F E (1986). US Commissioner of Food and Drugs. Letter to the 3M Company, 17 Oct. 1986. Quoted by Paul Motise of FDA in *PDA Letter,* April 1998.

Part Four

Documentation

14

Documentation: general

It is to be noted that when any part of this paper appears dull there is a design in it

Sir Richard Steele, *The Tatler*, No. 38, 1709

In many GMP guidelines, including the EC GMP Guide (EC, 1992), one of the longest sections is the one which covers that most powerfully soporific subject 'documentation'. It is surprising, however, to note that in the context of the great emphasis the FDA investigators place on document review, the US CGMPs (US FDA, 1990) have no separate section on documentation.

It would be a mistake to conclude that the general emphasis on 'the paperwork' (or its modern electronic equivalent) is just one more expression of the innate bureaucratic urges of the government departments which, by and large, are responsible for the publication of GMP guidelines. Documentation is, in fact, the main structural supporting member, indeed the backbone, of any system of quality assurance.

Documentation for quality assurance

In essence it is all very simple. It is about establishing written instructions for all significant activities, about following those instructions in practice, and about making records of those activities. The objectives are, in short:

1. To state clearly, in advance and in writing, what is to be done;
2. To do it – in accordance with those instructions; and
3. To record what was done, and the results of doing it.

Good reasons for documentation

There are a number of very good practical and patient-safety reasons for proceeding in this way. The reasons for documentation are:

1.   To be clear about what has to be done, by having formally approved instructions for each job, and then following them.
2.   To define standards for materials, equipment, premises, services and products.
3.   To confirm, as work proceeds, that each step has been carried out, and carried out correctly, using the correct materials and equipment.
4.   In the longer term, to keep for reference records of what has been done, for example manufacturing and test records, installation, commissioning, servicing and maintenance records.
5.   To enable investigation of complaints, defect reports and any other problems, and to permit observation of any drifts away from defined quality standards.
6.   To help decide on, and take, any necessary corrective action (including action to prevent re-occurrence) in the event of any complaint or defect report.

A further very good reason for documentation is to overcome a common human failing. The great majority of us are, like Hamlet, 'indifferent honest'. That is, we are pretty honest, pretty well most of the time. At opposite ends of the honesty spectrum are the few that are always totally honest, on the one hand, and the congenital liars, on the other. Both species are relatively rare. If a manufacturing instruction reads, for example, 'After 15 minutes, check that the temperature is between 42°C and 47°C', most people will conscientiously check that this is so – *on the first few occasions*, but may later drift into being less careful. If the instructions require that a temperature within the required range be confirmed by ticking and initialling in a box, the average 'indifferent honest' mind will be more acutely concentrated on ensuring that what is required is indeed done properly, but may well begin to lapse after the process has been performed scores, or even hundreds, of times. The best assurance is provided by an instruction which reads along the lines of: 'After 15 minutes, check the temperature, which should be between 42°C and 47°C. Record the temperature reading in the box, and initial. If the temperature is outside this range, report this immediately to the Section Head.' Few people will then be inclined to enter a completely false, or 'invented' reading. A more precise record will have been made, which may be used for later investigation or review.

Documentation helps to build up a detailed picture of what a manufacturing function has done in the past and what it is doing now, and thus provides a basis for planning what it is going to do in the future.

One common GMP recommendation is that manufacturers should, from time to time, carry out detailed reviews of their own operations – that is, perform 'self inspections', or 'internal quality audits'. Detailed reviews of past records and documents are a great aid in doing this. Certainly, government inspectors, during their inspections of manufacturing sites, often spend much time examining a company's documents and records. It has been suggested that some regulatory agencies adopt the official attitude that 'if there are not detailed instructions it will not be done, and if a written record has not been made and retained, it has not been done'. While this may be something of an extreme position, it is a useful thought to keep in mind. Another way of looking at it is that 'documentation is quality assurance made visible'.

The UK Orange Guide states as a principle (Sharp, 1983):

> Documentation is a prime necessity in Quality Assurance. Its purposes are to define the system of control, to reduce the risk of error inherent in purely oral communication, to ensure that personnel are instructed in the details of, and follow, the procedures concerned, and to permit investigation and tracing of defective products. The system of documentation should be such that the history of each batch of product, including the utilisation and disposal of starting materials, packaging materials, bulk and finished products may be determined.

The corresponding principle in the EC GMP Guide reads (EC, 1992):

> Good documentation constitutes an essential part of the quality assurance system. Clearly written documentation prevents errors from spoken communication, and permits tracing of batch history. Specifications, Manufacturing Formulae and Instructions, procedures and records must be free from errors and available in writing. The legibility of documents is of paramount importance.

One comment that might be made on this last statement is that it is dangerous to assume complacently that anything will *prevent* error. The safe attitude is that errors can, will and do occur. What we have to do is strive to reduce the chances of error to a minimum, and to minimise the severity of the consequences of errors if and when they do occur. Towards the achievement of that aim, sound documentation can make a big contribution.

Types of documentation

The different types of document may be classified broadly as:

- Specifications.
- Manufacturing instructions and packaging instructions.
- Standard operating procedures.
- Records.

Specifications

These are documents that state the standards which different materials and products should meet, and they describe the tests which should be carried out to show compliance with those standards. Thus, there are written specifications for:

- Starting materials.
- Packaging materials.
- Intermediates.
- Bulk products.
- Finished products.

Manufacturing instructions and packaging instructions

These are the documents that list the materials (with quantities) to be used in manufacture and/or packaging, and they provide stepwise instructions for carrying out the various manufacturing (or packaging) operations and in-process checks and controls.

It is customary for this type of document first to be set up as a carefully checked and formally authorised Master, a facsimile copy of which is issued to cover each specific batch manufacturing or packaging run.

The UK Orange Guide and the EC GMP Guide use the following terminology to distinguish between master and batch documentation of this type.

Master documents
UK – 'Master formula and method'
EC – 'Manufacturing formula and processing instructions'

UK – 'Master packaging instruction'
EC – 'Packaging instruction'

Batch documents
UK – 'Batch manufacturing record'
EC – 'Batch processing record'

UK – 'Batch packaging record'
EC – 'Batch packaging record'

The US CGMPs are somewhat less specific in their terminology, as well as being rather more diffuse in their coverage of documentation. They refer to 'written procedures', 'batch production and control records' 'appropriate master production or control records' and the like, all in a relatively non-specific fashion.

As is made quite clear in the UK and EC guidelines, the entirely sensible intention is that batch manufacturing records and batch packaging records should be compiled, as manufacturing or packaging proceeds, by making appropriate entries on the facsimile copy of the respective master document.

In this way, as a manufacturing or packaging operation proceeds, a complete record is built up of what happens, as it happens. If it is all done properly, operators will know precisely what they have to do, and it will be possible to determine later whether or not they have done it, and done it correctly. It will also be possible to determine, at any one time, the stage reached in a process, in case it becomes necessary to pause or break off, giving rise to a need to be absolutely sure just where to restart. Finally, when the process is completed, there will be a record of precisely what was done. If carefully kept, that record will, in the future, make it possible to carry out any necessary investigations, and take any necessary actions.

Standard operating procedures (SOPs)

These are commonly used to give instructions and information on how to carry out a wide range of operations which are not necessarily specific to any particular product or batch. There are many possible SOPs. Just a few examples are SOPs on:

- Receipt of materials
- General stores procedures
- Order picking, assembly and dispatch
- Dispensing procedures
- Issue of labels
- Issue of other packaging materials
- Calibrating and checking weighing equipment
- Calibration and maintenance of instruments
- Cleaning of areas and equipment
- Use of protective clothing
- Operator hygiene
- Operator training
- Set-up and operation of machines
- Machine and plant maintenance
- Packaging line clearance and start-up
- Complaints and recall procedures
- Process validation
- Analytical methods validation
- Computer systems validation.

The list of possibilities is almost endless.

Very often batch manufacturing instructions, or batch packaging instructions refer to one or more SOPs which need to be followed. It then of course becomes vital to ensure that the *correct current* SOP is, in fact, followed.

Records

Batch manufacturing and batch packaging records have already been mentioned above. There are a number of other records which need to be made, for example:

- Records of receiving and issuing materials
- Records of testing materials and products
- Distribution records
- Complaints records
- Training records
- Records of plant and equipment maintenance.

Making records

There are some important simple, and obvious, things to be remembered about making records, including entering a check signature or initials:

1. Records should always be made, or signatures, etc. entered, when (or immediately after) an action has been completed, a reading has been taken, or a check has been made. Records should always be made as things happen, not at the end of the shift, day or week. They should be about current, real-time, events not history.

2. A person entering a second check signature or initials is confirming that he or she actually saw what was done (for example, a weighing) and has personally checked that *everything* was correct (product, material, batch, quantity, reading or whatever). It is not good enough, and it could be very dangerous, for an operator to trust a 'mate' to have got it right, and write in second-check initials/signatures at, say, the end of the day or the shift.

3. Manuscript entries should always be neat and clear. They do not have to be beautiful, but operators need to be reminded that others may need to read these records in 5 or more years' time.

4. If a mistake is made when making a manuscript entry on a document, it should not be considered to be a crime. But if a mistake *is* made, it should not be obliterated or covered up. It should be crossed out neatly (so that it can still be read), the correction made and signed or initialled, and the date added, with any explanation that may be necessary.

Document control and revision

Issue and use of documents should be under formal control. They should be available to all who need them, and not available to those who do not. They should be kept up to date, but all revision should be formal and authorised, not haphazard. The documentation system overall should be subject to review. It is vital that systems exist for the removal from active use of outdated or superseded documents.

Retention of records

There is no point in making records unless they are retained for some useful period. How long that period should be will depend on the nature of the record and on what it will, or may be, used for, and here certain legal requirements come into play. Many national (and international) regulatory authorities require that records relating to manufacture, packaging (for some unfathomable reason referred to in UK regulations as 'assembly') and testing should be retained for specified minimum periods. In the UK it was originally 5 years. Article 22 (2) of Directive 75/319/EEC requires that 'the batch documentation shall be retained for at least one year after the expiry date of the batches to which it relates or for at least five years . . . (after release by a Qualified Person) . . . whichever is the longer'. Retained reference samples of products may also be regarded as 'records', and it is usually considered that they should be retained at least until 1 year after the expiry date of the batch of product concerned (EC requirement), or until such time as the batch may no longer be reasonably expected to be anywhere in stock or in use. The EC GMP Guide requires that samples of starting materials (other than solvents, gases and water) should be retained for at least 2 years after the release of the product(s) in which they were used.

Microfilm and electronic forms of data storage

Retaining large quantities of paper records can create storage space problems, and to overcome these, microfilm and microfiche records can be used. These are acceptable (both in a general sense, and to regulatory bodies) provided that the system will reproduce the data clearly, accurately and legibly. Care needs to be taken where interpretation of an original document depends on colour distinction. Thus, some form of annotation is needed where a black and white copy is made, say, of a multiple colour trace on a chart record. Original documents should be retained for at least 6 months, and not destroyed until the microfilm copies made from them have been checked for completeness and legibility.

Electronic document generation, data recording, storage and retrieval systems are increasingly being used. Given the usual provisos regarding system security, controlled access, system validation, back-up and ready availability of 'hard copy', such systems, if properly designed and implemented (and there, naturally, is the rub), can increase the level of assurance of quality that good documentation provides. Given these provisos, electronic documentation and data storage systems are generally accepted by regulatory authorities.

The EC GMP Guide Annex 11, on Computerized Systems, reads (in part):

> For quality auditing purposes, it should be possible to obtain clear printed copies of electronically stored data . . .
>
> Data should be secured by physical or electronic means against wilful or accidental damage. . . . Stored data should be checked for accessibility, durability and accuracy. If changes are proposed to the computer equipment or its programs, the above mentioned checks should be performed at a frequency appropriate to the storage medium being used . . .
>
> Data should be protected by backing-up at regular intervals. Back-up data should be stored as long as necessary at a separate and secure location.

Elsewhere (4.9) the EC GMP Guide also states:

> Data may be recorded by electronic data processing systems, photographic or other reliable means, but detailed procedures relating to the system in use should be available and the accuracy of the records should be checked. If documentation is handled by electronic data processing methods, only authorised persons should be able to enter or modify data in the computer and there should be a record of changes and deletions; access should be restricted by passwords or other means and the result of entry of critical data should be independently checked. Batch records electronically stored should be protected by back-up

transfer on magnetic tape, microfilm, paper or other means. It is particularly important that the data are readily available throughout the period of retention.

Details of the requirements for the content of the various different types of document or record, and of various other related matters, are to be found in the 'Documentation' section (No. 4) of the EC GMP Guide. Part 211.188 of the US CGMPs is shorter and much less detailed on this point.

Chapter 15 of this book provides some illustrations of key documents/records, indicative of appropriate content and in the form of suggested possible layouts.

Further considerations

Uninspiring topic though it may seem, documentation is a major element of quality assurance. Much attention needs to be given to the careful and effective design of documents so as to facilitate their proper use. Of particular importance is the need for unambiguous instructions, not only for the job in hand, but also for the use and/or completion of the document itself. Equally important is the need for careful control over revision and re-issue as required. There should be a system to ensure that obsolete documents are withdrawn, and cannot be (re)used.

All instructions to personnel should be clear, precise, unambiguous and written in numbered steps, in the imperative, and not as a general discursive essay in the passive mode. ('Weigh 500 grams of . . .' and *not* '500 grams is weighed'.) They should be written in a language, style and level of language that the user can readily understand.

Where a document requires the entry of data, sufficient space should be provided to permit the making of the entry in a clear and legible manner.

If a change is made to a process such that a particular step is no longer taken, or a record no longer made, this requirement should be formally removed from the relevant document immediately. To leave an instruction no longer followed, or a space (or 'box') for an entry no longer required, encourages the dangerous attitude that written instructions are not always mandatory.

Personnel should be trained in the use and completion of documents, record books and the like, and should be in no doubt about where and how they should record information, or the need to sign as having completed or checked an operation.

Importance of documentation

To conclude this chapter it is worth re-emphasising that, in the world of pharmaceutical and other healthcare manufacturing, documentation, far from being a drearily unnecessary bureaucratic exercise, is rightly to be considered as an important (indeed a major) element of quality assurance and good manufacturing practice.

Documentation is also to be accorded a similar importance in the manufacture of other products where quality is a crucial consideration. Certainly this is so on the evidence of the ISO 9000 Series, where documentation occupies a large part, perhaps even the major part, of this international 'quality systems' specification.

In addition to IS0 9000, virtually all texts on 'general quality', and its control, management, assurance, or whatever, indicate, explicitly or implicitly, a need for documentation in the form of specifications, manufacturing and test methods, various operating procedures, and a variety of records. Documentation is thus an essential quality tool, and this is particularly true of the manufacture of medicines and the like. There is however an important rider. Documentation is a means to an end, albeit a very vital end. Manufacturers, regulatory authorities, and others, should take care to ensure that it does not become an end in itself. Some regulatory authorities seem, regrettably, to have come to view it in that way.

References

EC (1992). *The Rules Governing Medicinal Products in the European Community, Vol. IV: Good Manufacturing Practice for Medicinal Products.* Luxembourg: Commission of the European Communities. Available from The Office for Official Publications of the European Communities, Luxembourg. Also available from The Stationery Office (HMSO), London, and The EC Information Service, Washington, USA. (Referred to as the EC GMP Guide.)

Sharp J, ed. (1983). *Guide to Good Pharmaceutical Manufacturing Practice,* 3rd edn. London: HMSO. (Referred to as the UK Orange Guide.)

US FDA (1990). *Code of Federal Regulations, Vol. 21, Ch. 1, Part 210,* Current good manufacturing practice in manufacturing, processing, packaging or holding of drugs, general; *CFR Vol. 21, Ch. 1, Part 211,* Current good manufacturing practice for finished pharmaceuticals; *CFR Vol. 21, Ch. 1, Part 820,* Good manufacturing practice for medical devices (revised 1995). Washington: US Food & Drug Administration. (Collectively referred to as the US CGMPs.)

15

Documentation in action

And enterprises of great pitch and moment . . . their currents turn awry,
and lose the name of action

W Shakespeare, *Hamlet*, Act 3, Sc. 1

The purpose of this chapter is to trace forward through a standard production cycle, from ordering and receipt of materials to despatch of finished product, illustrating this overall process with examples of key documents used, and the records maintained in quality-orientated manufacture. Illustrations will be given of major documentation and record types, with the exception of laboratory specifications, methods and records, which will be covered in Chapter 18 'Laboratory documentation'. It is important to keep in mind the purposes of documentation (see Chapter 14), and particularly to remember that the purpose is to ensure, and record, *correct action,* and not to be an end in itself.

The illustrative forms shown in this chapter are not intended to be immutably definitive, and are only to be taken as examples of possible layouts, with a form and content that are generally considered to be both suitable and acceptable. Individual manufacturers will have their own preferences, style and approach. It is also to be noted that this chapter was written at a time which might be said to be a turning point in the development of QA/GMP documentation. A number of manufacturers, particularly the larger ones, have turned, or are turning, to electronic documentation and record keeping. Nevertheless, worldwide, there is still a majority who relies largely upon manual/paper systems. For those who are not, this chapter may still serve as a basic indicator of what is required to be written in, and what data should be captured by, an electronic documentation system.

Starting materials: ordering, receipt, approval and issue

The term 'starting materials' is a European expression, defined as 'Any substance used in the production of a medicinal product but excluding packaging materials'. Other, more-or-less comparable expressions might be 'raw materials' or 'ingredients', although it should be noted that every starting material used in the manufacture of a product may well not remain as an ingredient of that product.

The US CGMPs use the term 'components' to refer to starting materials, and here there is a potential for confusion, for in the UK it is possible for 'component' to be taken as a shortened form of 'packaging component'. Other American expressions, now increasingly being used on the eastern side of the Atlantic, are 'bulk pharmaceutical chemicals' (BPCs) and 'active pharmaceutical ingredients' (APIs). Note: All APIs are BPCs, but not all BPCs are APIs.

Figure 15.1 is a flow diagram illustrating the ordering, receipt, sampling, approval (or rejection) and dispensing of starting materials, thus:

1. The Purchasing Department order the material on the basis of a starting material specification (see Chapter 18) provided to them by the Quality Control Department. Purchasing Department sends the order to an approved supplier, that is a company that has been approved, jointly by the Quality Control and Production Departments, to supply the material in question. (At the time of writing, the current expectation in the European Union is that requirements for compliance with GMP by, and inspection and approval of, starting materials' suppliers will become mandatory within the next year or so; then, depending on the form that this regulatory approval or certification takes, the supplier will need to be approved in a more formal regulatory sense.)

2. At the time of placing the order, the Purchasing Department sends a copy of the purchase order to the Goods Inwards (or Receiving) Department, where it is (accessibly) retained, pending the receipt of the goods.

3. On receipt, the goods are carefully examined by a responsible member of the Goods Inwards Department for amount/quantity and general condition, and to check for any signs of external damage, soiling or dampness. At the same time, the labelled identity of the delivered material is checked, and compared with the Goods Inwards copy of the purchase order, and with any supplier's delivery, or advice note, to confirm that the material delivered is, as far as its labelling is concerned, the material which was ordered. If there is any doubt about the nature or the quality of the goods delivered, the Quality Control Department is contacted immediately. A check is also made at this time on all the identity labels on the containers in a multi-container delivery. Different supplier's batches within one delivery are to be segregated, one from an other, with a different internal lot number for each entered on the Quarantine label now about to be applied to each container.

4. If all the containers in the delivery appear to be correct and in good condition, the Goods Inwards Department then place on each container a Quarantine label (see Fig. 15.2), with the entries for 'Code number', 'Name of material', 'Lot number' and 'Date received' completed. Notes:

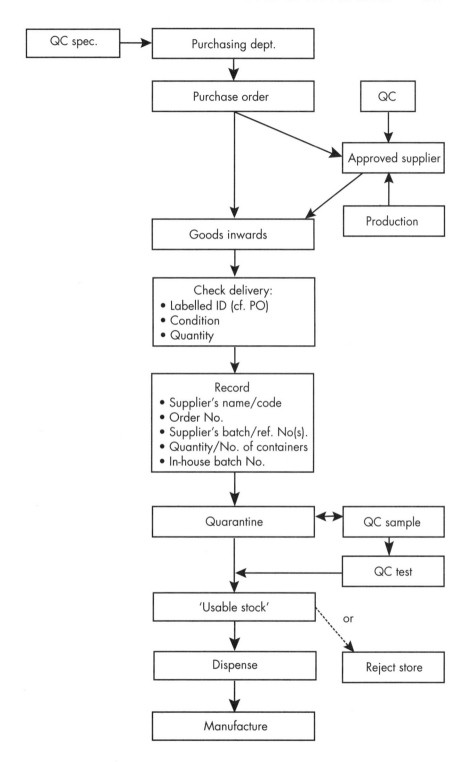

Figure 15.1   Pharmaceutical starting materials: documentation and process flow.

(a) It is useful to have the Quarantine label, and the Released and Rejected labels (see also Fig. 15.2) printed in different colours, for example, for 'Quarantine', black print on a yellow background, for 'Released' green print on a white background, and for 'Rejected' red print on a white background.

(b) In the examples shown, the intention is that the 'Released' (or 'Rejected') label, when the QC decision is made, should be applied just over the lower 'Quarantine' panel. This may seem an infringement of the golden rule about not applying new labels on top of old ones, but here (if the, say, Released label falls off, or is removed) the labelled status of the material reverts to Quarantine, i.e. it is fail-safe. The benefit of the labelling system illustrated is the elimination of any possible error in transcribing the information originally entered on the Quarantine label.

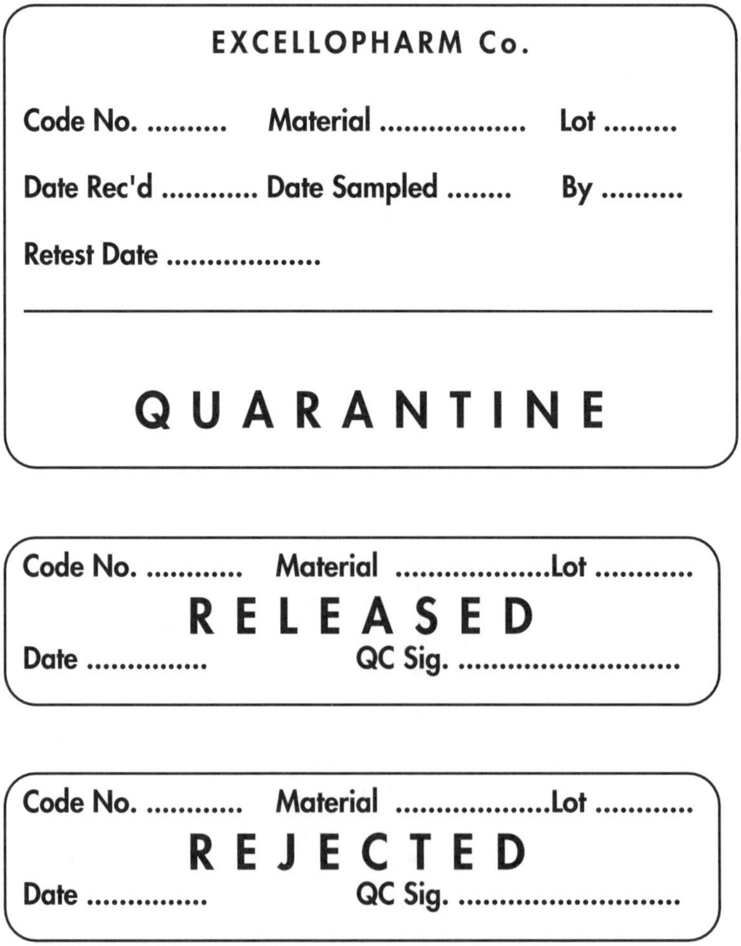

EXCELLOPHARM Co.

Code No. .... Material .... Lot ....

Date Rec'd .... Date Sampled .... By ....

Retest Date ....

QUARANTINE

Code No. .... Material ....Lot ....
RELEASED
Date .... QC Sig. ....

Code No. .... Material ....Lot ....
REJECTED
Date .... QC Sig. ....

Figure 15.2 Quarantine, Released and Rejected labels for pharmaceutical starting materials.

(c) It is important that at least the Quarantine label is in a recognisably 'house' style, with company name and/or logo, to avoid confusion with any other identity and status labels which may already be on the container(s).

5. Goods Inwards then complete a 'Materials Receiving Report' (Form 15.1) in four copies, retaining one copy and sending the other three to Quality Control. They then make the appropriate entries (except for entries in the last two columns) in a departmental running record – a 'Starting Materials Delivery Record' (see Form 15.2). This can be a printed sheet or card, or manually drawn up in a record book.

6. Receipt of the copies of the Materials Receiving Report alerts the Quality Control Department that the material has been delivered, and is required to be sampled. Following sampling ('Date sampled . . .' and 'By . . .' on the Quarantine label completed by sampler) and testing against the agreed specification, the QC decision is entered on the copies of Materials Receiving Report, one copy being sent to the Purchasing Department (for information), one to Materials Inventory Control (so, if material is released, it may be allocated to manufacturing batches), and one retained on QC file, with the full analytical report. An authorised member of the QC Department then places a Released (or Rejected as appropriate) label, over the Quarantine portion, with the necessary details entered and then enters a date at 'Retest date . . .' on the original label, to indicate when the material is due for re-examination. Note: Only the Quality Control Department should be authorised to hold stocks (securely), and apply, Released and Rejected labels.

7. On receipt of the QC decision, Goods Inwards either move the released goods into the usable stock area of the stores, or the rejected material to a secure reject store. The two last columns of the Starting Material Delivery Record (Form 15.2) are then completed ('Date approved by QC' and 'Location').

Packaging materials

The purchase, receipt, sampling, release and control of printed packaging materials and primary packaging materials (that is packaging materials which come into direct contact with the product, as compared with secondary packaging materials which do not) need to be accorded the same level of attention as given to starting materials. Documents, records and procedures analogous to those outlined above should be employed.

Standard operating procedures (SOPs)

The procedure to be followed will need to be defined in a standard operating procedure, an example of which is shown at Form 15.3. The content of

GOODS INWARDS – MATERIALS RECEIVING REPORT

Material .... **Code No** ....

INSTRUCTIONS: 1. Complete a separate Receiving Report for each delivery, and for each supplier's batch number within a delivery.
2. Retain one copy in Goods Inwards file, and send three copies to Quality Control.
3. **Quality Control:** On completion of testing, mark this report, where indicated, "RELEASED", "REJECTED", "HOLD" as appropriate, and send a copy to:
   Purchasing Department
   Materials Inventory Control

   Retain one copy on Quality Control files

Date goods received   ....

Supplier   ....

Supplier's batch No.   ....

Quantity received   ....

Number of containers   ....

Purchase Order No.   ....

Assigned Lot No.   ....

General condition/cleanliness of delivery   ....

....

....

....

Delivery examined by (Signed) .... Date ....

Remarks/Comments

QUALITY CONTROL DECISION

STARTING MATERIAL DELIVERY RECORD

Date of Delivery	Material	Code Number	Lot Number	Quantity	Number of Containers	Supplier	Delivery Note Number	Supplier's Batch No(s)	Supplier's Name for Material	Date Approved by QC	Location

Edition: 3-7-97

EXCELLOPHARM Co – Standard Operating Procedure

S.O.P. No:	Date Issued:	Supersedes S.O.P. No: New Document	Review Date:	Page 1 of 4

STARTING MATERIALS – GOODS INWARDS PROCEDURE

Contents	Page
1. PURPOSE	2
2. SCOPE	2
3. RESPONSIBILITY	2
4. REVISION	2
5. PROCEDURE	3

Written by:	Approved by:	Authorised by:
Date:	Date:	Date:

Edition: 3-7-97

S.O.P. No _____ **Page 2 of 4**

1. Purpose

To define the procedure to be followed on receipt of a delivery of starting material (ingredients or raw materials).

2. Scope

This S.O.P. applies to all deliveries of starting materials whatever their nature or source.

3. Responsibility

Routine responsibility for ensuring that this procedure is implemented as and when necessary rests with the Head of the Goods Inwards Department.

Writing and approval/authorisation of this procedure, and ensuring that it is revised and up-dated as necessary is the responsibility of ....

4. Revision

This procedure must be re-written, approved and authorised whenever any change in method of operation, or any other circumstance, indicates the need. It must be reviewed every 12 months from the date of issue, in the light of current practice, to determine whether any revision is necessary.

All copies of S.O.P.(s) which are superseded by any revision must be withdrawn from active use, and appropriate change-control records maintained to ensure effective implementation of this requirement.

Edition: 3-7-97

S.O.P. No   **Page 3 of 4**

5. Procedure

5.1 On receipt, all deliveries must be carefully examined by a responsible member of Goods Inwards personnel for general condition, and to check for any signs of external damage, soiling and dampness. At the same time, the labelled identity of the delivered material should be checked, and compared with the Goods Inwards copy of the Purchase Order and with any supplier's Delivery, or Advice, Note to confirm that the material delivered is, as far as its label(s) are concerned, the material that was ordered. If there is any doubt about the nature or the quality of the goods delivered, contact the Quality Control Department immediately.

5.2 At the same time, check the supplier's Batch (or Lot) numbers on the identity labels to confirm whether or not (in a delivery where there is more than one container) all containers contain material from the same supplier's batch. NOTE: Different supplier's batches within one delivery should be segregated, and a different internal LOT NUMBER for each entered on the QUARANTINE label.

5.3 If the material (**all** containers) appears to be correct and in good condition, label each container with a standard QUARANTINE label, with the required entries on the label completed. That is, enter on the label(s):

> Code number
> Name of material
> Lot number
> Date received

5.4 Complete a 'GOODS INWARDS – MATERIALS RECEIVING REPORT' (four-part set), retaining one copy on Goods Inwards files, and sending the other three copies to Quality Control.

5.5 At the same time, complete the columns of the STARTING MATERIALS DELIVERY RECORD as follows (NOTE – Make a separate series of entries for each internal Lot Number – see 5.2 above):

5.5.1 DATE – Enter date of delivery of the material

5.5.2 MATERIAL – Enter name of the material, as it appears on our Purchase Order.

5.5.3 CODE NUMBER – Enter our company code number for the material.

5.5.4 LOT NUMBER – Enter our internal Lot Number, which should be the same as the Lot Number which has been entered on the QUARANTINE label(s). NOTE: See 5.2 above.

Form 15.3 continues over

Edition: 3-7-97

S.O.P. No   **Page 4 of 4**

5.5.5 QUANTITY – Enter the quantity received.

5.5.6 NUMBER OF CONTAINERS – Enter the number of containers received per each Lot Number.

5.5.7 SUPPLIER – Enter the name of the supplier of the material.

5.5.8 DELIVERY NOTE NUMBER – Enter the reference number on the supplier's Delivery Note (or Invoice – or other delivery documentation).

5.5.9 SUPPLIER'S BATCH NUMBER – Enter the supplier's batch number for the material as it appears on the delivered container(s). See 5.2 above

5.5.10 SUPPLIER'S NAME FOR MATERIAL – Enter the name of the material as it appears on the supplier's label(s) and on the delivery note or invoice (etc.). If it is the same as the name already entered under 'Material', enter 'same'.

5.6 That completes the action necessary immediately on receipt of material. The material should be held safely and securely, taking note of any special storage requirements (see S.O.P. No.XXXX 'Special Storage Requirements for Starting Materials'), until it has been sampled by Quality Control, and a 'RELEASED' or 'REJECTED' decision has been made. An authorised member of the Quality Control Department will then apply 'RELEASED' (or 'REJECTED') labels to the Quarantined goods.

5.7 When the material is released for use by QC, enter the date in the 'DATE APPROVED BY QC' column of the Delivery Record, and move the approved goods into usable stock. Make note of its location (by pallet position) under 'LOCATION' in the Delivery Record.

5.8 If the material is rejected, enter 'REJECTED', plus date, under 'DATE APPROVED BY QC' and move the goods into the Reject Store, to await a decision on the disposition of the material.

this illustrative SOP is along the lines indicated above. It may also be taken as an example of general requirements for SOPs.

Features of SOPs

Standard features expected and required of SOPs in general, which this example illustrates, are as follows:

1. Each SOP should have a number, or alpha-numeric code, by which it can be specifically identified. To that number, or code, should be added a suffix (or an edition date displayed), so that it is possible to check that the currently approved version of the SOP is in use.
2. The 'Date issued' and 'Supersedes' entries also serve to aid this assurance, and to help make possible a document change control system.
3. The master copy should bear the (dated) signatures of the persons who wrote the document, who approved it (normally the production, or in this case the warehousing, manager) and who finally authorised it (normally a senior manager within the quality function).
4. All pages should be numbered, as indicated.
5. An SOP should commence with a clear and unequivocal statement of purpose and scope.
6. Responsibility for ensuring the implementation of the SOP, and for its revision and updating should be clearly stated.
7. The procedure to be followed should be stated in numbered steps in clear, simple and direct language.

Issue of materials for manufacture

In some manufacturing companies, the material dispensing and checking operation is recorded on a separate dispensing record sheet. It is more common, and conveniently reliable, for this operation to be covered by part of a copy of the Master Batch Manufacturing Formula, Method and Record (or some such similar title). This is the approach which is illustrated by the example document, Form 15.4.

In addition, the Starting Materials Store will need to keep a separate record, for each batch delivery, of receipts issues and balances. A possible layout is suggested in Form 15.5. This information could be recorded in a card index, in a book, or on a computer. The importance of such a record extends beyond materials inventory control and accounting. It enables comparisons to be made between 'book' and actual physical stocks. This could be invaluable in investigating, and perhaps preventing, manufacturing errors.

It is worth noting one or two special points regarding the Batch Manufacturing Formula, Method and Record (see Form 15.4):

1. On the first page (under the Formula and Weighing Record), provision is made for the entry of the names, in block capitals, of the dispenser,

Edition: 1-5-98
EXCELLOPHARM Co.
Page 1 of 4

BATCH MANUFACTURING FORMULA, METHOD and RECORD

OPPROBRIUM APOSTATE OINTMENT 2.5%	**BATCH NO.**
Form: ANHYDROUS OINTMENT	Batch Size: 2000 kg

PROCESS START AND COMPLETION TIMES
START: TIME: COMPLETION: TIME:
      DATE: DATE:

FORMULA and WEIGHING RECORD

MATERIAL	CODE	AMOUNT	LOT No.	DISPENSED BY	CHECKED BY
WHITE SOFT PARAFFIN UP	123	1750.00 kg			
HEAVY LIQUID PARAFFIN UP	130	200.00 kg			
OPPROBRIUM APOSTATE UP	1,376	50.00 kg			

Name of dispenser* .... Initials .... Name of checker* .... Initials ....
*Enter names in block capitals

MANUFACTURING LOCATION: Processing room no. 3b, Block B
MAJOR EQUIPMENT: Dedicated ointment manufacturing equipment –
                     OINTTECH KV2 MILL.
                     Steam-jacketed PZ/2 S/S MIXING VESSEL, fitted with HITECH 2 STIRRER
                     Mobile S/S holding tank.
                     Dedicated transfer pipework and pump.

Batch document issued by .... Date ....

MASTER DOCUMENT EFFECTIVE 1-5-98		**SUPERSEDES: 10-7-95**
Prepared by:	Approved by: QC:	Production:
Date:	Date:	Date:

Form 15.4 continues over

Edition: 1-5-98
Page 2 of 4

BMR: OPPROBRIUM APOSTATE OINTMENT 2.5%	**BATCH SIZE: 200 kg**

MANUFACTURING INSTRUCTIONS & RECORD

Name of operator* .... Initials .... Name of checker* .... Initials ....
*Enter names in block capitals

		DATE	TIME	OP'TOR	CHECK
1. Check the Plant Log, and enter details of following:					
1.1 Previous equipment use: Product					
B. No.					
Date					
1.2 Last equipment cleandown (SOP 03.16)					
Date					
2. Obtain clearance from Production supervisor and QC that equipment is clean and ready for use:					
PRODUCTION CLEARANCE					
QC CLEARANCE					
3. Add the 50.00 kg Opprobrium apostate to the 200.00 kg Heavy liquid paraffin in a clean stainless steel container and stir by hand, using a stainless steel rod.					
4. Immediately transfer the slurry to the KV2 mill.					
5. Mill at MEDIUM speed setting for 15 minutes					
Mill start time					
Mill stop time					
6. Open valve to supply steam to jacket of PZ/2 mixing vessel, and transfer the 1750.00 kg White soft paraffin to the mixing vessel.					
7. When the temperature of the molten White soft paraffin reaches 70 to 75°C close the steam valve and commence stirring at speed setting 5. Record the temperature of the melt: Temperature					
8. While stirring continues, add the slurry from the mill to the molten White soft paraffin in the mixing vessel.					
9. As mixture in mixing vessel cools, continue to stir for a total of 2.5 hours. Stirrer start time					
Stirrer stop time					

Etc. Etc. Etc.

Form 15.4 continues over

258

Edition: 1-5-98
Page 4 of 4

BMR: OPPROBRIUM APOSTATE OINTMENT 2.5%	BATCH SIZE: 200 kg

MANUFACTURING INSTRUCTIONS & RECORD (Contd.)

Etc. Etc. Etc.

	DATE	TIME	OP'TOR	CHECK
13. Pump ointment to tared mobile stainless steel holding tank.				
14. Weigh holding tank (and contents) on floor scales, record gross weight, and enter net yield of bulk ointment.				

13. Pump ointment to tared mobile stainless steel holding tank.

14. Weigh holding tank (and contents) on floor scales, record gross weight, and enter net yield of bulk ointment.

               Gross weight (tank + ointment)   ....

               Tare   ....

               Yield of bulk ointment   ....

STANDARD ACCEPTABLE BULK YIELD – 1950 to 2050 kg

14. Arrange for sample of bulk product to be taken by QC sampler

AUTHORISED DEVIATIONS FROM STANDARD PROCEDURE:

PRIOR AUTHORISATION: Production .... **Date** .... **QC** .... **Date** ....

NON-STANDARD EVENT RECORD (Include explanation of any non-standard yield):

PRODUCTION CERTIFICATION: Apart from any authorised deviations, or non-standard events, as recorded above, this batch has been manufactured in accordance with this BATCH MANUFACTURING FORMULA, METHOD and RECORD.

               Signed .... Production supervisor

               Date   ....

QUALITY CONTROL APPROVAL FOR PACKAGING

This bulk batch of OPPROBRIUM APOSTATE OINTMENT 2.5%, Batch No. ....
has been sampled and tested, and is RELEASED FOR PACKAGING.

               Signed .... Quality Control

               Date   ....

IF BATCH IS NOT RELEASED, FOR ANY REASON, BOLDLY DELETE THIS SECTION AND RECORD REASON

MATERIALS STOCK RECORD

Code No. ...... (a) .... Material .... (b) .... Supplier ....

Date received ....   Lot Number ....

Date released ....   Amount to stock .... (c) ....

Date ....   Amount issued ....
                                               Balance   ....

Date ....   Amount issued ....
                                               Balance   ....

Date ....   Amount issued ....
                                               Balance   ....

Date ....   Amount issued ....
                                               Balance   ....

Date ....   Amount issued ....
                                               Balance   ....

Date ....   Amount issued ....
                                               Balance   ....

Date ....   Amount issued ....
                                               Balance   ....

(a) i.e. Internal company code number for material
(b) i.e. Name of material as ordered
(c) i.e. Quantity of released material passed to usable stock.

and of the checker, against their respective initials. The same provision appears at the top of page 2, in relation to the manufacturing operator and checker. At the time of writing, this is not a common practice, but it deserves to be widely adopted. It overcomes the problem of attempting to interpret indecipherable signatures some time after the event. Perhaps more importantly, it also serves to concentrate the minds, before the event, of dispensers, operators and checkers on the importance of what they are doing, and their personal responsibility to do it properly.

2. Page 1 clearly indicates the manufacturing location, and the major items of equipment that are to be used.

3. Against each step in the manufacturing process, it may be necessary to record a date, time and a check, in addition to the operator initials. This requirement could well be variable, and this is illustrated, and catered for, by the way the various 'boxes' are arranged under each column heading, and against each instruction.

4. Before manufacture commences, a record is required of the previous product/batch which was manufactured using the equipment, plus confirmation that this equipment has been cleaned, plus confirmation that it is, in fact, clean (Instruction Nos. 1 and 2).

5. At completion of manufacture of the bulk product, provision is made for the recording of:

    (a) Authorised deviations.
    (b) Non-standard events.
    (c) Certification by Production that, apart from (a) or (b), the batch has been manufactured in accordance with these instructions.
    (d) Quality control approval for packaging.

Batch packaging

An illustrative example of Batch Packaging Instructions and Record is shown in Form 15.6, which should be largely self-explanatory. Noteworthy points are:

1. Provision for making and recording the crucially important line clearance and cleaning checks (page 2, A 1), and the on-line printing data (page 2, B 2).

2. The integral In-process Control Record (page 4).

3. The final provision for qualified person release for distribution.

Distribution

In the UK, it is a regulatory requirement that manufacturers of medicinal products shall keep such documents as will 'facilitate the withdrawal or

Edition: 2-7-98
EXCELLOPHARM Co.
Page 1 of 5

BATCH PACKAGING INSTRUCTIONS and RECORD

OPPROBRIUM APOSTATE OINTMENT 2.5% **20g Tubes**	**BATCH No.** Batch Size: 2000 kg Bulk Expected Yield: 95,200 20g tubes
PACKAGING START AND COMPLETION TIMES START: TIME: DATE:	COMPLETION: TIME: DATE:

BULK PRODUCT REQUIRED:

MATERIAL	AMOUNT	BATCH NO.	ISSUED BY	CHECKED BY
OPPROBRIUM APOSTATE 2.5% OINT.	2000 kg			

UNIT PACKAGING MATERIALS REQUIRED:

MATERIAL	CODE	AMOUNT	LOT NO.	ISSUED BY	CHECKED BY
PRINTED TUBES – 'OPPROBRIUM APOSTATE 2.5%'	PT 035	95,200			
LEAFLET	OA 014	95,200			
PRINTED UNIT CARTON	PC 021	95,200			

MULTIPLE PACKAGING MATERIALS: UNITS per MULTIPLE – 10× CARTONED TUBES

MATERIAL	AMOUNT	LOT NO.	ISSUED BY	CHECKED BY
PRINTED 10× 'OPPROBRIUM APOSTATE' OUTER CARTON	9,520			

PACKAGING LOCATION: Room no. 4, Block B
PACKAGING LINE: HUMBOLDT-SMITHERS AUTO. OINTMENT PACKAGING AND CARTONING
LINE NUMBER 2.

Batch document issued by ....   Date ....

MASTER DOCUMENT EFFECTIVE: 2-7-98   **SUPERSEDES: 10-8-95**

Prepared by:	Approved by: QC:	Production:
Date:	Date:	Date:

BATCH PACKAGING RECORD: **OPPROBRIUM APOSTATE OINTMENT 2.5%** **20g TUBES**	**BATCH SIZE:** 200 kg/ c. 95,200 20g tubes

PACKAGING INSTRUCTIONS

A. Line clearance and cleaning check

1. Check that the packaging line and equipment is clear of all previous, or any other product, packaging materials, labels, leaflets instructions and the like, and that the line and all associated equipment has been cleaned in accordance with SOP XXX "INSTRUCTIONS FOR CLEANING HUMBOLDT-SMITHERS AUTOMATIC OINTMENT PACKAGING AND CARTONING EQUIPMENT AND LINE"

LINE CLEARANCE and CLEANING CHECKED by.......................... CONFIRMED by.................
                                          TIME/DATE .... TIME/DATE   ....

2. Record details of previous product and batch packaged on this line:

   Previous product .... Batch Number .... Signed ....

B. On-line print data check

1. Check that the tube-crimper has been set up to print the correct batch code number on the tubes.

   Batch code to be printed on tubes is ....
   Checked by .... Time/Date ....

2. Check that the batch code, and other on-line printed information, to be printed on the unit cartons is as specified. Take a sample carton, printed with this information, and attach to the back of this record.

On-line carton printer set up to print required data. Checked by ....
                                          Time/Date ....

C. Packaging operation

1. Check that the general appearance/condition of the bulk ointment is satisfactory, and that its labelled identity and batch number is as entered under 'Bulk Product Required' on Page 1. Checked by ....

2. Set the ointment filler to fill 20.5 g per tube, and proceed to fill and package the ointment in accordance with SOP XXY 'INSTRUCTIONS FOR FILLING AND PACKAGING OINTMENTS, USING THE HUMBOLDT-SMITHERS AUTOMATIC LINE'.

Etc. Etc.

Form 15.6 continues over

BATCH PACKAGING RECORD: OPPROBRIUM APOSTATE OINTMENT 2.5% 20g TUBES	**BATCH SIZE:** 200 kg/ c. 95,200 20g tubes

IN-PROCESS CONTROL RECORD   **Batch Number** ....

TIME –													
Checks for ID, Clean, Defects	a. Tubes												
	b. Caps												
Fill Weight –													
Cap – Seal/Tightness	Sample 1												
	Sample 2												
	Sample 3												
	Sample 4												
	Tubes												
Checks for – ID & Defects	Leaflets												
	Cartons												
	Outers												
Tube print	B N												
Carton Overprint	BN												
	EXP												
	MFG												
Shipping Case Marking	BN												
	EXP												
	MFG												
Checked by													
Comment													

Form 15.6 continues over

Edition: 2-7-98
Page 5 of 5

BATCH PACKAGING RECORD: OPPROBRIUM APOSTATE OINTMENT 2.5% 20g TUBES	BATCH SIZE: 200 kg/ c. 95,200 20g tubes

Etc. Etc.

13. On receipt of QC/QP approval, send total yield of finished packaged goods to Finished Products Warehouse, obtaining a documented receipt for the batch and quantity supplied.

AUTHORISED DEVIATIONS FROM STANDARD PROCEDURE:

PRIOR AUTHORISATION: Production .... **Date**............ **QC**................ **Date**..........

NON-STANDARD EVENT RECORD (Include explanation of any non-standard yield):

PRODUCTION CERTIFICATION: Apart from any authorised deviations, or non-standard events, as recorded above, this batch has been manufactured in accordance with the relevant BATCH MANUFACTURING FORMULA, METHOD and RECORD, and packaged in accordance with this BATCH PACKAGING RECORD.

Signed .... Production Manager
Date ....

QUALIFIED PERSON RELEASE

This bulk batch of OPPROBRIUM APOSTATE OINTMENT 2.5%, Batch No. ....
has been sampled and tested, and found satisfactory, all documentation has been reviewed, and all relevant factors have been taken into consideration, and this batch is released for distribution.

Signed .... Quality Control
Date ....

IF BATCH IS NOT RELEASED, FOR ANY REASON, BOLDLY DELETE THIS SECTION AND RECORD REASON

recall from sale . . .'. The US CGMPs (211.196) are more explicit in requiring that (US FDA, 1990):

> Distribution records shall contain the name and strength of the product, and description of the dosage form, name and address of the consignee, date and quantity shipped, and lot or control number.

The most simple way of doing this is to record lot numbers on retained copies of customer invoices. This is perhaps easiest with computerised order processing and invoicing systems.

Complaints, defect report, and recall procedures

Concern for quality does not cease after products leave the manufacturer. Attention, for example, needs to be given to dealing with customer complaints, defect reports and recalls, which are to be regarded as the potential, or actual, consequences of quality failure. Proper provision to cover, act and record in such eventualities are a virtually global regulatory requirement. Examples of a 'Complaints and Defect Report Procedure', a 'Complaint/ Defect Report Record', and a 'Recall, or Freeze, Procedure' are shown in Forms 15.7, 15.8 and 15.9, respectively.

Reference

US FDA (1990). *Code of Federal Regulations, Vol. 21, Ch. 1, Part 210,* Current good manufacturing practice in manufacturing, processing, packaging or holding of drugs, general; *CFR Vol. 21, Ch. 1, Part 211,* Current good manufacturing practice for finished pharmaceuticals; *CFR Vol. 21, Ch. 1, Part 820,* Good manufacturing practice for medical devices (revised 1995). Washington: US Food & Drug Administration. (Collectively referred to as the US CGMPs.)

EXCELLOPHARM Co – Standard Operating Procedure

S.O.P. No:	Date Issued:	Supersedes S.O.P. No: New Document	Review Date:	Page 1 of 5

COMPLAINTS and DEFECT REPORT PROCEDURE

Contents   **Page**

Written by: Date:	Approved by: Date:	Authorised by: Date:

Form 15.7 continues over

S.O.P. No   **Page 2 of 5**

1. Purpose

To define the procedure to be followed on receipt of any product complaint or defect report.

2. Scope

This S.O.P. applies to all complaints and/or defect reports that are received or notified regarding products supplied/distributed by our Company, whatever their nature or source.

3. Responsibility

Routine responsibility for ensuring that this procedure is implemented as and when necessary rests with ....

Writing and approval/authorisation of this procedure, and ensuring that it is revised and up-dated as necessary is the responsibility of ....

4. Revision

This procedure must be re-written, approved and authorised whenever any change in method of operation, or any other circumstance, indicates the need. It must be reviewed every 12 months from the date of issue, in the light of current practice, to determine whether any revision is necessary.

All copies of S.O.P.(s) which are superseded by any revision must be withdrawn from active use, and appropriate change-control records maintained to ensure effective implementation of this requirement.

Form 15.7 continues over

5. Procedure

5.1 Complaints regarding product-quality, reports of defective products and the like, may be received in a number of formats (written or oral), at second or third hand, and from a number of sources, for example:

    a. From within the Company.
    b. From some point within the distribution chain.
    c. From customers, users or patients.
    d. From the UK (e.g. the Medicines Control Agency – MCA), or from some other National or International Regulatory Health Authority (e.g. the EU).

5.2 In all cases, the initial receipt of the complaint/defect report, whatever its nature, format or source, must be recorded **immediately** by the recipient on a 'COMPLAINT/DEFECT REPORT RECORD' form (see copy attached). Supplies of these forms will be available to, and held by, all those who are likely to receive such reports.

5.3 Overall responsibility for dealing with Complaints and Defect Reports will rest with (A). In the absence of (A) the deputies who will assume this responsibility are (B) (C)...................

5.4 Following receipt of a complaint/defect report, and on completion of parts 1 to 9 of the 'Complaint/Defect Report Record', the form, together with any relevant correspondence attached, must be passed immediately to (A) or in his/her absence to one of the designated deputies (see 5.3 above).

5.5 (A), or one of the designated deputies will review the report and decide whether any immediate action is necessary.

5.6 IMMEDIATE ACTION must be considered if the complaint/report is indicative of
    a. An actual or potential hazard to life, health or well-being of a user or consumer.
    b. A defect which, while not necessarily hazardous, could adversely affect the standing and reputation of our Company.

'Immediate action' may also be considered necessary where the defect renders the product difficult or inconvenient in use.

5.7 Immediate Actions to be considered, and implemented according to the actual or potential seriousness of the known or suspected hazard, include:

Form 15.7 continues over

S.O.P. No _____   **Page 4 of 5**

    a. 'Freezing' of all relevant Company stocks held on site.

    b. Reviewing distribution records, and requesting all points in the distribution chain to 'freeze' all relevant stocks, and not to use them or distribute them further.

    c. Initiation of a RECALL.

    e. Informing the Defective Medicines Report Centre (DMRC) of the Medicines Control Agency (MCA). (**NOTE**: It is a legal requirement that the DMRC must be informed of any defect in a medicinal product which could result in a recall or restriction on supply.)

5.8 If the decision is to 'freeze' (at any level) beyond Company stocks held on the Company site, or to recall, then reference must be made to the RECALL (or 'FREEZE') PROCEDURE, S.O.P. No. ...., which must be implemented immediately.

5.9 If the decision is made that it is necessary to freeze Company stocks only, pending further investigation, then those responsible for holding/maintaining in-house stocks should be informed orally immediately, with confirmation in writing as soon as possible. The information conveyed should include

    a. Name of Product(s)

    b. Batch Number(s)

    c. Nature of Defect (if and as appropriate)

    d. Precise action to be taken.

N.B. Particular care must be taken over any suspect goods which have been already assembled and are ready for dispatch.

5.10 If the complaint/defect report is not considered to be sufficiently serious as to warrant recall, freeze or any other emergency action, a letter of acknowledgement should be sent in response to all such reports received.

5.11 Whatever the action decided, arrangements must be made to have the complaint thoroughly investigated. Following these investigations, the remainder of the Complaint/Defect Report Record should be completed, and the person or body responsible for the original complaint informed of the results of the investigations, in writing.

5.12 The completed Complaint/Defect Report Record should be filed, along with all other relevant letters, papers and reports, and should be held in a filing system, such that they are readily retrievable for review and examination.

5.13 All records of complaints etc. should be periodically and formally reviewed in order to detect any adverse quality trends, 'common factors', etc.

Form 15.7 continues over

S.O.P. No   **Page 5 of 5**

MEDICINES CONTROL AGENCY: DEFECTIVE MEDICINES REPORT CENTRE

Address:

> Defective Medicines Report Centre,
> Medicines Control Agency,
> Room 1801, Market Towers,
> 1, Nine Elms Lane,
> LONDON SW8 5NQ.

Telephone Numbers:

Office Hours (08.30 to 17.45 Mon to Fri)	**0171 273 0574**
Other Times	**0171 210 5368/5371**
Fax. (Office Hours only)	**0171 273 0676**

(All telephone nos. checked as correct, as at ....)

COMPLAINT/DEFECT REPORT RECORD

1. **Date Complaint/Report received** .... **Time** ....

2. **Report received by** ....

3. **Received from:**
   - Name:
   - Address:

   - Telephone Number:
   - Fax. Number:

4. **Names/Addresses/Phone nos./Fax nos. of other Contacts/Persons/Organisations**

5. **Product(s) Concerned**

6. **Batch/Lot Number(s)**

7. **Nature of Complaint/Report**

8. **Have samples been returned for examination? (Give details)**

9. **Are samples available for collection/examination? (Give details)**

Page 1 of 2

Form 15.8 continues over

10. **Results of Investigations/Tests (Attach other sheets as necessary)**

11. **Conclusions, and Decision on Action to be Taken**

12. **Letter(s) Sent to:** **Date:**

13. **Also considered necessary to Inform:** **Done/Date:**

14. **Was Decision taken to FREEZE (beyond own on-site stocks) or RECALL?**

    (IF "YES", RECALL (and FREEZE) PROCEDURE SHOULD BE IMPLEMENTED)

    SIGNED..........................
    DATE   ....

Page 2 of 2

EXCELLOPHARM Co – Standard Operating Procedure

S.O.P. No:	Date Issued:	Supersedes S.O.P. No: New Document	Review Date:	Page 1 of 6

RECALL (or "FREEZE") PROCEDURE

Contents   **Page**

Written by: Date:	Approved by: Date:	Authorised by: Date:

S.O.P. No   **Page 2 of 6**

1. Purpose

To define the procedure to be followed in order to 'freeze' or recall products.
N.B. This S.O.P. should be read and followed in conjunction with S.O.P. No. ....'COMPLAINTS and DEFECT REPORT PROCEDURE'

2. Scope

This S.O.P. is to be implemented whenever a decision is taken to Recall, or 'freeze' any product(s), at any stage, for whatever reason.

3. Responsibility

Routine responsibility for ensuring that this procedure is implemented as and when necessary rests with ....

Writing and approval/authorisation of this procedure, and ensuring that it is revised and up-dated as necessary is the responsibility of ....

4. Revision

This procedure must be re-written, approved and authorised whenever any change in method of operation, or any other circumstance, indicates the need. It must be reviewed every 12 months from the date of issue, in the light of current practice, to determine whether any revision is necessary.

All copies of S.O.P.(s) which are superseded by any revision must be withdrawn from active use, and appropriate change-control records maintained to ensure effective implementation of this requirement.

5. Effectiveness of Procedure

This procedure should be practically evaluated from time-to-time (e.g. by performing internal 'dummy runs') to ensure that it is, and remains, capable of **prompt implementation at any time**, within or outside normal working hours.

Form 15.9 continues over

6. Procedure

6.1 An indication that a product, or product-batch, should be RECALLED, or placed on HOLD ('FROZEN') at some stage in the storage and/or distribution chain may arise from a number of sources, e.g.:

    a. From within the Company.

    b. From some point within the distribution chain.

    c. From customers, users or patients.

    d. From the UK (e.g. the Medicines Control Agency – MCA), or from some other national or International Regulatory Health Authority (e.g. the EU)

    e. From suppliers of products, materials or other goods.

    f. And/or via the COMPLAINTS and DEFECT REPORT RECORD(s) – See S.O.P. No...............

6.2 Overall responsibility for the co-ordination of all Recall or 'HOLD/FREEZE' will rest with (A). In the absence of (A) the deputies who will assume this responsibility are (B) (C) .... The decision to RECALL/FREEZE will be taken by the 'Recall Co-ordinator' in discussion with:

    ....

    ....

    ....

    ....

and with the Defective Medicines Report Centre (DMRC) of the Medicines Control Agency (MCA) and/or the local Medicines Inspectorate office, as necessary or appropriate.

6.3 Immediately the decision is taken to Recall/Freeze a product, or to issue any any other warnings outside the Company about the distribution or use of any product, the following Company Personnel (in addition to (A) and/or the designated deputies) must be informed at once:

    ....

    ....

    ....

    ....

6.4 At the same time, the Defective Medicines Report Centre (DMRC) of the MCA must also be informed of the incident, and of the action taken or proposed. (For telephone numbers etc. see Section 7 of this S.O.P. 'Contact Names, Telephone Numbers etc.').

Form 15.9 continues over

S.O.P. No   **Page 4 of 6**

6.5 The Recall Co-ordinator must immediately ensure (oral message, confirmed in writing) that all those, within the Company, concerned with the storage, packing and distribution of products and materials are aware of the problem and the action to be taken. The information conveyed should include:

    a. Name of Product(s)
    b. Batch Number(s)
    c. Nature of Defect
    d. Action to be taken.

6.6 All affected, or potentially affected, Kits and any other relevant stocks or materials must be securely segregated, and effectively quarantined so as to be sure they cannot be dispatched.

6.7 The Recall Co-ordinator (or his/her deputies) will arrange for the prompt preparation of a list of the recipients of the defective goods, down to the level at which the Recall or Freeze is to take place. He/she will then ensure that all the listed recipients are informed of:

    a. Name of Product(s)
    b. Batch Number(s)
    c. Nature of Defect
    d. Action to be taken.

According to the urgency/extent of potential hazard, this information should be conveyed by direct mailing, telephone call confirmed by mail, or fax. IF THE DEFECT IS CONSIDERED TO BE TOO SERIOUS TO PERMIT ANY DELAY, STEPS SHOULD BE TAKEN TO INFORM **ALL** POTENTIAL OR POSSIBLE RECIPIENTS WITHOUT NECESSARILY WAITING FOR THE COLLATION OF FULL DISTRIBUTION DATA.

6.8 If the defect is considered to represent a SERIOUS and IMMEDIATE HAZARD TO USERS or CONSUMERS, then consideration should be given (in consultation with MCA) to the use of the media to provide wider awareness of the problem.

6.9 When a Recall has been initiated, arrangements must be made by the Recall Co-ordinator to receive (or collect) the returned goods, and to ensure that they are securely segregated from other stock, such that there is no possibility that they could be re-distributed.

6.10 The progress of the Recall should be recorded and monitored, so that the

Form 15.9 continues over

S.O.P. No _____   **Page 5 of 6**

quantity of goods returned can be reconciled against the amount produced, distributed, and still held in stock.

6.11 When it is considered that the Recall/Freeze has been effected as completely as possible, a full report will be prepared by the Recall Co-ordinator (or deputy) detailing

     a. Reason for Recall/Freeze
     b. Results of full investigation into the cause(s) of the defective product.
     c. Action taken to Recall etc.
     d. Numerical details of the reconciliation exercise
     e. Action taken to prevent re-occurrence.

As required, a copy of this report should be sent to the DMRC of the MCA.

6.12 A list of contact names, addresses and telephone numbers, in and out of normal working hours follows on the next page. This information should be regularly checked for current accuracy, and amended as necessary.

Form 15.9 continues over

_____

7. CONTACT NAMES, TELEPHONE NUMBERS etc.
(For use in connection with Defect Reports, Recalls etc.)

COMPANY PERSONNEL

   Name: Extension: Home/Out-of-Hours No.:

MEDICINES CONTROL AGENCY: DEFECTIVE MEDICINES REPORT CENTRE

Address:

   Defective Medicines Report Centre,
   Medicines Control Agency,
   Room 1801, Market Towers,
   1, Nine Elms Lane,
   LONDON SW8 5NQ.

Telephone Numbers:

   Office Hours (08.30 to 17.45 Mon to Fri)   **0171 273 0574**
   Other Times   **0171 210 5368/5371**
   Fax. (Office Hours only)   **0171 273 0676**

   (All telephone nos. checked as correct, as at ....)

Part Five

Quality control

16

Quality control and good control laboratory practice (GCLP)

That lyf so short, the craft so long to lerne,
Th' assay so hard, so sharp the conquerynge
    G Chaucer (c. 1340–1400, *The Parliament of Fowls*

'Quality control' is not merely another term meaning more or less the same as 'quality assurance'. Quality assurance is a broader concept, which embraces quality control – plus a number of other factors (see Chapter 4). Quality control must nevertheless be considered as embracing rather more than just the laboratory testing of samples.

Quality control defined

There is however a very wide range of understanding of what precisely is meant by 'quality control'. Differences of opinion and interpretation still exist, both within the healthcare industry and between different regulatory bodies. Even wider differences have existed throughout the industrial world at large. For these present purposes, the definition will be taken as that which is given in the UK Orange Guide (Sharp, 1983):

> Quality Control – is that part of Good Manufacturing Practice which is concerned with sampling, specification and testing, and with the organisation, documentation and release procedures which ensure that the necessary and relevant tests are, in fact, carried out, and that materials are not released for use, nor products released for sale or supply, until their quality has been judged to be satisfactory. ('Quality Control' is sometimes used in the sense of the organisational entity which has responsibility for these functions.)

This same definition is repeated in the EC GMP Guide (EC, 1992), with only the substitution of 'actually' for 'in fact' and the deletion of the sentence in parenthesis.

So, quality control is about testing products, and the materials which are used in making those products, *but*, and it is a very important 'BUT', it is significantly more than that.

The wider aspects of quality control

There are many methods and techniques available to identify, to characterise, to isolate, to assay and to check the purity of the materials used, and
the products produced by, the industry. These techniques may be chemical,
physical, electronic, microbiological or biological. They can range from
simple, relatively crude, traditional volumetric or gravimetric methods, to
modern instrumental techniques (spectroscopic, chromatographic, calorimetric, voltametric, immunochemical, etc.) of ever-increasing sensitivity and
precision.

It is not the purpose of this chapter to deal with, or present a critique
of, these methods. They are all well described in the literature and in text-
books of analysis. Suffice it to say that a wide range of immensely powerful analytical tools is now available for use by the pharmaceutical quality
controller. It is however important to remember that, like all tools, their
ability to achieve the desired ends depends very largely on how they are
used. As is implicit in the definition quoted above, to be effective in controlling (and ultimately *assuring*) the quality of medicinal and like products,
these tools must be employed in the context of an organisation and a system
which embraces the sampling of materials and products, the establishment
of appropriate specifications and test methods, and well-controlled
release/reject mechanisms. In other words, quality control is laboratory
testing conducted in the context of good manufacturing practice (GMP),
and more specifically in accordance with good control laboratory practice
(GCLP).

A good, real-life example of a stark antithesis between a limited understanding of QC and true GCLP (and indeed of a failure of simple common
sense) is provided by an incident from the early days of inspection under the
UK Medicines Act (c. 1972). The Medicines Inspectorate received a report
from a regional hospital testing laboratory that a tablet product, from a
generics manufacturer, contained only around 60% of the claimed quantity
of active substance per tablet. This result was confirmed by further assays,
and an inspection of the manufacturer (at the time yet to be inspected) was
immediately scheduled. In a letter sent to this manufacturer, announcing the
inspection, the 60% potency issue was raised, with a comment to the effect
that 'there would appear to be something amiss with the company's quality
control'. An indignant reply was received from the managing director,
almost by return, protesting that there was nothing wrong with his
company's quality control. They had assayed samples of the product,
immediately following production, and they *knew* it assayed only 60% of
the stated potency. Their only error lay in their failure to inform production
of this result, and thus the batch was sent out on sale. But there was 'nothing
wrong with our quality control'. However, on inspection, a number of
defects were revealed, by comparison with which this particular incident
paled almost into insignificance.

Further cautionary tales, to be pondered by all who work in testing
laboratories or who may have an uncritical faith in the results which emerge

from them, are provided by an article which appeared in *The Times* (28 May 1996) on the hazards of unquestioning acceptance of forensic laboratory test results. Among the gems quoted are the well-known false 'positive' test for Semtex explosive found at the Government Forensic Explosives Laboratory which was later found to be due to previously contaminated test equipment, the hair sample found at the scene of a robbery, initially identified as coming from the prime suspect and later shown to have come from a dog, and the murder charge based on a lethal dose of barbiturate found in the body of the victim that was later found to have been reported as ten times higher than the amount actually present in the corpse due to the analyst having put a decimal point in the wrong place. It behoves all to maintain a healthily sceptical attitude.

Good control laboratory practice

The term 'good control laboratory practice' (GCLP) is used to mark a distinction from 'good laboratory practice' (GLP) which, for historical reasons now difficult to disentangle, is usually taken to refer to good practices in pharmacological/toxicity testing laboratories and the like. The EC GMP Guide uses the term 'good quality control laboratory practice' to mean the same as GCLP.

It is essential that control laboratories should have appropriate facilities, with properly trained, managed and motivated staff, in order that results obtained from any analytical or other test procedure may be considered to be both reliable and meaningful, whether the nature of the testing is chemical, physical, biological or microbiological. Steps should be taken to ensure the reliability of the laboratory's own systems and test methods. In other words, the basic principles of GMP apply to the laboratory just as much as to manufacturing areas.

Personnel – management

As ever, the most important single factor is the quality, training, management and motivation of the people working in the laboratory. It is important to recognise that this principle is just as crucial in the analytical laboratory as it is in the manufacturing environment. Clearly, the manager of the Quality Control Laboratory will need to have both the relevant academic/professional qualifications and experience in the science and practice of analytical chemistry, and if relevant, microbiology. This is not to say that the head of a laboratory, equipped and required to perform a wide range of analytical techniques, must be a complete expert in the theory and practice of all those techniques. This would hardly be possible, but he/she does need an understanding of the methods employed by the various experts under his/her command, sufficient to enable the making of valid and informed judgements on the results obtained by those experts. If, as recommended, for example, in the 'Code of Practice for Qualified Persons' (IoB, RPSGB and RSC, 1998), the head of quality control is also a/the Qualified Person, and the relevant qualification and experience requirements are quite comprehensively defined in official terms (see Chapter 11: Personnel – Management). It should not be overlooked, however, that the head of quality control will need to have the ability to *manage*; not only to manage people, but also to have the ability to manage a system which will ensure:

(a)   That materials and products which should be sampled are indeed sampled as specified.

(b)   That those samples are, in fact, tested in accordance with previously established and authorised procedures, using validated analytical methods (see Chapter 17).

(c)   That the test results on a given sample are properly collated, and evaluated against the test specification, and that an informed and authoritative decision is made on whether the sample does, or does not, comply with its specification.

(d)   That the correct messages ('Passed' [or 'Released], 'Rejected', 'Hold for Retest', etc.) are securely conveyed to those responsible for the storage, issue and use of the bulk material or product.

More than one instance has been encountered where the 'system' for conveying the 'Released/Rejected' message was notable more for its elegant simplicity than for its effectiveness as a contribution to the assurance of quality; the stores and production departments simply worked to the rule: 'If we have not heard from the laboratory within *n* days, it must be OK'.

With regard to point (c) above, it needs to be remembered that, although a sample which requires only simple 'classical' testing may well require no subdivision, increasingly (and with the development of ever more sophisticated methods) any given sample may well be subdivided for testing by different persons or laboratory sub-units, each with its own specialised equipment and expertise. (Samples which require both chemical and microbiological examination are an obvious and long-standing example.) It is thus crucially important that the identity and traceability of the sample remains secure, and that the test results (perhaps from several different sources) are securely brought together, to enable the final quality decision to be made on the basis of a reliable collation of all available relevant information.

Other staff

The establishment and maintenance of such a system is the responsibility of the Head of QC. Other QC laboratory staff will need to have the training, experience and, as relevant, the academic/professional qualifications appropriate to the tasks assigned to them. In a small QC laboratory, in a manufacturing company making only a limited range of products, there will perhaps be only a few or even only one person employed. In such cases, the management and training problem will be minimal. However, in any sizeable enterprise, experience, training and formal qualification requirements will vary from the relatively simple (in the case of junior laboratory technicians and laboratory support staff) to the complex and demanding in the case of those who are the leaders of the sub-units mentioned above, with the responsibility for performing specialist instrumental and other techniques. It is, however, worth re-emphasising that, whatever the level of complexity of the job, all staff should have the training/experience/qualifications required to perform that job effectively. In all but the smallest of QC laboratories, those jobs need to be defined in job descriptions, which define both technical and managerial responsibilities, with reporting relationships set out in an organisation chart.

Premises

Laboratories should be designed, equipped, maintained and have sufficient space to suit the work to be performed in them. Not only should there be adequate room and bench space for performing the analytical work itself, but there should be provision of adequate desk space to enable analysts to write reports and make records. If this is not provided, then one should not be surprised if the approach to laboratory documentation fails to rise above back-of-hand, sleeve-of-lab-coat scribbles. There should be working bench space for each analyst, sufficient to eliminate the possibility of mix-up between the samples, solutions and reagents of one analyst with those of another. There should also be sufficient space for the filing and storage of documents (specifications, methods, reports, etc.), and for the orderly holding, under suitable conditions, of retained samples of materials and products. Documents and retained samples should be readily recoverable when needed or requested. The introduction of electronic laboratory information systems (LIMS) may well reduce the space required for writing, calculating, reporting, and storing documentation, but the principles remain the same. Mistakes, mix-ups, transpositions, misreporting, etc. are more likely to occur in spatially inadequate, cluttered laboratories.

Chemical, biological and microbiological laboratories should normally be separated one from the other, and from manufacturing areas. In addition, separate rooms may be necessary to protect sensitive instruments from vibration, electrical interference, humidity, etc. Provision should be made for the safe storage of waste materials awaiting disposal, and all services (water, gas, electricity, compressed air, other gases, vacuum, etc.) should be clearly identifiable as to their nature.

In addition to ordinary running water, a supply of purified water will also normally be required. According to ambient climatic conditions, some form of air conditioning, or internal climate control may be necessary, both for the comfort of laboratory staff, and also to avoid ill effects on the performance of certain analytical techniques which can be influenced by temperature, humidity and exposure to direct sunlight and draughts (e.g. thin layer chromatography). Electrical outlets in instrument rooms should be fitted with voltage stabilisers where the local power supply is known to be variable, or subject to surges. Analytical balances should be placed upon vibration-damping tables.

Adequate provision should be made for the orderly and secure storage of reagents, reference materials and retained samples. Where controlled conditions (temperature, humidity) are required for such materials, they should be provided, and the conditions carefully monitored.

Equipment

Laboratory equipment and instrumentation should be appropriate to the testing procedures undertaken, that is, it should be the right 'kit' for the job. It should be serviced and calibrated at suitable specified intervals by persons or an organisation (under formal contract) of established competence, and readily available records maintained for each instrument or piece of equipment. These records should clearly indicate when the next calibration or servicing is due, and systems should be in place to ensure that calibration/servicing is *in fact* carried out on the due date.

Written operating instructions should be readily available for all instruments and other items of laboratory equipment of any complexity. Such equipment/instrumentation should only be operated by persons specifically trained to do so.

Where equipment, or services to equipment, are defective they should be marked as such, and any defective equipment should be withdrawn from use until the fault has been rectified. As appropriate, written analytical methods should require that steps are taken to verify that the equipment is functioning satisfactorily when being used in any determination.

Cleanliness

Control laboratories and equipment should be kept clean, in accordance with written cleaning schedules. Personnel should wear clean protective clothing appropriate to the work performed, and the disposal of waste material should be carefully and responsibly undertaken.

Reagents

Laboratory reagents should be marked with a date of receipt or preparation. Reagents made up in the laboratory should be prepared by persons competent to do so, following written procedures. As applicable, the labelling should indicate the concentration, standardisation factor, shelf life, and storage conditions. The label should be initialled or signed, and dated, by the person preparing the reagent. As relevant a date for re-standardisation should be recorded. If it is necessary to carry out tests to confirm that a reagent is suitable for the purpose for which it is to be used, a record of these tests should be maintained.

Reference standards, and any secondary standards prepared from them, should bear a date of preparation, and be stored, handled and used so as not to prejudice their quality.

Samples and sampling

Sampling is an activity which is of crucial significance to quality control in the pharmaceutical and other healthcare industries. It is necessary to take samples, because (a) it would be a totally impractical proposition to attempt to carry out tests on the entire bulk of a delivery of starting material, or on a complete batch of product, and (b) because most of the laboratory tests carried out are destructive. Thus, while any attempt to test a complete delivery lot, or an entire production batch might, potentially, yield sound and valuable information, the enormity of the task would be overwhelming, and the effect on profit would be disastrous. So, we take samples. That being so, we need to keep constantly in mind that if those samples are not valid, that is they do not adequately represent the batch, or lot, from which they were drawn, then any conclusions drawn from them, and indeed the entire system of quality control, will in turn be invalidated.

Surprisingly little of real value has been published on the theory and practice of taking samples for quality control purposes, *particularly in the healthcare industry*. A number of papers and books have indeed been published on the statistical approach to sampling in manufacturing industry generally. Although the approach expounded in such publications doubtless has value and application in some fields, it does not seem to have a lot of relevance to what is done in the production of pharmaceuticals. The difference lies in the fact that statistical sampling relies on the use of sampling tables (e.g. British Standard 6000 series and the US Military Standard Tables), which are based on assumptions that *some level of defective product is acceptable* (the Acceptable Quality Level or AQL), that the samples taken will be examined only for appearance and/or a few physical parameters, and that any *defects are distributed uniformly throughout the batch or lot*. Inevitably, the approach in the context of the production of pharmaceutical products must be different. While acknowledging that, in this imperfect world, it is a philosophical impossibility to produce products which are 100% free of defect, 100% of the time, it is difficult to accept *à priori* that there can be an agreed level of defective medicines. Certainly the patients who receive the defective products would find that difficult to accept. To illustrate the point: a common AQL in a number of manufacturing industries is 0.1%. This denotes an agreement that 0.1% defective items is acceptable, i.e. one defect in every thousand is OK.

Applying this notion to various fields of human activity, this would mean:

- Two aircraft crashes per day at Chicago Airport.
- 791 newborn babies sent home with the wrong mother per year in the UK.
- Over 100 000 microbially contaminated IV solutions infused per year in the world.
- 400 000 incorrectly dispensed prescriptions per year in the UK.

Clearly, there are a number of important areas of activity where the acceptance of a 0.1% level of defectives is **not** appropriate.

The way samples are taken, the quantity to be taken, and what (if any) sampling plan is used will depend upon:

1.   What exactly is the purpose of taking the sample? That is, what is it that the QC system requires to know?
2.   To what extent can that knowledge be acquired, or inferred, from other sources?

(The classic case of 'finding out from other sources' (point 2 above) is, of course, sterile production and the sterility test (see Chapters 19 and 20), which as is well known, from the sampling aspect, is a statistical non-event. There is, for example, a 12% chance of a batch passing the test when it is 10% contaminated. We are therefore forced to 'find out', to acquire our assurance of sterility, by other means, that is by careful *in-process control of previously validated processes*.)

Sampling requirements and guidelines

The conclusions drawn from the examination of samples will be affected by:

• The context in which they were taken.
• The nature of the sampling techniques, instruments and plans employed.
• The devices, instruments and methods used to examine/evaluate the sample.

The validity of those conclusions will depend upon:

• The quality of the sample (that is, its fitness for its intended purpose).
• The quality and the extent of the tests performed on it.
• The quality (including reliability) of the powers of inference of those drawing the conclusions.

Having discussed these perhaps more philosophical aspects of sampling, it is time to take a look at such practical instruction and guidance as is available in official guidelines and regulations.

The EC GMP Guide (EC, 1992) has a number of comments on sampling, in various different parts of its text. In its Chapter 4 'Documentation' (at paragraph 4.22) there is a general statement that there should be written procedures for sampling, which 'include the person(s) authorised to take samples, the methods and equipment to be used, the amounts to be taken and any precautions to be observed to avoid contamination of the material or any deterioration in its quality'.

In Chapter 6 'Quality control', this statement is expanded somewhat (para. 6.11), to require that samples should be taken:

> . . . in accordance with approved written procedures that describe:

— The method of sampling,
— The equipment to be used,
— The amount of the sample to be taken,
— Instructions for any required sub-division of the sample,
— The type and condition of the sample container to be used,
— The identification of the containers sampled,
— Any special precautions to be observed, especially with regard to the sampling of sterile or noxious materials,
— The storage conditions,
— Instruction for the cleaning and storage of sampling equipment.

A subsequent paragraph (6.13) declares that sample containers 'should bear a label indicating the contents, with the batch number, the date of sampling and the containers from which the samples have been drawn'.

In a similar context, the UK Orange Guide (Sharp, 1983), from which these above passages were clearly derived, is similarly worded, but the parallel statements on sampling (under 8. 'Good control laboratory practice') states that 'it should also be possible to identify the bulk containers from which samples have been drawn' and that:

> Care must be taken to avoid contamination, or causing deterioration, whenever a material or product is sampled. Special care is necessary when re-sealing sampled containers to prevent damage to, or contamination of or by the contents.

The EC GMP Guide has an Annex (No. 8) on 'Sampling of starting and packaging materials'. It opens with a statement of a general principle:

> Sampling is an important operation in which only a small fraction of a batch is taken. Valid conclusions on the whole cannot be based on tests which have been carried out on non-representative samples. Correct sampling is thus an essential part of a system of Quality Assurance.

This is followed by a sub-section on 'Personnel', where it is declared that 'Personnel who take samples should receive initial and ongoing regular training in the disciplines relevant to correct sampling . . .', with examples of the topics that should be included in this training:

— sampling plans,
— written sampling procedures,
— the techniques and equipment for sampling,
— the risks of cross-contamination,
— the precautions to be taken with regard to unstable and/or sterile substances,
— the importance of considering the visual appearance of materials, containers and labels,
— the importance of recording any unexpected or unusual circumstances.

Sampling of starting materials

There then follows another sub-section which deals specifically with the sampling of 'starting materials'. ('Starting material' is defined as 'any substance used in the production of a medicinal product but excluding packaging materials'. In effect it means the same thing as 'ingredient' or 'raw material', and may be considered to be synonymous with the term 'component', as used and defined in the US CGMPs – see below.) The first paragraph of this sub-section merits careful attention and discussion:

> The identity of a complete batch of starting material can normally only be ensured if individual samples are taken from all the containers and an identity test performed on each sample. It is permissible to sample only a proportion of the containers where a validated procedure has been established to ensure that no single container of starting material has been incorrectly labelled.

This is followed by a consideration of the factors which should be taken into account in this 'validated procedure', and thus of the circumstances under which it may be considered permissible to forego the sampling and identity testing of the contents of each container of a multi-container delivery of a staring material. To this we will be returning shortly. For the moment let us just concentrate on the paragraph quoted above. It has its genesis in Appendix 4 of the 1983 edition of the UK Orange Guide, where perhaps the point is made with greater clarity, and indication of purpose:

> The manufacturer of medicinal products must be aware of the possibility that containers of starting materials may be incorrectly labelled, and take steps to ensure that only the correct materials are used. Sampling and identity-testing the contents of each container can provide the necessary assurance.

The problem of mixed labels

In this same passage it is, however, acknowledged that that 'large deliveries in many containers can present practical and economic problems', and examples are given of circumstances under which 'it may be possible to relax the policy of identity-testing the contents of every container' to which, again, we will shortly return.

It is important to appreciate that, in both sets of guidelines (EC and UK) the sampling of every container in a delivery refers only to sampling for identification purposes, and not necessarily for the determination of quality and compliance with specification.

The background to this concern (in the UK at least) for the correct identity, as labelled, of starting materials was as follows. At some time in the mid-1970s, a highly reputable supplier of materials was discovered to have supplied a highly reputable pharmaceutical manufacturer with atropine mononitrate labelled as physostigmine sulphate, due to a labelling mix-up, and as a result of the same mix-up, to have supplied another equally reputable manufacturer with a similar quantity of physostigmine sulphate labelled as atropine mononitrate. Thus both manufacturers were confronted with the potential danger of producing eye-drops which would have the reverse of the intended physiological effect. In the event, both mis-labelled lots were recovered in time and no patient harm was done. The event did, however, concentrate official and industrial minds on the potential hazards of mis-labelled starting materials, the author recalling for example, from his days in industry, a delivery of containers labelled as citric acid which all contained oxalic acid, and a further delivery of one container labelled as strychnine alkaloid which in fact contained strychnine sulphate. At around this same time the Association of the British Pharmaceutical Industry (APBI) asked its member companies to report, with details, the incidence of incorrectly labelled starting material deliveries over the preceding 5 years. Replies were received from 65 companies, of which 35 were nil returns. The other 30 reported a total of 66 occasions where chemical materials had been received incorrectly labelled. Of these 66 incidents, the entire delivery had been incorrectly labelled as to identity on 46 occasions. The remaining 20 were instances where only *some* of the containers were wrongly labelled, and which might thus have escaped detection in any sampling scheme which left some containers unsampled. A few examples of the errors reported are listed in Table 16.1.

It is probably hardly necessary to note that the partial mis-labelling of a delivery represents a greater potential hazard, than a complete mis-labelling of all the containers in a delivery. If all the contents of all the containers are not as labelled, then it will be spotted even if only one container is sampled.

It was considerations such as these that gave rise to the recommendations that, on receipt of a multi-container delivery of a starting material, all containers in the delivery should be sampled and tested for identity, *unless adequate assurance against hazardous mis-identification by the supplier can be obtained by other means.*

Abstracting from the relevant passages in both the EC and the UK Guides, the 'other means' are:

Table 16.1   Incidence of wrongly labelled containers – case histories

Containers labelled	Contents	% containers
Chloroform	Ether	10%
Isopropanol	Acetone	3%
Sodium hydroxide	Ammonium chloride	100%
Prednisone	Prednisolone	100%
Theophyline	Aminophyline	50%
Hydrochlorothiazide	Hydrochlorethiazole	100%
Sulphaguanidine	Theobromine	100%
Chromium trioxide	Sodium dichromate	5%
Iron oxide	Brown organic dye	15%

- Where the source supplier, or plant, only produces and only supplies a single material, so there is no chance of mix-up.
- Where the material comes directly from its producer and/or in that producer's own sealed and unbroken container, and where the purchaser has built up a history, over a period, of supplier-reliability, and has been able to make a satisfactory assessment of the supplier's quality system through its own regular quality audits of that supplier.

(The EC GMP Guide, perhaps in anticipation of regulatory inspection of ingredient manufacturers, also accepts the possibility of such quality audits being performed by 'an officially accredited body'.)

The UK Orange Guide also allowed two 'other means', which are omitted from the EC GMP Guide. These were where:

> . . . a (manufacturing) process would self-evidently fail if the wrong material was used

and where,

> . . . the pharmaceutical manufacturer's own manufacturing and quality control procedures, including assays of the end-product, would reveal the use of a wrong material (e.g. where a material is assayed in the finished product and the assay is specific).

Note: in the latter example, exemption via this particular 'other means' suggests that, contrary to a frequently held view, it is just as, if not more, important, to assure the identity of inactive ingredients as it is active ingredients, since although the latter are usually assayed in the final product, the former rarely are.

Both sets of guidelines consider that, no matter the level of assurance of material identity that may be obtained by other means, every container of materials to be used in the manufacture of injectable products should be sampled for an identity test. This is based not on any suggestion that suppliers of materials to be used in injectables are more prone to labelling errors than other materials suppliers, but purely on a consideration of the relative patient hazards. The single example of potassium chloride will serve adequately to illustrate the point. Potassium chloride may be taken by mouth, without harm, in quantities which could prove fatal if injected in mistake for sodium chloride. Both guidelines also consider that adequate assurance of identity (other than that obtained by sampling and identifying the contents of every container) can*not* be obtained where the material is obtained via an intermediary (or series of intermediaries), particularly where the material is obtained from a broker who breaks bulk material and then repackages it in smaller quantities.

All this makes undeniably good sound sense. It does, however, create a problem for the manufacturer who obtains relatively large quantities of material in many separate containers, and is thus confronted with by no means insignificant materials-handling problems and cost implications. Many manufacturers will also look to purchase materials, at the 'best price' to themselves, in a world market. Indeed, some materials may only be obtainable from far distant lands. In such circumstances, 'regular quality audits' may be a somewhat less than economic proposition. The healthcare manufacturer will need to consider carefully whether or not the immediate cost advantages of obtaining materials from far-off, not too well-known sources, outweigh the costs of 100% container sampling, or of obtaining assurance by those 'other means', and also whether any patient hazard and/or commercial risk is justified. It is all a matter of balancing a number of different factors. The consideration of the 'safety, well-being and protection' of the ultimate consumer should always be paramount.

European guidelines and proposals for starting materials

Some help *may* be at hand, to assist the stressed European manufacturer of medicinal products in his efforts to assure the identity (and indeed the overall quality) of his starting materials. Moves are currently (late 1998) afoot to introduce formal inspection, with some form of certification, if not overt licensing, of the manufacture of the starting materials used in the manufacture of medicinal products. In July 1995 the European Commission issued a 'concept paper on a regulatory framework on GMP and certification of starting materials for the industrial manufacture of medicinal products', and in July 1996 a discussion document on the possible contents of a directive on the manufacture of starting materials. Since then the first draft of an EC 'proposal on GMP for starting materials and inspection of manufacturers of both medicinal products and their starting materials (amending Directives 75/319/EEC and 81/851/EEC)' has been circulated. This proposal was issued by the European Commission, together with an explanatory memorandum, in September 1997, for consultation and comment. The intention seems to be that, when implemented, the proposed amending requirements will apply to the manufacture of starting materials for clinical trial as well as marketed products.

In summary, the proposed amendments to Chapters IV and V of Directive 75/319 will mean that:

- Licensed manufacturers and importers must only use starting materials made in compliance with GMP for starting materials (although the holding of some form of authorisation or licence does not seem to be required).
- Manufacturers of starting materials (as listed in Annex II) must:

    (a) Obtain prior agreement of the medicinal product manufacturer before making any change to the starting materials supplied. (This is a very broad requirement, and it has to be wondered if it is indeed intended to apply to *any* change, no matter how trivial.)

    (b) Allow inspection by competent authority.

    (c) Provide samples to the European Pharmacopoeia on request.

Within the proposals are requirements that, subject to any arrangements between the Commission and third countries, a member state, the Commission, or the EMEA may require inspection of a third country starting material manufacturer, and that member states shall ensure that starting materials, when they are for use in medicinal products, are manufactured in compliance with GMP for starting materials.

Annex II to these EC draft proposals has two categories or lists of starting materials:

- List 1 – all active pharmaceutical ingredients (APIs) and intermediates.
- List 2 – gelatin and its derivatives; tallow and its derivatives.

The term 'intermediates' will need to be clarified. In the explanatory memorandum it is defined as applying to such things as granules intended for compression into tablets, thus providing considerable potential for confusion with 'intermediate' in the chemical synthesis sense.

These proposals define starting materials as:

> All the constituents of a medicinal product: the active ingredient(s) and the excipients as well as intermediate products, e.g. granules. For biological products it means all of the constituents as well as the source materials.

The expression 'manufacture of starting materials' would appear to embrace both total and partial manufacture, or importation, dividing up, packaging or presentation, including repackaging or relabelling – but wholesale distribution or brokering are not covered.

Other proposals include requirements that:

- Member states shall inspect starting materials manufacturers whenever they consider it necessary for the purposes of implementing the revised directive, or at the request of the starting material manufacturer, another member state, the Commission or the EMEA.
- Member states shall issue an inspection report to the starting material/medicinal product manufacturer.
- Member states shall issue a GMP Certificate, if appropriate, within 90 days of the inspection, the Certificates must be entered in a Community register. (A standard format is proposed, but has yet to be agreed.)
- If the starting material/medicinal product manufacturer does not comply with GMP, this must be entered in the Community register.

Further EC proposals on control of starting materials

It needs to be understood that, at the time of writing, these are only *draft* proposals. Furthermore, the decision of the European Commission *not* to produce an entirely new directive on starting materials, but rather to propose amendments to two existent directives (75/392 and 81/851) over 20 years old, and originally framed for other purposes, has already led to considerable difficulties in interpretation. Unless these difficulties are resolved, it will undoubtedly lead to serious problems in practical implementation. However, *if* these difficulties/problems are resolved, and the proposals effectively implemented, then this will add another layer to a manufacturer's confidence in the quality (including identity) of bought-in starting materials. But it will depend upon the confidence that may be had in whatever scheme of official inspection and monitoring is adopted, and of course upon the manufacturer obtaining starting materials from officially authorised, or certified, sources. It will also depend upon the general adoption, and serious (i.e. not 'token') implementation of GMP guidelines for the production and supply of starting materials. In this context, the draft proposals state that an annex to the EC GMP Guide for starting materials will be published. The explanatory memorandum states that this will draw upon PICS and WHO guidelines, and in September 1997 a working party of the Pharmaceutical Inspection Cooperation Scheme (PICS) issued a 'Draft internationally harmonised guide for active pharmaceutical ingredients (APIs) good manufacturing practice'.

US guidelines on sampling of starting materials

Guidance on sampling may also be obtained from the US 'Current Good Manufacturing Practice Regulations' (21 CFR, Parts 210 and 21; US FDA, 1990). Sub-part 211.84 is headed 'Testing and approval or rejection of components, drug product containers, and closures'. (For European English speakers it needs to be emphasised again that in the US CGMPs, 'component' is defined as 'any ingredient intended for use in the manufacture of a drug product, including those that may not appear in such drug product'. A 'drug product' is a finished dosage form, so 'component' is virtually synonymous with 'starting material'.) This sub-part 211.84 states:

(a) Each lot of components, drug product containers, and closures shall be withheld from use until the lot has been sampled, tested or examined, as appropriate, and released for use by the quality control unit.
(b) Representative samples of each shipment of each lot shall be collected for testing or examination. The number of containers to be sampled, and the amount of material to be taken from each container, shall be based upon appropriate criteria such as statistical criteria for component variability, confidence levels, and degree of precision desired, the past quality history of the supplier, and the quantity needed for analysis and reserve.
(c) Samples shall be collected in accordance with the following procedures:

(1) The containers of components selected shall be cleaned where necessary, by appropriate means.
(2) The containers shall be opened, sampled, and resealed in a manner designed to prevent contamination of their contents and contamination of other components, drug product containers, or closures.

(3)   Sterile equipment and aseptic sampling techniques shall be used when necessary.

(4)   If it is necessary to sample a component from the top, middle and bottom of its container, such sample subdivisions shall not be composited for testing.

(5)   Sample containers shall be identified so that the following information can be determined: name of the material sampled, the lot number, the container from which the sample was taken, the data [presumably 'date' is intended] and the name of the person who collected the sample.

(6)   Containers from which samples have been taken shall be marked to show that samples have been removed from them.

(d)   Samples shall be examined and tested as follows:

(1)   At least one test shall be conducted to verify the identity of each component of a drug product. Specific identity tests, if they exist, shall be used.

(2)   Each component shall be tested for conformity with all appropriate written specifications for purity, strength and quality. In lieu of such testing by the manufacturer, a report of analysis may be accepted from the supplier of a component, provided that at least one specific identity test on such component by the manufacturer, and provided that the manufacturer establishes the reliability of the supplier's analyses through appropriate validation of the supplier's test results at appropriate intervals.

(3)   Containers and closures shall be tested for conformance with all appropriate written procedures. In lieu of such testing by the manufacturer, a certificate of testing may be accepted from the supplier, provided that at least a visual identification is conducted on such containers/closures by the manufacturer and provided that the manufacturer establishes the reliability of the supplier's test results through appropriate validation of the supplier's test results at appropriate intervals.

(4)   When appropriate, components shall be microscopically examined.

(5)   Each lot of a component, drug product container, or closure that is liable to contamination with filth, insect infestation, or other extraneous adulterant shall be examined against established specifications for such contamination.

(6)   Each lot of a component, drug product container, or closure that is liable to microbiological contamination that is objectionable in view of its intended use shall be subjected to microbiological tests before use.

(e)   Any lot of components, drug product containers, or closures that meets the appropriate written specifications of identity, strength, quality and purity and related tests under paragraph (d) of this section may be approved and released for use. Any lot of such material that does not meet such specifications shall be rejected.

The diligent reader of the above extract from the US CGMPs will have noted a number of ambiguities and a few redundancies. That, however, is what the US Federal Regulations have to say about sampling of components (equals 'starting materials') and primary packaging materials. Concerning the sampling of finished dosage forms, or of manufacturing intermediates such as powder mixes or granules, the US CGMPs offer relatively meagre fare, confined to statements (under 'Subpart I – Laboratory controls') that sampling plans 'shall be drafted by the appropriate organisational unit and approved by the quality control unit', that 'For each batch of drug product there shall be appropriate laboratory determination of satisfactory conformance to final specifications for the drug product' and that 'Any sampling and testing plans shall be described in written procedures that shall include the method of sampling and the number of units per batch to be tested; such written procedure shall be followed.'

Both the US CGMP Regulations on Good Manufacturing Practices for Medical Devices (Part 820 CFR) and the EC Device Directive yield little, if anything, in the way of further 'solid' information on the act of taking samples.

Assessment of guidance on sampling

This fairly lengthy excursion into 'official' statements on taking samples for testing purposes has been a necessary preliminary to the extraction of what are generally agreed to be the essential features of this activity, and to the discovery of what it is that remains that manufacturers, zealously concerned for the quality of their products, still need to know.

These essential features may be summarised as:

1. Samples need to be taken, for test purposes, from deliveries of materials for use in manufacture (including packaging), and of the products produced by the process of manufacture.
2. Sampling is unquestionably an important activity, to be conducted with care and skill, and with a full awareness of all the implications of this activity.
3. Samples should be in some way 'representative' of the total lot from which they are taken.
4. In some way, not clearly defined, sampling plans and 'statistical criteria' have an important significance.
5. Precautions are necessary, when taking samples, to avoid contamination (chemical, microbial – or any other form) *of* the material being sampled, or of any other goods *by* the material being sampled.
6. Records need to be made, on labels or by other means, which will ensure traceability of any given sample to not only the lot, but also to the individual container from which the sample was taken. Records also need to be made of date of sampling, and of the name of the person who took the sample.
7. If the supplier of the material also supplies an analytical or test

certificate of known reliability, it may not be necessary to take samples of delivered goods, other than those taken to confirm the identity of lots of starting materials (or 'components' in US terminology).

As far as the 'real life' approach to actually taking samples is concerned, some important things seem to be missing from all this regulatory guidance. This is not to criticise the regulators, who would generally declare that their job is to set down *what* should be done, not to define *how* to do it; a view which many manufacturers, wishing to avoid increasingly prescriptive regulation, would applaud. So, having accepted these 'essential features', what more does one need to know in order to establish and implement a rational and effective sampling policy? Well, in addition to information on the actual mechanics of sampling, the tools to be used, etc., what *are* the relevant 'statistical criteria'? How may a suitable sampling plan be devised? In short, how many samples should be taken, from what number of (and which) containers of bulk material or product, and should or should not these individual samples be pooled ('composited') for testing purposes, and if so, in what way?

As already suggested, the standard statistical sampling tables (e.g. the BS 6000 series, or the US 'Military Standard 105E Tables') are hardly applicable to the sampling of pharmaceutical ingredients or finished products, depending as they do:

1. On the dubious premise of a predefined acceptable level of defective material or product, the 'Acceptable Quality Level' or AQL; and
2. On an assumption that the purpose of taking the sample is to examine the articles present in the sample either for various measurable physical properties such as weight, length, diameter, resistance (either electrical, or to stress) and the like – the 'variables' – or for non-quantifiable properties, such as appearance, finish, 'feel', freedom from burrs, flashing, or surface oil and suchlike – the 'attributes'. Separate tables are to be used in sampling for variables, as compared to sampling for attributes. However, neither seems relevant to the sampling of pharmaceutical ingredients and finished products, although they may have some application in the sampling of incoming supplies of packaging materials.

If we turn again to Annex 8 ('Sampling of starting and packaging materials') of the EC GMP Guide, paragraph 4 initially seems to be offering some promise:

> The quality of a batch of starting materials may be assessed by taking and testing a representative sample. The samples taken for identity testing could be used for this purpose. The number of samples taken for the preparation of a representative sample should be determined statistically and specified in a sampling plan. The number of individual samples which may be blended to form a composite sample should also be defined, taking into account the nature of the material, knowledge of the supplier and the homogeneity of the composite sample.

Unfortunately, as can be seen, this turns out to be just another example of donning a mantle of spurious statistical authority, only to duck the crucial issue.

WHO guidelines on sampling of starting materials

A World Health Organisation document (WHO, 1997), in a section (8.2) on 'Sampling plans for consignments of starting materials supplied in several sampling units' (for 'sampling units' read 'bulk containers'), at least attempts to offer some sampling plans. Three of them are given below.

The n-plan

This 'should be used with great caution and then only when the material is considered uniform and is supplied from a well-known source':

$$n = \sqrt{N}$$

where N is the number of possible sampling units in the consignment. The value of n samples is rounded up to the next highest integer. Under this plan, original samples are take from n sampling units selected at random, and each placed in a separate sample container. The control laboratory then inspects the appearance, and tests the identity, of the material in each original sample. 'If the results are concordant', the original samples are pooled into a final sample from which an analytical sample is prepared, the remaining part being kept as a retention sample. 'The n plan is not recommended for use by control laboratories of manufacturers who are required to analyse and release or reject each received consignment of the starting materials used to produce a drug product.'

The p-plan

This 'may be used when the material is uniform and is received from a source that is well known and where the main purpose is to check the identity':

$$p = 0.4 \sqrt{N}$$

where N is the number of sampling units. Under this plan, samples are taken from each of the N sampling units in the delivery, and each placed in a separate sample container. These original samples are each then visually inspected and tested for identity in the laboratory, and ('if the results are concordant') p final samples are formed by 'appropriate pooling of the original samples'.

The r-plan

This 'may be used when the material is suspected to be non-uniform and/or is received from a source that is not well known':

$$r = 1.5 \sqrt{N}$$

where N is the number of sampling units. Under this plan, samples are taken from each of the N sampling units in the delivery, and each placed in a separate sample container. These original samples are then tested for identity in the laboratory. 'If the results are concordant', r samples are randomly selected and 'individually subjected to testing'. If the results are concordant the r samples are pooled for the retention sample.

Notes on the WHO guidelines

Under both the p-plan and the r-plan, samples taken from every container in a delivery are tested for identity. No statistical basis is offered for any of these three plans. Nor would there appear to be one, any more than there is for that old favourite:

$$n = \sqrt{N} + 1$$

Sampling – summary and conclusions

Given that the advice that may be obtained from the official national and international regulations and guidelines is somewhat less than complete, what directions can be given to the pharmaceutical manufacturer? The following, although somewhat short of being fully comprehensive, may be offered.

General

1. Sampling, of any sort of material or product, is not something to be undertaken as a casual, menial job, by persons who have had no specific training in the task. It must be conducted in accordance with written procedures (prepared and/or approved by the Quality Control Department), by persons who have been trained in the task and *who have a full understanding of the importance and also the potential hazards of what they are doing*, both to themselves and to the ultimate consumer of the company's products.
2. The training given to samplers should cover, at least:

    — Sampling plans.
    — Application of the written sampling procedure(s).
    — The techniques and equipment for sampling.
    — The risks, and prevention, of cross-contamination.
    — Special precautions to be taken when sampling unstable sterile or hazardous substances.
    — The importance of noting the visual appearance of materials, containers and labels.
    — The importance of recording any unexpected or unusual appearance, odour, etc.

3. The written sampling procedure should clearly define:

    — The method of sampling.

— The equipment to be used.

— The amount of each sample to be taken.

— The number of samples to be taken.

— Instructions for any sub-division of the sample(s).

— The type and condition of the sample container to be used.

— The identification of the containers sampled.

— Any special precautions to be observed, especially with regard to the sampling of sterile or hazardous materials.

— Storage conditions for the sample(s).

— Instruction for the cleaning and storage of sampling equipment.

4. Sampling should be performed (preferably) by QC personnel, or by other trained persons (e.g. production staff) who have been approved by QC and who are following the QC written procedures.

5. Great care needs to be taken to ensure that the act of sampling does not allow contamination, either *of* the material or product being sampled, or of other goods *by* that material or product. The written procedure should clearly define the precautions necessary to avoid any such contamination. Attention needs to be directed at the environment in which the sample is taken (for incoming supplies of starting materials, a separate dedicated sampling room is to be preferred), also at the external cleanliness of the container holding the bulk material or product, of the sample containers, and of the sampling equipment.

6. Sampling devices and other equipment need to be scrupulously clean before, during and after use. They should be stored, pending further use, in a manner which will maintain them in a clean condition. In many cases the best, and ultimately most cost-effective, solution will probably be to use single-use disposable sampling implements (scoops, spatulas, pipettes, dip-tubes and the like).

7. The importance of the sampler carefully examining the general appearance of the bulk from which the sample is taken, and of recording and drawing attention to anything unusual or untoward, should not be underestimated.

8. Statistics-based sampling plans, and simple 'rule of thumb' sampling formulae of the '$n = \sqrt{N} + 1$' type must, unfortunately, be considered as having little relevance or application to many of the requirements for sampling in the manufacture of pharmaceutical and similar products. Indeed, it may well be necessary to warn of the potential hazard of the sense of false security that a statistical sampling plan may engender, and to emphasise that even the most splendidly sophisticated sampling plan, used to select a proportion of containers to be sampled, will tell absolutely nothing about the quality (including identity) of the contents of the unsampled containers.

Starting materials

1. The importance of 'knowing your supplier', and of establishing a good working relationship generally with suppliers is, rightly, much stressed. It is, as a prime necessity, vital to ensure that a supplier knows precisely

what is needed, the form and the containers in which it is to be delivered, and the purpose (in general terms at least) for which it is required. That is, a detailed and agreed specification should form part of the order or contract. 'Knowing the supplier' means a thorough understanding of the supplier's practices and quality systems, gained through diligent quality audits (see Chapter 24).

2.   Goods Inwards personnel have an important role to play in the assurance of the quality of incoming materials. They should be required (by written procedures) and trained to examine carefully all incoming shipments for appearance, damage, spoilage, integrity of seals, labelling, and indeed for any and all signs that there is anything untoward – and to report anything which seems amiss.

3.   The extent of sampling, and the number of samples taken, will depend upon the confidence gained through genuine knowledge of the supplier. The more slight the knowledge, the more remote the supplier, and the greater the number of hands through which the material has passed, the greater is the need for extensive sampling and testing.

4.   It is impossible to disagree with official guidance that (with exceptions) 'the identity of a complete batch of starting material can normally only be ensured if individual samples are taken from all the containers and an identity test performed on each sample' (EC GMP Guide). This must be particularly so in these days where the possibility of deliberate contamination or 'switching' must, regrettably, be added to the purely inadvertent. However, the sheer handling problems which can be presented by large multi-container deliveries cannot be denied. Reliable, rapid techniques which are easy to apply are clearly much to be desired. Near infra-red (NIR) techniques, which can be simply applied in the warehouse itself, directly to material in the container (as delivered), without the need to take a sample and send it to the laboratory, and without the need for highly specialised expertise (at the implementation stage) is now finding increasing application in pharmaceutical and other industries, and may well prove to be the answer (Higgins, 1997a,b). Smaller companies may be deterred by initial capital and set-up costs, but they are, by the very nature of their business as small companies, unlikely to receive many large deliveries in many containers. Larger companies have found that savings accruing from reductions in the overall supply time (from placing of order to supply of dispensed material to production) more than compensate for the initial investment.

Products

1.   Well stirred bulk liquid products in the form of readily soluble materials dissolved in a solvent vehicle (e.g. water) may be considered to be homogeneous, given that the manufacturing process has been adequately validated to that end, and that the validated process has been followed. Thus any sample of the bulk liquid may reasonably be taken

to be representative. A manufacturer may wish to sample from a bulk manufactured liquid, as a guard against the cost of filling and labelling a product which is later rejected for inhomogeneity. Even so, it clearly makes good sense to take samples for assay from the filling line, at the beginning, the middle and the end of the filling run.

2. Sampling of liquid suspensions, emulsions and the like may be more problematic. Process validation should have established that, at the completion of the bulk batch the active ingredient(s) is/are uniformly and homogeneously distributed. However, against the possibility of separation during holding and transfer to filling, sampling from the filling line (beginning/middle/end) must surely be obligatory. Similar considerations also apply to the sampling of creams and ointments.

3. Unit dose solids (tablets and capsules). The commonly employed in-process controls on tablet weights and thickness, and on capsule fill-weights, will contribute towards the assurance of the uniformity of these products. For an impressive analysis of the problems of sampling bulk powder mixtures, with comprehensive guidance on sampling filled capsules and compressed tablets, see PDA Technical Report No. 25 (PDA, 1997). An original impetus for this report was the so-called 'Wolin decision' (that is, the judgement of Judge Wolin in the US versus Barr Laboratories case). The report clearly shows that, despite the great store that the US FDA placed upon it, the judge's decision was fundamentally flawed, in both practical and statistical terms.

Related issues

Retained (or reference) samples

The EC GMP Guide requires that reference samples (in their normal final packaging) from each product batch shall be retained until 1 year after the expiry date of the batch.

Samples of starting materials are required to be retained for at least 2 years after the release of the product in which they were used, 'if their stability allows'. The EC GMP Guide also states that 'reference samples of materials and products should be of a size sufficient to permit at least a full re-examination'. (For reasons which should be obvious, the prudent manufacturer will, where practicable, retain sufficient samples to permit *several* 'full re-examinations'.)

Testing

The persons responsible for laboratory management should ensure that suitable test methods, validated in the context of available facilities and equipment (see later), are adopted or developed.

Samples should be tested in accordance with the test methods referred to, or detailed, in the relevant specifications. The validity of the results obtained should be checked (and as necessary, any calculations checked) before the material is released or rejected.

Any in-process control work carried out by production staff should proceed in accordance with methods approved by the person responsible for quality control.

Contract analysis

Although it is by no means an uncommon, and a perfectly acceptable, practice for analysis and testing to be undertaken by an external Contract Analyst, the ultimate responsibility for quality control (still less for quality assurance) cannot be thus delegated to any external body, organisation or laboratory. The nature and extent of any such contract analysis should be formally agreed by both parties, clearly defined in writing, and procedures for taking samples should be established as set out above. The contract analyst should be supplied with full details of the test methods relevant to the material or product under examination. These will need to be validated as suitable for use by the contract laboratory. Formal arrangements will also need to be made for the retention of samples, and of records of test results.

Certificates of analysis

It is quite a common practice for deliveries of starting materials to be released for use in manufacture, substantially on the evidence of a certificate of analysis received from the supplier. This may be an acceptable procedure, provided that the document purporting to be a 'Certificate of Analysis' is indeed genuinely just that, and not merely a copy of a standard specification, a statement of compliance with a specification, or a 'typical batch analysis'.

A true certificate of analysis should:

- Clearly indicate the laboratory, or organisation, issuing it.
- Be authorised (i.e. by signature, or by comparable electronic means) by a person demonstrably competent to do so.
- Clearly state the material, and the specific batch number to which it refers.
- Clearly indicate by whom the material was tested, and when.
- Clearly indicate the specification (e.g. Pharm. Eur., USP, Purchaser's Specification Reference) and methods against which, and by which, the tests were performed.
- State the test results obtained, or assert that the results showed compliance with the stated specification.

It is up to the Quality Control Department of the receiving company to satisfy itself that the person, or persons, issuing the certificate are competent to do so.

It needs to be firmly understood that the possession of a certificate of analysis does not (a) preclude the possibilities of a labelling mix-up, or of damage to (or contamination of) the material in transit, or (b) absolve the purchasing company from the ultimate responsibility for the quality (including identity) of the material to which the certificate refers, and as used in manufacture. Careful visual examination, and tests for identity are therefore (perhaps more than ever) necessary.

References

EC (1992). *The Rules Governing Medicinal Products in the European Community, Vol. IV: Good Manufacturing Practice for Medicinal Products.* Luxembourg: Commission of the European Communities. Available from The Office for Official Publications of the European Communities, Luxembourg. Also available from The Stationery Office (HMSO), London, and The EC Information Service, Washington, USA. (Referred to as the EC GMP Guide.)

Higgins M (1997a). Pinpointing production problems with NIR analysis. *Manuf Chem* **68** (4), 38–39.

Higgins M (1997b). Near infra-red spectroscopy applied in the cosmetics industry. *Chimica Oggi* **15** (5), 30–33.

IoB, RPSGB, RSC (1998). *Joint Register of Qualified Persons.* Appendix: Code of Practice for Qualified Persons. London: Institute of Biology, Royal Pharmaceutical Society of Great Britain and Royal Society of Chemistry.

PDA (1997). Technical Report No. 25. Blend uniformity analysis: validation and in-process testing. *PDA J Pharm Sci Technol* **51** (Suppl 3), Nov/Dec.

Sharp J, ed. (1983). *Guide to Good Pharmaceutical Manufacturing Practice,* 3rd edn. London: HMSO. (Referred to as the UK Orange Guide.)

WHO (1997). *Quality Assurance of Pharmaceuticals, a Compendium of Guidelines and Related Materials, Vol. 1.* Geneva: World Health Organisation.

US FDA (1990). *Code of Federal Regulations, Vol. 21, Ch. 1, Part 210,* Current good manufacturing practice in manufacturing, processing, packaging or holding of drugs, general; *CFR Vol. 21, Ch. 1, Part 211,* Current good manufacturing practice for finished pharmaceuticals; *CFR Vol. 21, Ch. 1, Part 820,* Good manufacturing practice for medical devices (revised 1995). Washington: US Food & Drug Administration. (Collectively referred to as the US CGMPs.)

17

Analytical validation

Sweet Analytics, 'tis thou has ravished me
    Christopher Marlowe, *Doctor Faustus*, 1604, Act 1, Sc. 1

Any analytical method worthy of the name must be scientifically sound, and, when used by different operators, with similar apparatus in different laboratories, must be capable of giving reliable and (within limits) consistent results. In other words, it should have a rational basis, and it should 'work', (i.e. it should be adequate for its stated purpose). The process of demonstrating that such a method 'works' is called 'analytical validation' or the 'validation of analytical methods'.

The EC GMP Guide (EC, 1992) (Section 6.15) requires, somewhat baldly, that 'analytical methods should be validated'. In this chapter we will be attempting to add a little more substance to that bald statement. We will be considering the differing criteria for analytical validation, how they may be defined, and the methodology used to establish these criteria.

Defining test methods and conditions

It is generally accepted, for example by the EC quality guideline on analytical validation (July 1990), that official pharmacopoeial methods (e.g. BP, Ph. Eur., USP) *when applied to pharmacopoeial materials or products*, may be taken as validated. Other methods, or pharmacopoeial methods applied to non-pharmacopoeial materials, should be validated. Certainly, such validation will be expected by regulatory bodies when considering applications for Marketing Authorisations (in UK terminology, 'Product Licences'). In the USA, the FDA requires details of the validation of analytical methodology to be submitted with New Drug Applications (NDAs), and to a greater or lesser extent (depending on the quality and extent of the data submitted) will conduct method validation studies, on samples of the new drug, in their own laboratories.

Regulatory bodies will require sufficient descriptive detail of the method to allow its repetition by the regulatory authorities themselves. They will normally require, for example, adequate information on the preparation of the sample, on any reference materials required, on the use of the apparatus and its calibration, on the number of replicates to be carried out, and on the methods of calculation of the results (together with details of any necessary statistical analysis).

Thus, as a preliminary to any analytical validation study, the test method and conditions will need to be precisely and formally defined. This formal definition should include:

- Sampling details (e.g. size and number of samples, method of sampling, sample container, any necessary pretreatment of sample).
- Any special sample-storage conditions.
- Details of reagents and equipment to be used.
- Description of the apparatus.
- Any tests necessary to determine the satisfactory function of the apparatus.
- System suitability tests (e.g. separating power of chromatographic columns).
- Exact test conditions, including reaction conditions and use of reagents for preparation of any derivatives.
- Any precautions to be taken.
- Method of calculation of the results, and any necessary statistical analyses.

The definition of reference materials may also need particular attention. In-house reference materials should be characterised and evaluated for their suitability for their intended uses and any working standards should be characterised against an authentic reference material.

Criteria for analytical validation

The following are the main criteria to be considered for validation studies. Their relative importance will depend on the use to which the method is to be put:

- Accuracy
- Precision
  - — Repeatability
  - — Reproducibility
- Specificity
- Sensitivity
- Limit of detection
- Limit of quantitation
- Linearity
- Range.

The ICH guideline on the validation of analytical procedures (ICH, 1993, 1995) introduces a further sub-class (in addition to repeatability and reliability) of the more general class 'precision' which it terms 'intermediate precision'.

Not all of these criteria will need to be considered in all cases. Thus, for example, with an identity test, specificity will obviously be a key factor to be established. For an impurity control test not only the specificity, but also the limit of detection and the limit of quantitation will also need to be confirmed. With quantitative assay procedures, the specificity, precision, accuracy, linearity, range and sensitivity will all need to be considered.

The ICH *Draft Consensus Text on Validation of Analytical Procedures* (ICH, 1993) contains a table illustrating 'those validation characteristics regarded as the most important for the validation of different analytical procedures'. A version of that table is shown in Table 17.1. Others, for example, Carr & Wahlich (1990, 1994) and Hovsepian (1996) have considered that this, and other similarly skeletal tables, fall somewhat short of complete adequacy, and have suggested something rather more comprehensive and specific along the lines of Tables 17.2 and 17.3, which are relevant to the analysis of chemical materials and finished products, respectively.

Demonstrable accuracy

Accuracy may be defined as the closeness of an experimental result to the true value. This raises the philosophical question of what *is* the true value, and in

Table 17.1   Analytical validation characteristics

Analytical validation criteria	Identification	Impurities tests		Assay (content/ potency/ dissolution)
		Quantitative determination	Limit test	
Accuracy	–	+	–	+
Precision –				
Repeatability	–	+	–	+
Reproducibility	–	+(1)	–	?*
Specificity	+	+	+	+ (2)
Detection limit	–	+	+	–
Quantitation limit	–	+	–	–
Linearity	–	+	–	+
Range	–	+	–	+

Adapted from the table listing 'those validation characteristics regarded as the most important for the validation of different types of analytical procedures', in ICH (1993).

–, Signifies that this parameter is not normally evaluated; +, signifies that this parameter is normally evaluated; (1), may be needed in some cases; (2), may not be needed in some cases. The ICH document introduces the further concept of 'intermediate precision', which is considered redundant and is therefore omitted here.

*The ICH table has no entry (neither + nor –) under 'Assay', against 'Reproducibility'. Presumably this is an error of omission, and there should be a '+'.

Table 17.2 Analytical validation criteria – bulk chemical substances

	Accuracy	Linearity	Repeatability	Reproducibility	Specificity	Detection limit	Quantitation limit	Analyte and system stability	Robustness
Identification	–	–	–	–	+	–	–	–	–
Physico-chemical									
M.Pt.	–	–	–	–	–	–	–	–	–
B.Pt.	–	–	–	–	–	–	–	–	–
Light absorption	–	–	+	–	–	–	–	–	–
O.R.	–	–	+	–	–	–	–	–	–
Particle size	–	–	+	–	–	–	–	–	–
Impurities									
Sulphated ash, heavy metals	–	–	–	–	–	–	–	–	–
Cations/anions									
Solution tests	+	–	+	–	+	+	+	–	–
Ion select. electrode	+	+	+	–	+	+	+	–	–
Atomic spectroscopy	+	+	+	–	+	+	+	–	–
Related substances									
TLC	+	–	+	+	+	+	–	+	+
HPLC	+	+	+	+	+	+	+	+	+
GC	+	+	+	+	+	+	+	+	+
Water									
Loss on drying	+	–	+	–	–	–	–	–	–
Karl Fischer	+	–	+	–	–	–	–	–	–
Assay									
Titration	+	–	+	+	–	–	–	+	–
Light absorption	+	+	+	+	–	–	–	+	–
Chromatography	+	+	+	+	+	–	–	+	+
Residual solvents									
Gas chromatography	+	+	+	+	+	+	+	+	+

Table 17.3 Analytical validation criteria – finished products

	Accuracy	Linearity/ sensitivity	Repeatability	Reproducibility	Specificity	Detection limit	Quantitation limit	Analyte and system stability
Identification	–	–	–	–	+	–	–	–
Dissolution								
Non-modified release	+	+	+	+	+	–	–	+
Modified release	+	+	+	+	+	–	–	+
Related substances								
TLC	+	–	+	+	+	+	–	+
HPLC	+	+	+	+	+	+	+	+
GC	+	+	+	+	+	+	+	+
Preservative assays								
Light absorbtion	+	+	+	+	–	–	–	+
Chromatographic	+	+	+	+	+	–	–	+
Assay for active substance								
Light absorbtion	+	+	+	+	–	–	–	+
Chromatographic	+	+	+	+	+	–	–	+

practical terms it is usually taken to represent the closeness of the mean value found using a number of repeat analyses to the 'conventional true value', i.e. that attributed to an in-house standard, or to an accepted reference value such as that attributed to a pharmacopoeial reference material.

Clearly, it is necessary to carefully evaluate the accuracy of most, if not all, assay methods. One approach is to compare the results obtained with the proposed new test procedure with those obtained using a previously validated or reference method (e.g. a pharmacopoeial method). This approach is often adopted when validating analytical methods used for ingredients and raw materials. With finished products, the test procedure can be evaluated by using samples or mixtures which have been 'spiked' with known amounts of pure added analyte (that is, the substance, ion, functional group, etc. that is under test). Added confidence in the accuracy of a method can be obtained by taking the demonstrably pure analyte substance and spiking it with excipients and/or impurities and demonstrating that the assay result, in comparison with results on unspiked pure samples, is unaffected by the presence of the added materials.

The results of such tests can give a measure of the systematic errors associated with the method. Accuracy may be improved by studying and eliminating as many sources of systematic error as possible (for example, those due to interference, imprecise calibration, faulty equipment settings and so on).

Chromatographic methods of impurity testing

The determination of the accuracy of quantitative impurity tests using thin layer chromatography (TLC) – as in a test for related substances – may be approached by spiking a sample with the known, or suspected impurities, at the proposed specification limit, and/or at a series of levels up to that limit. After development, the plate should be examined by each of the proposed methods of detection. For a satisfactory validation, the impurity zones in the spiked sample should display similar responses to those generated in adjacent zones, by standard applications of the impurities.

A similar approach is suitable for high performance liquid chromatography (HPLC) and gas chromatography (GC) methods of quantitative determination of impurities. Here, however, the test results will normally be calculated by electronic integration of detector responses, based on peak heights or areas. Validation is then based on comparison of integrator values for impurities in the spiked samples, with those generated by known levels of pure samples of the known or suspected impurities. Carr & Wahlich (1994) hold that, for impurity levels in the range 0.1–1.0%, using modern chromatographic equipment, recoveries in the range 80–120% may be expected.

The accuracy of other methods for the quantitative determination of impurities (e.g. ion-selective electrode, potentiometric and atomic spectroscopic methods) can also be evaluated by recovery experiments, using samples spiked with known quantities of impurities.

Assay

A variety of analytical methods are used in the assay of bulk drug substances (or 'APIs'), and thus the approach to evaluating accuracy must be selected accordingly, as appropriate to the analytical method concerned. For titrimetric methods, expected equivalence points can be calculated theoretically, taking into account the number of titratable functions and the molecular weight. It is however necessary to ensure that the expected stoichiometric relationships do indeed apply in practice, and this is best determined by performing the proposed titration procedure on a well-characterised reference standard. Recalling the relatively narrow assay tolerances common in specifications for bulk synthetic drug substances (often of the order of 99.5–100.5%), it is necessary to establish that this range is still valid in the presence of impurities at their proposed maximum limits, as these may significantly influence results due to additional titratable functional groups and/or large molecular weight differences.

In the determination of the accuracy of a UV light absorption assay of a bulk drug substance, based on a specific absorbance (A1%, 1 cm) value, it is essential to ensure that the value selected is the appropriate one for the purpose. This may be verified by examination of the results achieved, using the selected A1%, 1 cm value in the assay of a well-characterised reference sample. It is also important to consider the potential effects of the presence of impurities at their maximum limits, which could compromise the accuracy of the assay method.

The accuracy of assays of bulk substances by HPLC may be evaluated by methods analogous to those outlined above in relation to quantitative impurity determinations.

In the determination of the accuracy of assays of active content in a finished product, a prime consideration is that of the introduction of the further complicating factor of the common need to extract the analyte from the sample matrix. Thus, demonstration of the accuracy of the assay method *per se* may, on its own, be insufficient. What is needed is a demonstration of the accuracy of the 'total package' – extraction plus assay. A spectrophotometric assay (say) of a solution of an analyte, extracted from (say) a tablet may well have a high level of accuracy. But it is of no avail if only a portion of the analyte has been extracted from the product, and/or if other interfering substances have been extracted with it.

A common approach to determination of the accuracy of assays for the active component of a finished product is to perform what are commonly termed 'recovery experiments', in which the assay is performed on mixtures of excipients which have been spiked with accurately measured amounts of the pure active substance. Rational selection of the spiking range is important. For example, in the determination of the accuracy of an assay method used as a basis for product release, against a specification of 95–105%, then a spiking range of 80–120% should be employed, with the excipient mixture spiked with, say, five levels of the analyte equivalent to 80, 90, 100, 110 and 120% of the theoretical content. Errors at each level of not more than ± 2% would normally be considered to be an adequate demonstration of the accuracy of the assay. For the assay used in a stability study, particularly when the product samples are subject to more than usual stress, and may thus be expected to degrade to below 80%, then accuracy validation over a wider spiking range is obviously appropriate.

In this type of accuracy validation, it may be that the relevant excipient mixtures are not available. Nevertheless recovery experiments are still possible by spiking the actual product with pure active substance at carefully measured levels of, say, 5, 10, 15 and 20% above the theoretical level and assaying the samples 'as is' (i.e. 100%) and at the 105, 110, 115 and 120% levels.

As an alternative approach, where recovery experiments as outlined above may not be possible, Carr & Wahlich (1990) have suggested 'recovery efficiency experiments'. This is most appropriate for HPLC and GC methods, and requires an internal standard. In this approach to determination of the accuracy of a finished product assay, the sample is extracted with the solvent intended in the assay procedure, but with the addition of an internal standard. After centrifuging or filtering, about 75% of the supernatant (or the filtrate) is taken and subjected to the remainder of the assay procedure and the ratio of the analyte response to the internal standard response noted. The sample residue (including the approximately 25% supernatant from the first extract) is then re-extracted with a further volume of solvent, without internal standard. Following centrifuging (or filtration) this second extract is subjected to the remainder of the assay procedure, as before, and the ratio of analyte response to internal standard response is again noted. The variance between the two ratios should not be greater than ± 2%. If after the second extraction the peak response ratio remains unchanged, this indicates that no further analyte has been extracted, and the method may therefore be considered to be efficient. If the response ratio increases, this indicates that the extraction procedure was not efficient, as additional analyte has now been extracted. It does however need to be noted that if the active drug substance(s) is so strongly absorbed on to the excipient(s) that it is not extracted by the second solvent treatment, the two response ratios will remain equal, and the problem will not be identified.

A further factor is the issue of sample ageing. Analytical methods for products tend to be developed and validated using samples which have been freshly prepared, but it should be demonstrated that the method will remain accurate when applied to older samples. This is particularly relevant to the assay of samples of stability study materials which have been stored under stress conditions.

Precision with repeatability and reproducibility

Precision is the closeness of the agreement, one with another, of a series of separate measurements or determinations made when applying a prescribed method to a series of samples all taken from the one homogeneous lot of material. It is a measure of the closeness of the 'grouping' (or the wideness of the 'scatter') of a series of results. It is thus possible for a method to be precise, without necessarily being very accurate. Tests for precision also reveal the random errors associated with the method.

The question arises of whether a method which is very precise, but notably inaccurate, is of any value – and the answer is it can be if the inaccuracy is quantifiable and always in 'the same direction'. Then a systematic correction can be applied, to yield results which may be considered to be accurate.

Precision validation needs to be directed at the two sub-classes of precision: determination of repeatability and of reproducibility. An ICH text, *Note for Guidance on Validation of Analytical Procedures: Methodology* (ICH, 1995), introduces a third sub-class of precision, which it terms 'intermediate precision'.

Repeatability involves the evaluation of the results obtained by the same analyst, working under the same operating conditions, repeatedly using the same equipment, with identical reagents, over a relatively short time period. That is, it is about precision under the same, or very closely similar, conditions. The results may be expressed in terms of a repeatability standard deviation, repeatability coefficient of variation/relative standard deviation, and confidence interval of the mean value. The ICH text recommends that repeatability should be assessed by either (a) using a minimum of nine determinations covering the specified range for the procedure (e.g. three concentrations/three replicates each), or (b) a minimum of six determinations at 100% of the test concentration.

Reproducibility refers to variation between laboratories using different reagent sources and different analysts on different days and apparatus from different suppliers. That is, it is about precision under different conditions, and is assessed by a series of inter-laboratory trials. The results may be expressed in terms of the reproducibility standard deviation, reproducibility coefficient of variation/relative standard deviation, and confidence interval of the mean value.

Validation

The precision of virtually all quantitative methods needs to be validated. Clearly, the validation of repeatability is crucial. However, it becomes something of a philosophical question as to when and how the reproducibility of an analytical method should be validated, and it has to be wondered if a method intended only to be used in one laboratory, under standard and consistent conditions, requires reproducibility validation. However it does need to be noted that, in a 'new product cycle' from R&D, via scale-up, to full-scale production, the new assay method may well be employed, even within the one company, in a series of different laboratories, from the analytical development laboratory, via pilot plant and (possibly) clinical trials manufacturing laboratory to routine production QC laboratory. So, even though the original intention is that a method is intended for use within the one organisation, it may well be prudent, from a Quality viewpoint, to validate reproducibility in the context of different laboratories, analysts, times, equipment and sources of reagents.

When validating a finished product test-method for precision, it is important that 'real' samples, as distinct from spiked excipient mixes, are tested, as this can lead to apparently satisfactory results which cannot then be achieved in real life. Furthermore, the complete procedure should be applied to each replicate analysis, although it may be useful to examine separately the precision of the various stages of the analytical procedure in order to reveal any steps which may be critical to the precision of the procedure.

Assuming that, in a repeatability test, x_n results are obtained from n replicate tests, then the mean (m), standard deviation (σ) and relative standard deviation (RSD) should be calculated as follows:

$$m = \frac{(x_1 + x_2 + x_3.....x_n)}{n}$$

$$\sigma = \frac{\sum\limits_{x=1}^{x=n}(x - m)^2}{(n - 1)}$$

$$RSD = \frac{100\sigma}{m}$$

The RSD value is an index of the scatter that may be expected in the results obtained from an assay procedure. An assay result x may, for example, be taken (with (96% confidence) to be within the range $x \pm 2RSD$. Such considerations bear significantly on the relationship between an assay method and the limits set in the specification for the material to be assayed. It is both useless and pointless, for example, to employ an assay procedure with a precision RSD of 2, when the specification limits are $\pm1\%$. There are two alternatives: select a more precise method of assay, or adopt wider limits. Compendial limits for the assay of bulk drug substances are often of the order of 98.5–100.5%. For an assay method to be valid in the context of limits such as these, a high degree of precision (and thus a low RSD) is required. Thus the assays recommended in official compendia are often titrimetric methods, which can function at RSD values well below 1%. On the other hand, chromatographic methods, although generally more specific, are usually less precise. Generally they can be demonstrated as having RSD values of under 2%. They are thus well suited to finished product assays, where specification limits of the order of 95–105% are common.

The precision of a method also bears upon its value for use in stability studies. It might, for example, be expected that a product will degrade less than 1% during its anticipated (or simulated) shelf-life. Even an HPLC method which is considered to be stability-indicating will not be able to discriminate, with 96% confidence, between samples at 99% and 100% of original potency, after a period of storage. It is thus necessary to monitor the test samples for individual degradation products, both for this reason as well as from the aspect of patient safety.

The determination of that other aspect of precision, *reproducibility,* requires a number of different repeatability studies (as discussed above) to be performed under the various different conditions, i.e. different laboratories, different analysts, different equipment, different times, different batches (or suppliers) of reagents. It may not be necessary to involve all these variables, which should be selected as best to model the range of circumstances under which the method will be applied in routine use. From the results obtained in each set of circumstances, the mean, standard deviation and RSD should be calculated, from whence it can be determined whether or not the different sets of values indicate acceptable reproducibility. A Student's t-test can be used to compare mean values, and an F-test to compare standard deviations. Reference to standard statistical tables for these values will indicate whether or not there are any significant differences when the method is performed under the various different circumstances.

Specificity (selectivity)

The term 'selectivity' often appears in the literature, used as if synonymous with 'specificity'. However, a distinction has been drawn between the two terms in the CPMP guidelines on analytical validation (CPMP, 1990) thus:

- *Specificity* is a term to be applied to a method designed to make a quantitative determination of an analyte in a mixture with one or more other substances.
- *Selectivity* is a term to be applied to a method designed to detect qualitatively the analyte in the presence of other substances, functional groups etc.

In more simple terms, the distinction has been expressed (Carr & Wahlich, 1994) as: *specificity* is the ability of a non-separative method to distinguish between different compounds, whereas *selectivity* is the ability of a separative method to resolve different compounds.

The importance and significance of the validation of method specificity vary according to the use to which the test is put. For an identity test, the method should ensure the identity of the analyte. That is, the method should demonstrably be capable of specifically identifying the substance, compound, group, ion etc. that it is intended to identify. With impurity control tests it may be possible to consider the totality of the control methods and their *overall* adequacy in controlling factors such as related substances, impurities, degradation products, heavy metals and catalyst residues, organic solvent residues, etc.

The assay used for stability studies should be capable of detecting the signal from the analyte alone, without interference from excipients, degradation products or other impurities. That is, it should provide a specific indication of the stability of the substance under study. On the other hand, for routine batch analysis, such a degree of specificity for the assay procedure may not be necessary, provided that additional tests adequately control such things as related substances and degradation products, which might otherwise interfere.

Validation of method specificity can be performed by spiking experiments, using known (or expected) impurities, degradation products or excipients, and then analysing the spiked sample against an unspiked sample to demonstrate an adequate response from the specific analyte of interest, and a lack of interference from the other substances present.

Method selectivity may be confirmed by spiking experiments. For example, when using a chromatographic method, if the 'spike' substance appears clearly in the chromatogram, the method may be considered to be selective. If, on the other hand, it does not appear, it may have been co-eluted with another substance in the sample mix, it may not be detectable by the method selected, or it may have been retained on the column. Applying the same chromatographic method to the pure substance alone should reveal which of these factors is operating. The selectivity of a method for finished product analysis can be established by comparing the results obtained when applying the method to the pure drug substance with those obtained on samples of the drug substance plus excipients.

Sensitivity/linearity

Sensitivity may be defined as the capacity of an analytical method to record small variations in the concentration of the analyte. It may be determined by applying the method to samples containing increasingly small differences in the concentration of the analyte.

The linearity of a test procedure is a measure of its ability, within a given range, to yield results directly proportional to the amount (or concentration) in the sample of the substance under test (the analyte). Analytical procedures which are not strictly linear may be acceptable if some other mathematical relationship, or proportionality factor, is determined and applied.

For the establishment of linearity, a minimum of five different known concentrations of the analyte should be assayed, and the results obtained plotted against the known concentrations, to determine if the relationship between the known concentration and the assay response is linear, and if extrapolated back to zero concentration, the intercept passes through the origin. The range of concentrations over which linearity is determined should be selected with care, and in relation to the intended application of the analytical method. The ranges recommended by Carr & Wahlich (1994) are given in Table 17.4.

Table 17.4   Linearity verification

Intended application	Typical spec. range (%)	Validation range (%)
Release spec. assay	95–105	80–120
Assay of active in a stability study	90–105	80–120
Content uniformity test	75–125	60–140
Assay of preservative in stability study	50–110	40–120
Assay of degradation products in stability study	0–10	0–20

Limit of detection

This is the lowest amount of the analyte that can be detected, but not necessarily quantified, by the method. It is a parameter mainly of significance in the context of limit tests for impurities. It is determined by the analysis of samples with differing known concentrations of the pure analyte, and thus establishing the minimum level at which the analyte can be detected.

Limit of quantitation (limit of quantification)

This is the lowest level at which a quantitative determination can be undertaken with a stated precision and accuracy under stated experimental conditions. That is, it is the lowest amount of an analyte in a sample which can be quantitatively determined (with suitable accuracy and precision). It is particularly relevant to the quantitative determination of low levels of impurities and/or degradation products in a sample. It is generally determined by the analysis of a series of samples with differing, and decreasing, low concentrations of the analyte, thereby establishing the minimum level at which the analyte can be quantified with acceptable accuracy and precision.

Range

This is the interval between the upper and lower level of the amount of an analyte which can be demonstrated with suitable precision, accuracy and linearity. It is normally derived from linearity studies.

Robustness

A further term which appears in the literature (e.g. ICH, 1993) is 'robustness'. The term 'ruggedness' is also often used synonymously.

The robustness of an analytical procedure is a measure of its capacity to remain unaffected by small, but deliberate variations in method parameters, and thus provides an indication of the reliability of the method during normal usage, under various conditions.

If the results of an analytical procedure are susceptible to variations in the analytical conditions, such conditions must be properly controlled, and an appropriate cautionary statement included in the written specification/method.

Typical variations which may need to be evaluated include:

- Different makes of equipment.
- Different analysts.
- Instability of analytical reagents.

In the case of liquid chromatography:

- Influence of variations of pH in a mobile phase.
- Influence of variations in mobile phase composition.

- Different columns (different lots and/or suppliers).
- Flow rate.
- Temperature.

In the case of gas chromatography:

- Different columns (lots and/or suppliers).
- Flow rate.
- Temperature.

Afterthought

It might be useful to conclude this section with a caution against excess of analytical zeal, and to do so in the words of the late, great C A ('Johnny') Johnson, long-time Scientific Director and Secretary of the BP, speaking from the chair of the Science Sessions at the British Pharmaceutical Conference, 1974:

> The enthusiasm of the analyst for the power and wonder of the tools at his command is understandable but must not be allowed to cloud the real purpose of his work, which is to ensure that the medicines he examines are adequately pure, but not necessarily devoid of all detectable traces of foreign substances. The mere existence of a test is not of itself a justification for applying it; as with everything else in life we must keep things in perspective.

References

Carr G P R, Wahlich J C (1990). A practical approach to method validation in pharmaceutical analysis. *J Pharm Biomed Anal* 8, 613–618.

Carr G P R, Wahlich J C (1994). Analytical validation. In: Cartwright and Matthews (eds), *International Pharmaceutical Product Registration – Aspects Of Quality, Safety and Efficacy.* London: Ellis Horwood.

CPMP (1990). CPMP Notes for Guidance: Analytical Validation. Addendum 1990 to Volume III of *Rules Governing Medicinal Products in the European Community.* Committee on Proprietary Medical Products. Available from the Office for Official Publications of the European Community, Luxembourg.

Hovsepian P K (1996). Bulk drug substances and finished products. In: Relay and Rosanske (eds), *Development and Validation of Analytical Methods.* London: Pergamon.

ICH (1993). *Draft consensus text on validation of analytical procedures.* International conference on Harmonisation, 27 October 1993.

ICH (1995) *Note for Guidance on Validation of Analytical Methods: Methodology.* International conference on Harmonisation, 29 November 1995.

Johnson C A (1974). The influence of chromatography on the purity of medicines. *Pharm J* 213 (7 Sept), 199–201.

18

Laboratory documentation and records

To the last syllable of recorded time
W Shakespeare, *Macbeth*, Act 5, Sc. 5

The *raisons d'etre* for laboratory documentation, and its basic objectives, are the same as discussed in Part Four, in the context of manufacturing operations. Laboratory documentation should be designed and used so as to be in line with the general principles outlined. In particular, test results should be recorded in a manner that will facilitate comparative reviews of those results and thus the detection of trends.

Laboratory records

The details recorded should include:

- Name of product or material, and code reference.
- Date of receipt and sampling.
- Source of product or material.
- Date of testing.
- Batch or lot number.
- Indication of tests performed.
- Reference to the method used.
- Results obtained.
- Decision regarding release, rejection or other status.
- Signature or initials of analyst, and signature of person taking this decision.

In addition to the records in this format, analysts' laboratory records (e.g. laboratory notebooks) should also be retained, with the raw data and calculations from which the test results were derived. Often notebooks with preprinted page numbers are used to demonstrate that all notes, and data, have been retained.

Laboratory documentation

The EC GMP Guide (EC, 1992) states requirements for the following types of document:

- Specifications.
- Sampling procedures.
- Testing procedures and records (including analytical worksheets and/or laboratory notebooks).
- Analytical reports and/or certificates.
- Data from environmental monitoring, where required.
- Validation records of test methods, where applicable.
- Procedures for and records of the calibration of instruments and maintenance of equipment.

It also adds a recommendation that analytical test results (and certain other data) 'be kept in a manner permitting trend evaluation', and that '. . . original data such as laboratory notebooks . . . should be retained and readily available.'

Specifications

Written specifications, prepared and authorised by Quality Control should be established and maintained for all starting materials, packaging materials, and bulk, intermediate and finished products. Materials and products should be tested against the relevant specification and the results recorded. A system should be in place to ensure that a formal decision is made, on the basis of the test results, by an appropriately authorised person (e.g., in the case of products, the designated Qualified Person), and that this decision is securely and unequivocally conveyed to the persons (or organisational unit) who have to act upon it.

An illustrative example of a starting material specification is shown at Form 18.1. The same format will serve also for bulk, intermediate and finished products.

In the example shown, a compendial material is assumed, and the majority of the test procedures to be employed are those of the relevant pharmacopoeia (the 'UP', or 'Universal Pharmacopoeia'). In the case of tests which are not pharmacopoeial, or cannot be defined by reference to other official standards, reference to an internal house procedure is necessary. For example, in Form 18.1, for the bulk density test there is a reference to an in-house procedure (ASOP – 'Analytical Standard Operating Procedure' – No. 142). Note, too, the listing of suppliers approved to supply this material.

As the testing of the sample against this written specification proceeds, the raw data are commonly noted in the analyst's laboratory notebook. As the result of each test is obtained, it is entered on an analytical

EXCELLOPHARM Co. – STARTING MATERIAL SPECIFICATION

Opprobrium apostate UP – Code no. 1376

Molecular formula. $C_nH_yN_xP_z$, $2H_2O$

Relative molecular mass. 187.2

Pharmacopoeial Tests:
Description. Pale yellow fine crystalline powder
Solubility. Slightly soluble in water. Readily soluble in ethanol and acetone to give clear, faintly yellow solution.
Identification. Complies with the UP tests.
Melting Point. 168 to 172°C
Loss on drying. Not more than 0.5%
Heavy metals. Not more than 15 ppm
Sulphated ash. Not more than 0.1%
Related substances. Complies with the UP test
Assay. 99.9 to 101% as the dihydrate, calculated with reference to the dried material (UP method)

Additional tests:

Bulk density: 1.7 to 2.3 ml/g (ASOP no. 142)

Approved suppliers:
>   Chemolux Ltd.
>   Apimatic Inc.
>   Pharming Corp

Spec. No.	Supersedes	Prepared by:	Approved by:	Effective date:	Page 1 of 1

report form. Form 18.2 shows an example of a format much to be recommended. This type of analytical report requires the preparation and printing of a series of report forms which are specific to a given material or product. The great advantage is that the printing of a summary of the specification, against which each result is entered, permits an easy, rapid and relatively secure evaluation of the compliance of the test results with the specification. In the example shown, the form has been completed manually and the decision (to release) taken and formally entered.

At the same time, the test results should be entered on a summary report sheet, or card. An example is shown at Form 18.3, with a manual entry made for the same lot of opprobrium apostate 15927. A record in this format facilitates checking for quality trends, and comparison of the standards attained by different suppliers. Indeed it makes these useful quality tactics a rapid and ongoing, rather than a tedious occasional, activity.

Note that as this is not a primary record, and space is probably limited, a little 'shorthand' (ticks, 'complies', 'OK', etc.) is usually considered acceptable.

The message that the material is released (or rejected) is conveyed to those who need to know, by means of the materials receiving report, previously shown in Chapter 15, but now re-shown in Form 18.4 as completed by Goods Inwards, and now stamped 'Released' and signed. The concept illustrated presupposes that the allocation of starting materials to manufacturing batches is the responsibility of a Materials Inventory Control unit, who are only able to allocate materials which have been released by QC. It is also at this stage that an authorised QC person applies the completed 'Released' labels to the quarantine goods. For completeness, he/she can, at the same time, stamp 'Released' and sign the GI copy of the Receiving Report, and GI can now complete the last two columns of the Starting Material Delivery Record (see Chapter 15, especially Form 15.2).

These four documents (Forms 18.1 to 18.4), together with variations suitably adapted to cover intermediate and finished products, can be regarded as the key documents in the quality control of routine manufacture, with the 'release' message in relation to finished products being conveyed by the Qualified Person on the final page of the Batch Packaging Record (see Form 15.6).

Written sampling procedures, stating amounts of sample to be taken, from whence and how, will be required in relation to both starting materials and products. These should be laid down as for SOPs (see Chapter 15). The same applies to testing procedures which are not as given in a pharmacopoeia or other official compendium, and to procedures and programmes for the calibration and maintenance of laboratory instruments, including balances. Records of such calibration and maintenance need to be maintained. This is probably most conveniently done by means of ruled hardback notebooks held with, or close to, the equipment in question. Whatever system is employed, it should clearly 'flag' when the next calibration, or maintenance service, is due.

EXCELLOPHARM Co. – ANALYTICAL REPORT

Opprobrium apostate UP – Code no. 1376

Lot no. ...*15927*... Date received ...*19/8/98*... Date sampled ...*20/8/98*... Supplier ...*Apimatic*...

	Specification (No. 168/B)	Result
Description	Pale yellow crystalline powder	*pale yellow crystal. powder*
Solubility	Sl. soluble in water Readily soluble in ethanol and in acetone	*complies*
Solution	Clear, faintly yellow	*clear, almost colourless (just yellow)*
Identification	Complies with UP tests	*complies*
Melting Point	168 to 172°C	*169.5°C*
Loss on drying	Not more than 0.5%	*<0.25%*
Heavy metals	Not more than 15 ppm	*5 ppm*
Sulphated ash	Not more than 0.1%	*0.06%*
Related substances	Complies with UP test	*complies*
Bulk density	1.7 to 2.3 ml/g	*1.9 ml/g*
Assay	99.9 to 101.0% (as dihydrate, with ref. to the dried material)	*100.30%*

Report compiled by (Sign.) ...*G. Dipper*... **Date** ...*24/8/98*...

Release/Reject decision ...*Released*... **Signed** ...*C. Chemist*... **Date** ...*25/8/98*...

Comments

ANALYTICAL REPORT SUMMARY: 1367 Opprobrium apostate

Lot No.	Supplier	Description	Solubility	Solution	Ident.	M.Pt.	Loss on drying	Heavy metals	Sulphated ash	Related subs.	Bulk density	Assay	Decision	Date
15927	Apimatic	✓	Complies	Complies	Complies	169.5°C	<0.25%	5 ppm	0.06%	Complies	1.9 ml/g	100.3%	RELEASE	25/8/99

GOODS INWARDS – MATERIALS RECEIVING REPORT

Material ...... *Opprobrium apostate* .... **Code No.** .... *1376* ....

INSTRUCTIONS: 1. Complete a separate Receiving Report for each delivery, and for each supplier's batch number within a delivery.
2. Retain one copy in Goods Inwards file, and send three copies to Quality Control.
3. **Quality Control**: On completion of testing, mark this report, where indicated, "RELEASED", "REJECTED", "HOLD" as appropriate, and send a copy to:
    Purchasing Department
    Materials Inventory Control

    Retain one copy on Quality Control files

Date goods received ...... *19 Aug. 1998* ......

Supplier ...... *Apimatic* ......

Supplier's batch no. ...... *1375/1* ......

Quantity received ...... *100 kg* ......

Number of containers ...... *10* ......

Purchase Order No. ...... *02956* ......

Assigned Lot No. ...... *15927* ......

General condition/cleanliness of delivery

...... *satisfactory* ......

Delivery examined by (Signed) ...... *J. Reynolds* ...... Date ...... *19/8/98* ......

Remarks/Comments

QUALITY CONTROL DECISION

> # QC RELEASED
> Signed ...... *R. Smithers* ......
> Date ...... *24/8/98* ......

Reference

EC (1992). *The Rules Governing Medicinal Products in the European Community, Vol. IV: Good Manufacturing Practice for Medicinal Products.* Luxembourg: Commission of the European Communities. Available from The Office for Official Publications of the European Communities, Luxembourg. Also available from The Stationery Office (HMSO), London, and the EC Information Service, Washington, USA. (Referred to as the EC GMP Guide.)

Part Six

Sterile and other products

19

Sterile products: basic concepts and principles

This goodly frame, the earth, seems to me a sterile promontory
W Shakespeare, *Hamlet*, Act 2, Sc. 2

Sterile products are very significantly different from non-sterile products. The reason for this difference lies quite simply in the obvious and banal truism that they are, or are intended to be, sterile. This raises a whole raft of manufacturing, control and quality issues, additional to those which are relevant to non-sterile products. The same quality and GMP considerations which apply to non-sterile products, apply equally to sterile products. But the attainment and maintenance of the sterile state imposes additional quality assuring demands. The special requirements (ethical, professional and regulatory) for sterile products manufacture are additional to, rather than separate from, those which apply to products in general. It is noteworthy that most major statements on GMP, throughout the world, with the surprising exception of the US CGMPs, have substantial separate sections on sterile products. The 'Sterile medicinal products' annex of the EC GMP Guide is, for example, the largest single section in that publication. Before looking further at those special quality-assuring requirements it is necessary to establish some basic concepts and principles and to look at the various methods of sterile products manufacture.

Definition of sterility

'Sterility' is such an important word, so central a concept in the context of products used for parenteral administration (and similarly critical applications) that it is surprising there has been so much variation, laxity and confusion in its use.

First, two obviously inadequate definitions which have been proposed in the past:

1. A sterile product is one that is free from living micro-organisms.
2. Sterility is the absence of organisms able to reproduce themselves.

The former would permit the presence of goldfish, tadpoles and newts, and the latter the presence of living micro-organisms, still potentially dangerous, but which had had their reproductive processes inhibited (for example, by sub-lethal doses of radiation). It would also permit the presence of several monkeys, swimming about in a 'sterile' bulk solution, provided they had been neutered, or were all of the same sex.

A totally uncompromised, and uncompromising, definition was given in the UK Orange Guide (Sharp, 1983):

> Sterility: The complete absence of living organisms.
> [Note: The state of sterility is an absolute – there are no degrees of sterility.]

There have, however, been those who seem to find such a definition *too* uncompromising – and who prefer a concept of a state of 'near' or 'almost' sterility, where apparently the odd organism, here and there, is acceptable.

The first official statement along these lines appeared in an amendment to the Nordic Pharmacopoeia in 1970:

> Sterile drugs must be prepared and sterilised under conditions which aim at such a result that in one million units there will be no more than one living micro-organism.

This same broad general line was also followed by the United States Pharmacopoeia (USP XXI):

> [It is] . . . generally accepted that . . . injectable articles or . . . devices purporting to be sterile . . . (when autoclaved) attain a 10^{-6} microbial survivor probability, i.e. assurance less than one chance in a million that viable organisms are present in the sterilised article or dosage form.

The British Pharmacopoeia (BP) in 1988 adopted a similar (but note, only an *approximately* similar) stance, in considering sterility to be:

> . . . a theoretical level of not more than one living micro-organism in 10^{6} containers in the final product.

Setting aside this strange concept of a 'theoretical' level of micro-organisms (surely here, of all places, we should be thinking of what is, or is not, *really* present), it needs to be noted that there are subtle but very real differences between these two pharmacopoeial definitions. The USP considered sterility to be a less-than-one-in-a-million chance that one, or any number (?) of containers, are contaminated with one or any number of organisms, whereas the BP permits, to qualify as sterile, no more than one organism in only one out of a million containers. The potential problems (for patients) need to be considered before any unquestioning acceptance of such definitions. Consider for example a large volume parenteral infusion (LVP). As real life events have tragically illustrated, in such products even normally non-pathogenic organisms can kill. In many such products, one organism today can become many millions tomorrow. Over 100 million units of LVP solutions are administered annually throughout the world. Are we really happy to accept that one in every million of those may contain organisms?

For if we are, then we must also logically be happy to accept 100+ unnecessarily dead patients per year worldwide.

However, more recent editions of the USP and BP have evidenced a degree of backing away from the 'less-than-one-in-a-million' position, possibly as a result of a dawning realisation of the potential practical consequences of adopting such a position.

The current edition of the USP (XXIII, 1995) states:

> Within the strictest definition of sterility, a specimen would be deemed sterile only when there is complete absence of viable organisms from it. However, this absolute definition cannot currently be applied to finished compendial articles because of limitations in testing. Absolute sterility cannot be practically demonstrated. . . . The sterility of a lot purported to be sterile is therefore defined in probability terms, where the likelihood of a contaminated unit or article is acceptably remote.

What is, in fact, 'acceptably remote' the USP XXIII does not explicitly state. It is, however, implicit in a later comment in the same edition (in fact, an extended version of the statement quoted above) that:

> It is generally accepted that terminally sterilised injectable articles or critical devices purporting to be sterile when processed in the autoclave attain a 10^{-6} microbial survivor level, i.e. assurance of less than one chance in one million that viable micro-organisms are present in the sterilised article or dosage form. With heat-stable articles, the approach often is to considerably exceed the critical time necessary to achieve the 10^{-6} microbial survivor probability (overkill). However, with an article where an extensive heat exposure may have a damaging effect, it may not be possible to employ the overkill approach. In this latter instance the development of the sterilisation cycle depends heavily on knowledge of the microbial burden of the product, based on examination over a suitable time period of a substantial number of lots of the pre-sterilised product.

This latter comment is somewhat dubious, in conveying the idea that a sort of 'mean pre-sterilisation bioburden' figure be established by the examination of a finite number of batches over a finite period of time. In fact, as many would agree, the sound quality-assuring approach is to determine and record the bioburden in/on each lot, or load, each and every time, immediately prior to the sterilisation process.

The current BP unequivocally states 'Sterility is the absence of viable organisms'. It however adds later in the same appendix (XVIII):

> The achievement of sterility within any one item in a population submitted to a sterilisation process cannot be guaranteed, nor can it be demonstrated. . . . The SAL (Sterility Assurance Level) for a given process is expressed as the probability of a non-sterile item in that population. An SAL of 10^{-6}, for example, denotes a probability of not more than one viable micro-organism in 1×10^6 sterilised items of the final product. The SAL of a process for a given product is established by appropriate validation studies.

The question thus arises of what, in practice, is an acceptable SAL? The BP 1998 provides answers in relation to some, but not all, types of sterilisation process. For steam sterilisation it is stated that 'the procedures and precautions employed are such as to give a SAL of 10^{-6} or better'. This same statement is also made in relation to dry heat, and to radiation sterilisation. No comparable comment is made in relation to gaseous or to filtration sterilisation, doubtless in recognition that the SAL concept is not applicable to these latter two methods of sterilisation.

The French definition

It is interesting to note that the second edition of the French GMP guidelines *Bonnes Pratiques de Fabrication* (BPF, 1985) played a variation on both the 'one in a million' and the 'theoretical' themes, thus:

> *Stérile (état):* Etat défini en théori par l'absence de microrganisme vivant, en pratique par la proabilité d'avoir au maximum une unite non-sterile sur un million d'unites.
>
> *Sterile (state):* State defined in theory by the absence of living organisms, [and] in practice by the probability of having a maximum of one non-sterile unit in a million units.

Note the reversal of the earlier BP concept. In France, it was the total absence which was considered to be theoretical, and the probability of 1 non-sterile unit in 10^6 which was deemed to be practical.

Thus, from these few examples alone (and there are others) the range of conflicting definitions which have been offered, with their various ambiguities and imprecisions, becomes all too apparent. There can be no more crucial quality characteristic than the sterility of a parenteral product, yet just precisely what 'sterile' *means* seems to have been not at all clear in a number of minds.

When one makes these sort of comments the cry can often be heard: 'That is not what it really means. *Nobody* could really think or believe that one organism in 10^6 containers is acceptable.' But, they could and they *do*. To quote one more example, this time from a Professor of Pharmaceutical Technology, and a former chairman of the European Pharmacopoeia Commission (Polderman, 1990):

> Out of a batch of one million units only one container may contain an organism (Statistically maximally 3 at a 95% confidence level).

US FDA definition

Of all the 'quantitative/probability' definitions of sterility the one that perhaps gives the most comfort is the one implied in the US 'Compliance guideline on parametric release' (US FDA, 1987) which requires, as one of a number of preconditions, that the sterilisation process has been:

> ... validated to achieve ... bioburden reduction to 10^0 [unity], with a minimum safety factor of an additional six logarithm reduction.

The EC definition

It is both interesting and relevant to consider how the European Community (EC) defines 'sterility' (EC GMP Guide, English Edition, 1992):

> Sterility is the absence of living organisms. The conditions of the sterility test are given in the European Pharmacopoeia.

With the first clause there can be no argument. However, the whole statement is undermined by the immediately following implication that the so-called 'sterility test' has relevance to the establishment of a state of sterility throughout a batch of product.

Most, if not all, of the statements on sterility so far considered appear to be based on an assumption, explicit or implied, that the method used to achieve that state is some form of heat sterilisation process. A fairly recent FDA guide creates the impression that its author believes that moist heat is the *only* method (US FDA, 1993):

> Sterilization: the use of steam and pressure to kill any bacteria that may be able to contaminate that environment or vessel.

This definition may also be criticised on a number of other counts, not least the implication that the pressure kills bacteria, and that sterilisation can only be achieved by *killing* bacteria.

There are, of course, methods of sterilisation other than by steam. How has 'sterility' been defined in relation to these? What, for example, of filtration with subsequent aseptic filling? An early official statement on this subject appeared in the WHO's *General Requirement for the Sterility of Biological Substances* (1973):

> The operations where liquid preparations are filled should be checked. This may be done, e.g. at least twice a year, by filling not less than 1000 containers with nutrient medium . . . and incubating. If the containers . . . show a contamination rate above 0.3% some countries do not consider the procedure acceptable.

It is to be hoped that *all* countries would consider such a high contamination rate unacceptable!

In the US Parenteral Drug Association's (PDA) monograph 'Validation of Aseptic Filling for Solution Drug Products' (PDA, 1980), the comment is made that the WHO (1973) level of 0.3% is 'widely accepted', but 'a manufacturer should strive for a contamination level of less than 0.1%'.

This last document has been replaced by the PDA's technical report 'Process Simulation Testing of Aseptically Filled Products' (PDA, 1996), where under 'Interpretation of results and acceptance criteria' it is stated that:

> . . . the ultimate goal for the number of positives in any process simulation test should be zero. A sterile product is, after all, one which contains no viable organisms. . . . There are, however, numerous technical problems in achieving this goal. . . . The selection of acceptance criteria for aseptic processing validation is the central issue to be resolved in the conduct of process simulation tests.

Disappointingly, or perhaps inevitably, the report then offers little, if anything, in the way of quantitative advice on how to solve the technical problems, or to resolve the central issue. Nevertheless, in the field of aseptic processing, positions seem to shift from considerations of acceptable contamination levels of 3 in 1000, to 1 in 1000, to more recently expressed views that the target should be no more than 1 in 10,000. And these aims have to be compared with the 1 in a million, for heat sterilisation processes, which appears to be acceptable, in some form or other, to some authorities. Is 'sterility' therefore to be considered as a moving target?

Flawed thinking over the definition of sterility

Sufficient examples have been given to demonstrate a range of variable (and indeed, often ambiguous) views on what is meant by the word 'sterility'. In so many statements on the subject (and the original UK Orange Guide was a notable exception) there is an element of compromise. Sterility tends to be regarded by some, very wrongly, as a *conditional*, rather than an *absolute* state.

What is the problem? Why this indecision and ambiguity over so fundamental an issue? The answer is a very simple, albeit philosophical, one. It is that there is a fundamental flaw at the heart of much thinking and writing about sterility, and *that flaw resides in a confusion between the nature of a concept or a state, and the probability of the existence of that state*.

The point was well made in an insufficiently noticed paper by Brown & Gilbert (1977):

> The concept of sterility is absolute. Whether or not a medicinal product is sterile is inevitably a matter of probability.

If this distinction were universally noted and adopted, the problem would cease to exist. The *only possible* definition of 'sterility' is the uncompromised, unconditional and absolute one given in the UK Orange Guide (Sharp, 1983). The question of the existence of such an absolute, negative state must, inevitably, be a matter of probability, not of absolute certainty. But what is odd or new about that? We have long been aware that we do not live in a grand, simple, predictable, deterministic, Newtonian universe. We inhabit an Einsteinian, quantum mechanical, *probabilistic* universe (or, at least for the present we think we do). In such a universe, the question of the existence of the absolute state of sterility is, of course, a matter of probability, just as the existence (or chances of happening) of any other state, event, thing or occurrence is a matter of probability (not certainty).

This does not preclude our *aiming* to achieve this (or any other) absolute state. In the case of sterility, our concern should be over whether we have in fact achieved that state at an acceptable level of probability, and it is not unreasonable to suggest that what may be regarded as an acceptable level of probability could well be considered to vary according to circumstances.

Compare, for example, two different types of terminally heat-sterilised product:

1.   A small volume (say, 0.5 or 1.0 ml) injection of a *non*-growth supporting liquid, intended for intramuscular or subcutaneous injection.
2.   A large volume parenteral (LVP), say 1 litre of dextrose/saline solution for intravenous infusion.

That both should be sterile there can be no question. However, one could well consider that the *level of assurance of the probability of attainment of that state* is more critical in the latter than the former.

Assuming a low pre-sterilisation bioburden, and a validated sterilisation cycle, the chance of the presence of even a single heat-resistant pathogenic organism in a unit of the first product is remote, probably extremely remote. The non-growth promoting solution will not encourage the proliferation of organisms, and non-pathogenic organisms, although undesirable and indeed objectionable, are not likely in these circumstances to be a matter of life or death.

Now compare the second product, the LVP. As real life events have tragically illustrated, in such products even normally non-pathogenic organisms can kill. In such solutions, one organism today can become many millions tomorrow. As already noted, well over 100 million LVP units are administered annually throughout the world. Can anyone (particularly the 100+ doomed patients) be really happy to accept that one in every million of those may contain organisms?

Two different products, and the *absolute* requirement that they should be sterile applies to both of them. But the *degree of probability* required for the achievement of that state could well be considered to be different.

Why sterility?

There are a number of different methods of sterilisation, which will be considered shortly. Before we do, it is worth raising the question of why certain products have to be sterile.

The most important, simple and obvious, reason is that there are special dangers of causing serious infections if they are not.

In the case of orally administered products such as tablets, capsules, syrups, etc., the body has certain natural defences against at least low levels of contamination, although it is obviously not a good idea that even these products should be contaminated with dangerous organisms. Products required to be given in, or through, more sensitive areas must be sterile.

Injected products by-pass the body's natural defences against micro-organisms, and the consequences of injecting even slightly contaminated products can be very serious. Injection of products contaminated with micro-organisms can cause, and has caused, death. The same applies to things like devices, instruments and implants which are intended to be inserted into blood vessels, muscles or other parts of the body.

For the same reason, products intended for use in the eye (drops, ointments, lotions), for application to wounds, sores or broken skin (liquids, creams, ointments or dressings) or used in operations to irrigate body cavities, must be sterile. It is also usually considered necessary that ear drops should be sterile, and some consider that nose drops should be sterile as well.

So, the sort of products which need to be sterile include:

- Injections, e.g.

    — Antibiotics
    — Large volume infusions ('drips')
    — Vaccines

- Eye products (ophthalmics), e.g.

    — Eye drops
    — Eye lotions
    — Eye ointments

- Ear drops.
- Some skin preparations, e.g.

    — Lotions, creams and ointments for application to broken skin

- Irrigation solutions, e.g.

    — Wound irrigations
    — Bladder irrigations

- Implants.
- Dressings.
- Medical and surgical devices and instruments.
- Diagnostic products.

In addition, *materials, equipment, containers, closures,* etc. used in the manufacture of sterile product, and for use in microbiological/pathological laboratory procedures will need to be sterile.

There is thus a wide range of uses, and routes of administration, of sterile products and materials. For parenteral products alone there are a number of different injection routes, e.g. subcutaneous, intradermal, intramuscular, intravenous, intrathecal, intra-articular, intracardial, intraperitoneal, intracisternal, peridural. It will be apparent that parenteral routes of administration, all other things being equal, present a significantly higher level of potential patient risk than, for example, oral administration, and the question inevitably arises, 'Why inject if this is such a potentially dangerous route of administration?' There are a number of possible reasons for choosing this route. They include:

1. When the active substance in the product is destroyed when it is taken by mouth. (For example, some substances are inactivated by the digestive fluids in the gut, yet retain their activity when injected into the bloodstream or into the muscles.)
2. When very rapid action is required, for example in an emergency, after

injury, or in the case of a severe infection. (Action following an injection is usually much quicker than when a product is swallowed.)

3.   When it is necessary to 'target' the part of the body where the action of the medicine is required more accurately than is usually possible with products taken by mouth. For example, injection into the heart, brain or spinal canal.

4.   When the patient is unable to take the medicine in any other way, for example, he or she cannot swallow or is unconscious.

Sterilisation – fundamental concepts

Not infrequently there is talk of 'sterilisation' as if it were one single, discrete type of operation. This is just not so. There are a number of different methods of sterilisation. They include:

- Heat (steam or dry heat).
- Radiation (e.g. gamma ray or electron beam).
- Gas (e.g. ethylene oxide).
- Filtration (with subsequent aseptic handling).

These are not mere variations on a basic theme. These processes are all very different, one from another. Each has its own technology, mode of action and application. It is no exaggeration to state that the technological difference between the manufacture of sterile products using (a) steam sterilisation and (b) filtration and aseptic processing is as great, if not greater, as the difference between the manufacture of tablets and the manufacture of ointments. Thoughtlessly to 'lump-together' all possible types of sterile manufacture as if they were all essentially the same is but one of a number of possible errors of judgement.

A feature which *is* common to all the types of process is, obviously, the objective of making a product which is, in fact, sterile. Concomitantly, the products should also, in many cases, be free of particles and of pyrogens. The attributes of freedom from organisms, from non-viable particles and from pyrogenic substances may be said to be interconnected. Some micro-organism species can release toxic metabolites, or endotoxins, which can render parenteral products highly dangerous to patients. From a human point of view, the most significant of these are pyrogens. They largely consist of poly-liposaccharide components of Gram-negative bacterial cell walls. They are relatively heat-stable, and can be present when the bacteria have been destroyed or removed. They can cause acute febrile reactions when introduced directly into the bloodstream.

Another fundamental point, which is common to all types of sterilisation, and which it is absolutely vital to grasp is that *sole reliance cannot be placed on the sterilisation process alone, in isolation, to achieve sterility.* Much depends on:

- The microbial condition of the materials, or articles, as they are presented to the sterilisation process.
- How they are prepared and handled *before* the actual sterilisation, by whom and under what conditions.
- The pre-established validity of the sterilisation process itself.
- The careful control of that process during the sterilisation.
- What happens after the sterilisation process to confirm its efficacy and to prevent product recontamination.

The achievement of sterility requires the application of disciplines and techniques additional to those required in the manufacture of all other medicinal products. As has been noted, the requirement that a product should be sterile imposes additional, not merely alternative, demands.

A further fundamental issue which bears balefully on all types of sterilisation process is the fragile fallibility of the only end-product test available to us as weak support in the assurance of that most crucial quality characteristic – the *de facto* sterility of a purportedly sterile product. Table 19.1 (Russel, 1983) shows the chances of passing the standard pharmacopoeial sterility test, for various levels of contamination (statistical probability considerations only; no account taken of microbiological limitations).

Not exactly confidence-inspiring, even for those who have faith in end-product testing as a determinant of quality. Compared with the sterility test, an assay (for example) to determine the content of active ingredient of a tablet by HPLC is a powerfully quality-assuring tool. The very fact of the sheer poverty of this test must colour all thought and action in this field, and necessitates more disciplined approaches and higher orders of care and attention. Crucial to success are:

- The *people* involved and their *training*.
- The *premises* used, and the *environmental standards* therein.
- The *equipment* and its *commissioning/cleaning/sterilisation*.
- The quality of the *materials* used (including *water*).
- *Validation* of the sterilisation process.
- *In-process control* of the process, and *in-process control* of the manufacturing environment.

Table 19.1   Statistical probability of passing a standard sterility test

No. of units contaminated (%)	Chance of passing test (%)
0.1	98
1.0	82
5.0	36
10.0	12

Data from Russel (1983).

Following the actual sterilisation process, it is vital to guard against mix-up with non-sterile product and/or recontamination, for example by the air entering a steriliser, or by water used for spray cooling a sterilised load.

Methods of sterilisation

A distinction may be drawn between two main approaches to the manufacture of sterile products: terminal sterilisation and processes where the sterilisation is not 'terminal' and where some form of aseptic processing must follow the actual sterilisation stage. The two approaches may be compared as follows.

A *terminal sterilisation* process usually involves:

1. Taking a clean, low bioburden (but not necessarily sterile) bulk product, containers and closures.
2. Filling and sealing the product in what we may term in a generalised sense a 'high quality environment'.
3. Sterilising the filled and sealed product.

In contrast, *aseptic production* involves:

1. Taking previously sterilised bulk product, containers and closures.
2. Filling and sealing the product in an 'extremely high quality environment', protecting all the while against recontamination.

Thus, in comparison with terminal sterilisation, aseptic processing:

*   Has more variables;
*   Usually involves more than one type of sterilisation process (e.g. dry heat for glass containers, steam for rubber closures, filtration for a liquid product);
*   Is very environment sensitive;
*   Is very operator dependent.

Another important distinction between terminal heat sterilisation, and filtration followed by aseptic filling, and one which has perhaps not received the emphasis it requires, is that terminal heat sterilisation is an 'all in' batch-wise process, whereas the filtration of a liquid and filling it aseptically is a sequential, or serial, process. Although, through temperature variations within the chamber (which should, in any event, have been investigated and controlled), there may be variations in heat input in different parts of the load, it is still reasonable to regard a load as one (putatively homogeneous) batch. A filtered and aseptically filled product cannot by any means be regarded in the same light. The filtration takes place over a period of time. It cannot be asserted that the first runnings through the filter are exactly the same as the last. Similarly, the filling operation continues over a period of time, a period during which conditions can change, either through accident, inadvertence or carelessness. Total homogeneity throughout the run cannot be assumed. Some items, but not all, in the run may become contaminated through operator intervention, coughing/sneezing, hairy arms over open sterilised vials and the like. This leads to a strange and inexplicable paradox. Although it can be acceptable to eschew sterility testing when products or materials have been terminally sterilised, experts generally hold that the sterility test should be performed on samples of aseptically processed products. Yet it is fundamental to the drawing of conclusions about a population, on the basis of the examination of samples drawn from that population, that it may be assumed to be homogeneous, with any faults or defects evenly or randomly distributed. It is entirely impossible to make such an assumption about aseptically processed products.

To recap: the main methods of sterilisation may be classified as follows:

— Heat: steam or dry.
— Radiation (e.g. gamma ray or electron beam).
— Gas (e.g. ethylene oxide).
— Filtration (plus aseptic handling).

As noted, these processes are all very different one from another, and it is therefore a mistake to think that sterilisation is just 'one thing'. For example, filtration differs from all the others in that sterilisation by heat, radiation, or gas *kills* organisms. Filtration *removes* them. There is a difference.

Heat sterilisation

Sterilisation by heat is generally considered to be the most reliable method, and the one to choose if possible. The question thus arises – in what circumstances would it *not* be possible to use a heat sterilisation process?

The main reason is when the product or material cannot stand the heat required and would therefore break down or deteriorate.

Steam sterilisation

Of the two possible forms of heat sterilisation, steam sterilisation is more effective than dry heat at the same temperature. The reasons for this are the better contact (and thus heat-transfer) that the steam provides, and the fact that steam has a greater heat energy content than, say, water or air at the same temperature. Steam has:

• Sensible heat, that is the heat required to raise the temperature of a mass of water to its boiling point.
• Latent heat of vaporisation, that is the additional heat absorbed when a liquid (e.g. water) at its boiling point is converted to steam.

Both these forms of heat energy are transferred from the steam to the objects being sterilised, and it is heat energy which kills the organisms. Approximately 80% of the total heat energy in saturated steam is the latent heat, and this is released when the steam makes contact with a cooler surface and condenses. This condensation leads to an immediate contraction of the steam and a localised lower pressure region, into which more steam will flow.

Steam sterilisation is used, for example, to sterilise aqueous solutions in sealed containers where the steam acts as a heat transfer medium to raise the temperature of the solution to the desired sterilising temperature. Here it is crucial that the integrity of the container seals are assuredly validated, to avoid entry of the condensed steam. Water-wettable articles such as empty containers, container seals, instruments, machine and equipment parts are steam sterilised by direct contact. Here the quality of the steam is crucial. It must be pure, or 'clean steam', for otherwise the contact surfaces will suffer contamination by impurities in the steam. Where items other than sealed containers containing water, or aqueous solutions, are steam sterilised it is essential that precautions are taken to prevent recontamination after the process has been completed. This may be done, for example, by wrapping the item to be sterilised in a material which allows the removal of air and the penetration of steam, but which provides a barrier against entry of micro-organisms after the sterilisation. Sheets and bags of suitable wrapping material (treated paper, etc.) are available commercially. Often two layers of the material are used (the 'double wrapping' technique). This enables successive removal of the two layers, while for example the sterilised article is passed through a hatchway into a clean room, with the inner wrapping removed only when the sterilised item is under some form of protection against recontamination.

Steam sterilisation is not a suitable method for the sterilisation of sealed containers of oily solutions or suspensions. The reason is that the special effectiveness of steam sterilisation is due to the *moist*, not dry, heat. Oily material in a sealed container may reach the temperature of the steam sterilising chamber, but the heat will only be dry heat and that (at the temperatures usually used for steam sterilisation) will not be sufficient.

It is important to note that boiling water (or steam) at normal atmospheric pressure (that is, water or steam at 100°C) will not kill all organisms. It will kill many, even most, of them. But some micro-organisms are extraordinarily resistant to heat, particularly those which form spores, and can survive boiling water for long periods. Therefore, whilst in certain cases it may be considered safe to drink water which is only lightly contaminated after boiling, higher temperatures are needed to ensure sterilisation. To achieve these higher steam temperatures it is of course necessary to operate under pressure, that is in autoclaves.

The British Pharmacopoeia states that 'the preferred combination of temperature and time is 121°C *maintained throughout the load* [author's emphasis] during a holding period of 15 minutes', and adds that other combinations of temperature and time may be used provided that they have been shown to achieve the desired result.

Commonly accepted as effective combinations (and the over-pressure

Table 19.2   Effective combinations of temperature and time for steam sterilisation

Temperature (°C)	Pressure (psi)	Time (min)
115–118	10	30
121–124	15	15
126–129	20	10
134–138	32	3

which is required to achieve the corresponding steam temperature) are given in Table 19.2.

It is generally considered that temperatures below 115°C do not provide a sufficient level of sterility assurance. Important points to note:

- As the temperature increases the time required reduces significantly.
- The temperature must be achieved throughout the load for the time required. That is, for example, a temperature of 121°C must be achieved at the coldest part, of the coldest item, in the coldest section of the load, for at least 15 mins. It is NOT sufficient that at some point, or at a few points only, this temperature is achieved for the specified time.
- The pressure is only used to achieve the required temperature, and contributes nothing to the sterilisation process. It is the temperature which must be used to control and monitor the process.

Autoclaves

Autoclaves are sealable pressure vessels, specially designed for use in the sterilisation of materials, products, devices and equipment by steam under pressure. They come in a great range of shapes and sizes, from small bench-top laboratory models, to large industrial autoclaves, free standing or inserted through walls. They may be single-ended (that is, with just one door at one end) or double-ended (that is with a door at each end). The advantage of a double-ended autoclave is that it makes for more effective segregation of sterilised items from non-sterilised items, especially if one end is on one side of a wall, and the other end on the other side. Unless very great care is taken, there is always a risk with single-ended autoclaves, of mix-up between items being removed from the chamber after sterilisation, and the next (unsterilised) load waiting to go in. Double-ended autoclaves also allow the direct passage of a sterilised load into a clean, or aseptic, area.

At one time autoclave cycles were controlled manually. Today, in all but the simplest laboratory units, autoclaves (once loaded and with the doors closed) function automatically in accordance with a pre-set time/temperature cycle. Heat sensors within the chamber detect when the required temperature has been reached. It is essential that there is complete surety that this temperature has been reached throughout the entire load. The load is then held at the required temperature for the predetermined period of time, for example 15 minutes at 121°C. There then follows a cooling down period before the door(s) of the chamber can be re-opened and the sterilised items unloaded. One reason for this cooling phase is obvious. The load immediately following sterilisation will be dangerously hot. But there is another very important safety reason. When containers of fluid are being sterilised, high pressure builds up inside the containers. They do not burst during the process because the pressure inside the containers is balanced by the pressure outside them, within the autoclave chamber. If, however, the autoclave doors are opened (thus allowing the pressure in the chamber to drop suddenly) before the load has cooled, then there could be some very nasty explosions. Fortunately, most modern autoclaves are designed so that the doors **cannot** be opened until the cooling part of the overall cycle is completed.

Thus, there are three main stages to an autoclave sterilisation cycle to consider:

1.   Heating up
2.   Holding period
3.   Cooling down.

There are also a variety of preheating phases, depending on the type of autoclave, and various measures have also been introduced to speed up the cooling phase, and thus increase autoclave throughput.

Types of autoclave   When the chamber of an autoclave contains only saturated steam under pressure, there is a direct linear relationship between the temperature of the steam and the pressure. The higher the pressure, the higher the temperature. Elementary though it may seem, it needs to be stressed that the pressure is used solely to obtain the temperature required (micro-organisms are killed by the heat and are not crushed to death, as some people still seem to think). Also, the direct relationship between the temperature and the pressure does not hold if there is both steam and air, or some other gas, in the chamber. Worse still, unless special steps are taken, there is a strong possibility that in some parts of the chamber or load there will be 'layers' or 'pockets' of air trapped within the chamber. Normally, since steam has a lower density than air, it is the steam which will rise to the top of the chamber. This could, and has, caused serious problems. The steam and air could well be at different temperatures, and items which are surrounded by air (and not steam) would only be subjected to *dry* heat which is far less effective (at a given temperature, for a given time) than steam.

This *is* a serious problem. Patients have been killed due to administration of drips which failed to be sterilised because of a layer of air in an autoclave.

A major feature of autoclave design concerns the measures taken to overcome the problem of air in the chamber. Various types which tackle this problem in various ways include:

- *Downward displacement autoclaves.* When using earlier and simpler autoclave models it is necessary to displace the air in the chamber, through a pressure-regulated drain, or vent, at the bottom of the chamber, before the sterilisation cycle proper begins. This displacement is effected by allowing steam to enter at the top of the chamber for what is called a period of 'free steaming'. Because the steam displaces and forces the air out through the drain at the bottom, this type of autoclave has been called a 'downward displacement autoclave'.

- *Vacuum purged (or assisted) autoclaves.* These are autoclaves fitted with vacuum pumps to remove the air, from the bottom of the chamber, before or as the steam enters at the top. This can have an additional useful function. At the end of a sterilisation cycle the pump can be used again to evacuate the chamber, remove the steam, and thus allow more rapid drying of the contents.

- *Fan-assisted autoclaves.* Another way of overcoming the problem of air in an autoclave chamber is to ensure that there is a complete mixture of the steam and air. That is, it becomes a question not of removing the air, but of mixing it thoroughly. The important point is to ensure that it *is* thoroughly mixed, and that the entire load is held at the required temperature for the required time. It is thus even more critical that the sterilisation cycle is controlled via internal temperature, and not pressure. Various designs of internal fans, and similar devices, have been used to ensure this mixing.

- *Porous load autoclaves.* In addition to the problem of layering of air and steam, there is the possibility of trapped pockets of air. These can occur, for example, within packs of dressings, inside wrapped articles, equipment and tubing. To overcome this problem, autoclaves used for sterilising such articles are equipped so that they can run a 'porous load cycle', the essential feature of which is a repeating or pulsing application of the vacuum – an alternating series of pulling and releasing the vacuum, before the heating begins. This vacuum pulsing can also be used to dry the load at the end of the cycle. In a typical porous load cycle the internal chamber is first reduced to around 2.5 kPa absolute pressure. This is followed by alternating steam injection and evacuation (pulsing) to dilute and remove any residual air. When this has been removed, steam is admitted rapidly so as to reach sterilising temperature (and pressure), which is maintained for the required time. Finally there is a rapid evacuation to around 6–7 kPa absolute, to remove the steam and dry the load. Air is then admitted to the chamber through a bacteria retaining filter.

- *Air ballasted autoclaves.* When plastic containers (bags, bottles, vials, ampoules) are sterilised in an autoclave, at the temperatures required for sterilisation, such containers soften and can distort. When the steam pressure drops at the end of the sterilisation phase, the internal pressure can cause the containers to 'balloon' or even burst. Some autoclaves are designed to compensate for this, by pumping in air under pressure. This over-pressure within the autoclave chamber prevents the 'ballooning' etc., and can be held until the temperature has dropped below the softening point of the plastic, when the over-pressure can be reduced. In such autoclaves initial air removal is usually unnecessary, but a good circulating fan system is essential to ensure thorough mixing of steam and air.

- *Spray-cooled autoclaves.* As a means of reducing the time taken for the load to cool down (and thus increase throughput, and also reduce the possible deleterious effects that prolonged heat may have on products or materials) a number of autoclaves are fitted with a rapid or spray-cooling facility. Following the heating phase, the load is subjected to a fine spray or mist of cold water. This can reduce the time taken to cool a load from a matter of hours to a matter of minutes. Pumping air into an autoclave chamber for ballasting, and spraying water in for cooling can give rise to further potential contamination problems, as can the air which will also enter as the autoclave cools, and when the doors are opened. When sterilising liquid products in well-sealed containers, and if there is no concern about the sterility of the *outsides* of the containers, then there is no problem, *if* there is absolute surety that there is no chance that the water or air can enter the cooling container. If there is not this assurance (and serious infections have been caused by contaminated cooling water penetrating bottle 'seals'), or if, when attempting to sterilise the surfaces of any items which can come into contact with the entering air or water, then this air or water must itself be sterile (and, of course, free from chemical impurities or additives).

- *Continuous sterilisers.* The need for the large-scale cost-effective industrial production of sterile fluids has led to the development of continuous sterilisers. These take the form of substantial tower-like structures, up to 20 m or more high. They typically contain three interconnected chambers: a water-filled preheating chamber, a central steam sterilisation chamber, and a water cooling chamber. The hydrostatic pressure in the preheating and cooling chambers seals and counterbalances the steam pressure in the sterilising chamber. Filled containers move through the chambers on an ascending and descending conveyor belt system. The holding time in each chamber is governed by the speed of the conveyor belt. Sequential spray cooling and drying may also be incorporated in the system.

These different types of autoclave are not all mutually exclusive, and any one autoclave can have more than one of the features discussed. For example, a particular autoclave can be vacuum purged, air ballasted, and spray cooled and fitted to run a porous load cycle if required. It is then possible to select the combination of features required for a specific sterilisation process.

Steam sterilisation: sterilisation in place (SIP)

A traditional method for the connecting of vessels, pipework, tubing, and filter assemblies has been to separately sterilise each component part, and then to assemble them together using aseptic technique, that is by making 'aseptic connections'. This sort of approach is not all that practical in large-scale high-throughput production, and it introduces a further element of risk of contamination when the connections are made. A more modern, practical approach is to use 'sterilisation in place' (SIP). To apply this technique, it is first necessary to design and install all the manufacturing equipment, pipework etc. so that it is possible to use SIP – sealable stainless steel vessels, capable of withstanding steam pressure, stainless steel pipework, all connected up by sanitary fittings and so on. The whole setup (e.g. sealed pressure mixing tank with stirrer, connected to pump, connected to filter assembly, connected to filling machine, etc.) is assembled in a clean but not necessarily sterile state, and the whole sterilised internally by feeding in steam under pressure, at the required temperature for the required time. The whole setup must be designed so that it is possible to do this, with entry point(s) for the steam, drainage points for condensate, and places to insert temperature sensing probes. SIP as a 'bolt-on modification' is neither a practical nor sensible proposition.

Dry heat

This is a process used, in, for example, hot air ovens or sterilising tunnels.

Because dry heat is less effective than steam, higher temperatures and longer exposure times are required. Again, it is vital that *all* parts of *all* items being sterilised reach at least the required temperature for at least the required time.

Generally accepted as effective time/temperature combinations for *dry heat* sterilisation are shown in Table 19.3.

Other time/temperature combinations are possible and acceptable, if they are demonstrably capable of achieving the desired and intended effect.

Dry heat sterilisation is used for articles that are thermostable, but which are either moisture sensitive or impermeable to steam. It is used for equipment, containers (e.g. glass) and other packaging components, dry chemical substances (i.e. BPCs or APIs which can stand the heat), and for non-aqueous solutions and suspensions. Oils, fats, waxes and silicone lubricants can be sterilised by dry heat. It thus can be used to sterilise oily injections, implants, ointment bases, certain surgical dressings and absorbable gelatin sponge. Dry heat temperatures of 250°C and above can be used to both sterilise and depyrogenate glass containers and other glassware.

Table 19.3 Effective sterilising times for dry heat sterilisation

Temperature (°C)	Time (min)
180	30
170	60
160	120

Hot air ovens

The most common form of dry heat steriliser is the hot air oven. These are usually constructed of stainless steel, with electrical heating elements placed around the internal wall of the insulated chamber, and arranged so as to minimise localised over-heating. Heat is delivered to the load mainly by convection and radiation and fans are fitted for efficient internal air circulation and optimum heat distribution. To this end, shelves within the chamber are constructed of perforated steel, or of steel mesh. Internal temperature is thermostatically controlled, and monitored by thermocouples.

Overall cycle times in hot air ovens can be lengthy, and when, say, glass vials are being sterilised for aseptic filling, the vial sterilisation process is decoupled from the filling process. The filling phase must wait for the availability of a batch of sterilised vials. There is also the contamination-risking handling that is necessary in transporting the vials from the oven to the filling line. These problems, of course, can be, and regularly are overcome.

Sterilisation tunnels

A more efficient, and effective, solution (where production volume justifies the cost) is the on-line sterilisation tunnel, which has the additional advantage that it can also effect depyrogenation. Clean vials are loaded on to the conveyor which passes through the tunnel, from outside the aseptic filling room. The conveyor belt transports the vials through the tunnel, where they are exposed to high temperature, sterile filtered, laminar flow air. Before they leave the tunnel, and on to the aseptic filling line, the vials are cooled rapidly by a sterile filtered laminar air flow. Some designs utilise internal infrared heaters in addition to the filtered air flows. Differential pressures, and the internal air flows, prevent entrance of contamination into the filling room from the entrance of the tunnel.

Radiation sterilisation

Radiation sterilisation can be used to sterilise materials that are heat sensitive, but are able to withstand the relatively high radiation levels required. The most common forms of radiation employed are gamma rays and accelerated electron beams. Other forms of radiation have been suggested, for example ultraviolet light, which cannot be recommended for product sterilisation, due to its poor penetrating power and its extensive absorption by glass, plastics, particles and turbid liquids. Recently the use of pulsed 'pure bright light' as a sterilant has been proposed. Initial results look very promising, but more independent work needs to be done (Dunn, 1998). The use of high frequency microwave continuous sterilisers has also been proposed (Ebara, 1998).

The usual source of gamma radiation is cobalt-60, although some irradiation plants use caesium-137. Electron beams are generated by high energy electron accelerators. Radiation sterilisation is not the sort of process that is usually carried out in a standard pharmaceutical or device manufacturing facility. Specialised plants, with elaborate precautionary systems, are necessary to protect both operators and the environment. Thus radiation sterilisation tends very largely to be an operation contracted out by manufacturers. Radiation sterilisation has been performed as a batch or a continuous process. Generally preferable is the continuous process in which a conveyor system takes the individual items (containers, sealed cartons, bags, etc.) through the irradiation chamber in such a manner as to ensure that the orientation of the load in relation to the source varies so that all parts of the load receive the same dose. The dose delivered depends upon the strength of the source, the distance from the source, the resistance of materials between the articles to be sterilised and the source, and the time of exposure. Exposure time must be adjusted to allow for any decay of the source. In the UK and in most of Europe a minimum absorbed dose of 25 kGy has normally been accepted as the standard for radiation sterilisation. However, as an interesting example of discordance within a harmonised community, in Scandinavia doses of up to 35 kGy have been specified. In the USA, the Association for the Advancement of Medical Instrumentation has developed dose-setting guidelines based upon the extent and resistance of the pre-sterilisation bioburden present in and/or on the load.

It is necessary to monitor dose received during radiation sterilisation. To this end, dosimeters (usually of the 'red Perspex' type) are used, in sufficient number, and in packages sufficiently close to one another, so as to ensure that in a continuous process there will always be at least two dosimeters in the chamber, exposed to the source. Biological indicators may also be used as an additional control measure.

Sterilisation by irradiation can be very effective, especially since it can be used to sterilise products and materials which are already packaged, provided the radiation can penetrate the package. (Radiation is not used to sterilise just the surface of a product, material, device or article, given that the radiation is able to penetrate that product, etc.) It thus provides a means of terminal sterilisation without the use of heat, but it needs to be recognised that it can have serious deleterious effects on a number of products, materials, compounds and containers. Further, expensive and complex plant and equipment are required, such as are usually not found in a normal pharmaceutical or device manufacturing factory.

Some materials such as natural rubber, styrene (and styrene derivatives such as ABS), polyethylene, polycarbonate, polysulphones, silicones, cellulose compounds and nylon show little if any change after gamma irradiation, but many other materials can be adversely affected. Some glasses, and plastics (such as polyvinyl chloride, polytetrafluoroethylene and polypropylene) may be discoloured, and this discolourisation may continue after the sterilisation process has finished. Gas may be liberated; for example hydrogen chloride from polyvinyl chloride. Mechanical properties (such as increased brittleness or hardness) may be altered. Many chemical compounds can be degraded by having their molecules rearranged, and this effect is greatest in the presence of water. This severely limits the use of radiation for the sterilisation of aqueous solutions. However, radiation has been used successfully for the sterilisation of a wide range of pharmaceutical products and materials, including enzymes, vitamins, minerals, antibiotics, monoclonal antibodies and peptides. It can also be used to sterilise some containers and closures. Plasma, tissue and bone grafts can be sterilised by gamma irradiation. Perhaps, in sheer volume, the major use of gamma radiation is in the sterilisation of medical equipment devices, including surgical gowns, hoods and masks, dressings, catheters, syringes, needles, surgical blades, prosthetic implants and the like.

Gas sterilisation

Many chemical substances are toxic to micro-organisms, but only a very limited number of them have any use as sterilising agents (as distinct from the considerable range of chemical compounds which can be effectively used as disinfectants).

While other substances in a gaseous state have been proposed and tried (for example formaldehyde, propylene oxide, vapour phase hydrogen peroxide) in practice the substance which has been by far the most widely used as a gas sterilant is ethylene oxide (commonly, and unscientifically, abbreviated to 'EtO').

Ethylene oxide can only be used to sterilise surfaces. That is, unlike heat or radiation it cannot penetrate through the walls of many containers to the product inside. It is therefore not possible, for example, to sterilise sealed vials or ampoules of liquid products by EtO, although it will penetrate certain plastic films and bags.

Amongst the *dis*advantages of ethylene oxide is that it is highly explosive (it is usually diluted with an inert gas, such as a fluorinated hydrocarbon, or carbon dioxide) and is highly toxic both acutely and chronically. (Acute toxic reactions resulting from inhalation include headache, nausea, vomiting and respiratory and conjunctival irritation. Contact with the skin causes burns and sensitisation. Chronic exposure can result in neurological, ocular and haematological reactions.) Ethylene oxide is mutagenic, and a suspected human carcinogen. For these, and other reasons (for example the dependence for the success of this method on a number of critical operational parameters, all of which need to be most carefully controlled and monitored) its use is declining. Certainly, where possible, other methods are to be preferred. Factors that affect the efficacy of EtO as a sterilant include:

- Concentration of the gas.
- Temperature.
- Gas pressure.
- Humidity (some moisture must be present, but with an excess, activity declines).
- Time of exposure.
- Gas distribution and penetration.

All of the above must be carefully controlled and monitored.

Failure to attain the required conditions in relation to any single process parameter can result in failure to sterilise the load, in whole or in part. For this reason it is generally considered necessary to include biological indicators in each load. Furthermore, because of the complex interrelationships between these various factors, there is no universally accepted standard cycle for ethylene oxide sterilisation. Cycles used have included ethylene oxide gas concentrations of 250 mg/l to 1500 mg/l, relative humidity from 30% to 90%, temperatures from 30°C to 65°C, and exposure times from 1 h to 30 h. Thus a sterilisation cycle must be designed, developed and validated for each specific product and product load configuration.

Ethylene oxide sterilisation is carried out in a purpose-built EtO steriliser, with a gas-tight jacketed stainless steel chamber, built to withstand high pressure and vacuum. The product, or material is loaded into the chamber in a predefined configuration. This configuration must remain consistently the same as the configuration adopted when the process was validated, otherwise the validation can no longer be considered to be valid. A vacuum is drawn on the chamber to about 2 kPa, to remove air and thus to facilitate later EtO penetration. Pulses of steam then enter the chamber to moisturise the load, and to raise it to the required sterilisation temperature. Ethylene oxide gas is then admitted through a heated vaporiser. The gas is circulated within the chamber, using internal fans or external recirculation loops, to ensure even internal gas distribution. At the end of the exposure time the gas mixture is exhausted from the chamber, and rendered harmless by acid hydrolysis or catalytic oxidation.

A further problem is the reaction products left as residues after the sterilisation. These include such toxic substances as ethylene chlorohydrin and ethylene glycol. Thus the load must be held under controlled airflow and temperature conditions for a further de-gassing period of up to ten days. Precautions are, obviously, necessary to prevent microbial recontamination of the load.

Ethylene oxide is mainly used to sterilise dressings, catheters, infusion and giving sets, syringes, prostheses and similar devices. It can also be used to sterilise some plastic containers and closures, and also some thermolabile powders (provided the required humidity does not present a problem).

Another form of gaseous sterilisation which has been developed is sterilisation by low temperature steam and formaldehyde (LTSF). Formaldehyde is acutely toxic to human beings. It is also mutagenic, and possibly carcinogenic. It has been widely used to disinfect clean rooms. In admixture with steam, at temperatures between 60°C and 80°C (at pressures below atmospheric) it has been used for a range of medical devices.

Filtration sterilisation

Although all the different sterilisation processes so far discussed are significantly different one from the other, in terms of technology, mode of action and applications, filtration is 'more different' than all the rest:

- It removes organisms rather than kills them.
- It is only applicable to fluids (liquids and gases).

Furthermore, it cannot be used as a terminal sterilisation process. Any sterile-filtered bulk product which is not going to be subjected to a further terminal sterilisation, must be filled and sealed into final containers observing special aseptic precautions to prevent recontamination. Thus a further element of risk of contamination is inevitably involved. Hence it is generally considered that where it is possible to terminally heat-sterilise products (particularly injections) this should be done, with filtration sterilisation restricted to uses where the product cannot withstand heating. However, more modern and automated techniques such as barrier (or isolator) or blow/fill/seal technology are becoming increasingly refined and being used to significantly reduce the risks of recontamination following sterilisation by filtration. Some impressive claims have been made for the advantages of blow/fill/seal (Jones, 1995; Leo, 1990; Sharp, 1987, 1988, 1990) and isolator technology (Coles, 1998) in providing greater confidence of sterility in aseptic processing. Not, it would seem without justice, although it has to be acknowledged that some regulatory bodies have not embraced these two technologies with the utmost of enthusiasm (Hargreaves, 1990).

In essence the process of filtration sterilisation is a simple one. A liquid is forced, under moderate pressure, through a filter in the form of a membrane or a cartridge, the filter itself and the assembly in which it is mounted having first been sterilised. Various types, sizes, grades and porosities of filter are available from a number of specialist manufacturers, and for effective sterilisation a pore size of not more than 0.22 micrometres (μm or 'microns') is required. Given the right filter for the job, properly assembled, fitted and sterilised, and with confirmation that the filter is not damaged before use (or has not become damaged in use), a very high level of assurance of the sterility of the liquid *as it emerges through the filter* is possible, especially if the fluid is passed through two filters, connected in series. The main problem is ensuring that the liquid does not become recontaminated after the filtration (e.g. in the filling process). And that is not easy, particularly when and where people are involved. Aseptic filling involving human operators is a highly skilled operation, requiring an excellent aseptic technique.

Sterilising grade filters have been made from sintered glass or sintered metal, but the most commonly used filter media today are polymeric membranes, either as sheets or discs, or as one or more layers of the filter material supported on an inert and relatively rigid matrix to form a 'cartridge filter'. A wide range of types, sizes and porosity of such filters are available from specialist suppliers. Filter manufacture and supply is a relatively large, competitive business, and filter manufacturers are generally more than ready to provide details on their range, and to give advice on applications and to offer technical back-up.

It needs to be noted that although filters are designated as having 'nominal' or 'absolute' pore size ratings (e.g. of 0.22 μm), it is not correct to view a filter as a sort of sieve plate, pierced by holes all of identical size (of, say, 0.22 μm). The pores in a membrane, in fact, consist of a range of sizes, characterised by pore size distribution. It is thus preferable to refer to a given type and make of filter in terms of its organism-retentive properties (numbers and dimensions of organisms). A number of filter manufacturers provide this information, and in the USA guidelines (HIMA, 1982) have been issued which specify, for a sterilising grade filter, a minimum challenge of 10^7 *Pseudomonas diminuta* (0.5×1.0–4.0 μm) per square centimetre of filter surface, with no passage of these organisms through the filter, into the filtrate.

Summary of sterilisation methods

The following list and Table 19.4 briefly summarise the different major methods of sterilisation, their applications, advantages and disadvantages.

Steam

- Heating in an autoclave by steam under pressure, or sterilisation in place (SIP).
- Steam is effective at lower temperatures for shorter times than dry heat, because of its latent heat in addition to its sensible heat.
- Kills, but does not remove organisms.
- Typical temperature/times: 121°C for 15 minutes; 134°C for 3 minutes. (Other time/temperature combinations are possible.)

Dry heat

- Hot air ovens or sterilising tunnels.
- Less effective than steam (at a given temperature).
- Kills but does not remove organisms.
- Typical temperature/times: 180°C for 30 minutes; 160°C for 120 minutes.

Radiation

- Exposure to gamma radiation or high speed electrons.
- Typical required dose 25 kGy.

Ethylene oxide

- Usually used as a mixture of ethylene oxide with an inert gas (carbon dioxide, CFCs).
- Concentration, pressure, humidity, temperature and the nature of the material and its packaging all influence effectiveness as a sterilant.

Filtration

- Fluid is passed through a sterile filter (membrane or cartridge) with a pore size of 0.22 μm, or one known to have equivalent bacteria-retaining properties.

Table 19.4 Major methods of sterilisation

Sterilisation method	Applications	Advantages	Disadvantages
Steam	• Aqueous preparations in sealed containers • Equipment, instruments • Dressings • Manufacturing vessels/pipework/tubing • Filter assemblies • Surgical gowns, drapes and dressings made of cellulosic materials • Some medical devices	• A process for terminal sterilisation • Can provide a very high margin of safety • Can destroy viruses as well as bacteria, etc. • Relatively short process time	• Unsuitable for materials or articles damaged by heat • Only suitable for water-wettable materials or sealed aqueous solutions (e.g. not oils or powders) • Expensive (capital and energy costs)
Dry heat	• Non-aqueous products (e.g. oils, powders) in sealed containers • Glass and metal articles, equipment, parts, etc. • Some plastics • Oils, fats and waxes • Silicone lubricants	• Can be used for terminal sterilisation • Kills viruses • Can be used for depyrogenation • Can be used for non-aqueous and/or non-wettable materials • Can be less damaging to metals than steam	• Can only be used for items that can withstand the necessary heat input • Unsuitable for most dressings, plastics and rubber materials
Radiation	• Some heat-sensitive materials but not those which are radiation-sensitive • Dressings • Surgical instruments • Some chemical compounds	• No heat effects • Can be used for terminal sterilisation • Can be accurately controlled	• Expensive specialist plant and equipment • Most manufacturers have to contract out • Elaborate safety precautions necessary • Has deleterious effects on a number of chemicals, products and containers (e.g. plastics)

Table 19.4 (Continued)

Sterilisation method	Applications	Advantages	Disadvantages
Ethylene oxide	• Heat-sensitive materials • Rubber and plastics • Dressings and fabrics	• No heat damage • Effective at low temperatures • Effective against many organisms	• Toxic • Explosive • Expensive • Slow • Needs time for dispersal of residual gas and reaction products
Filtration	• Liquids and solutions that cannot withstand heat-treatment • Gases	• No heat effect • Removes dead as well as living organisms • Clarifies as well as sterilises	• Not a terminal process • Requires additional aseptic handling/ filling following sterilisation • Will not remove or inactivate viruses • Requires skilled techniques • Some substances may be absorbed by filter • Cannot be used for suspensions • Filter-integrity tests must be performed • Very operator and environment sensitive

References

BPF (1985). *Bonnes Pratiques de Fabrication,* 2nd edn. Paris: Ministère des Affaires Sociales et de la Societé Direction de la Pharmacie et du Medicament.

Brown M R W, Gilbert P (1977). Increasing the probability of sterility of medicinal products. *J Pharm Pharmacol* **29**, 517–523.

Coles T (1998). *Isolation Technology – a Practical Guide.* Illinois: Interpharm Press.

Dunn J *et al.* (1998). Pure bright pulsed light processing and sterilisation. *Eur J Parenter Sci* **3** (4), 105–114.

Ebara T *et al.* (1998). Development and practical application of high-frequency wave (microwave) continuous steriliser. *Eur J Parenter Sci* **3** (2), 39–47.

Hargreaves D P (1990). Good manufacturing practice in the control of contamination. In: Denyer S and Baird R (eds), *Guide to Microbiological Control in Pharmaceuticals.* Chichester: Ellis Horwood.

HIMA (1982). Microbiological evaluation of filters, HIMA Document No. 3, Vol. 14. Washington DC: Health Industries Manufacturers Association.

Jones D, Topping P, Sharp J (1995). Environmental microbial challenges to an aseptic blow-fill-seal process. *PDA J Pharm Sci Technol* **49** (3), 226–234.

Leo F (1990). In: Olson and Groves (eds), *Aseptic Pharmaceutical Manufacturing – Technology for the 1990s.* Illinois: Interpharm Press.

PDA (1980). Validation of aseptic filling for solution drug products. The US Parenteral Drug Association's Monograph No. 2.

PDA (1996). Process simulation testing of aseptically filled products. Technical Report No. 22. *PDA J Pharm Sci Technol* **50** (Suppl).

Polderman J (1990). *Introduction to Pharmaceutical Production.* The Hague: Novib.

Russel A D (1983). Chapter 22. In: Hugo and Russel (eds), *Pharmaceutical Microbiology,* 3rd edn. Oxford: Blackwell.

Sharp J, ed. (1983). *Guide to Good Pharmaceutical Manufacturing Practice,* 3rd edn. London: HMSO. (Referred to as the UK Orange Guide.)

Sharp J R (1987). Manufacture of sterile pharmaceutical products using 'blow-fill-seal' technology. *Pharm J* **239**, 106–108.

Sharp J R (1988). Validation of a new form-fill-seal installation. *Manuf Chem* **59** (Feb.), 22.

Sharp J (1990). Aseptic validation of a form-fill-seal installation: principles and practices. *J Parenter Sci Technol* **44** (5).

US FDA (1987). *Compliance Guideline on Parametric Release.* Washington: US Food and Drug Administration.

US FDA (1993). *Guide to Inspection of Lyophilization of Parenterals.* Washington: US Food and Drug Administration.

WHO (1973). *General Requirements for the Sterility of Biological Substances.* Geneva: World Health Organisation.

20

Assurance of quality in the manufacture of sterile products

Too many people believe that sterilisation of fluids is easily achieved with simple plant operated by men of little skill under a minimum of supervision, a view of the task which is wrong in every respect

Clothier Report, 1972

A fundamental prerequisite for the manufacture of sterile products, as with other pharmaceutical and healthcare products, is the research and development of a product which is demonstrably efficacious and acceptably safe. The additional requirement for a sterile product is that a suitable, fit for purpose, sterilisation process has also been both established and validated as part of the product development phase. There is no point whatsoever in developing a product which can be shown to be splendidly efficacious and safe from an 'ordinary' pharmacological/ toxicological aspect, but which, if intended for injection, cannot, for example, be reliably sterilised when manufactured on a commercial scale.

The wider aspects of sterile assurance

It needs always to be remembered that mere passing of a sterility test is far from being an adequate determinant of sterility. Further, the need is not only for a valid sterilisation process, vital though that is. What happens both before and after the sterilisation process must also be regarded as crucially important.

Every effort must be made to ensure that the items to be sterilised present the lowest possible microbial challenge to the sterilisation process. This is to (a) reduce the risk of failure in part of the load or batch and (b) to guard against the presence of dangerous levels of pyrogenic substances which will not be destroyed or removed by most sterilisation processes. The standard, or pharmacopoeial, sterilisation cycles are not designed to ensure the sterilisation of very highly contaminated materials, and careful control and monitoring of pre-sterilisation bioburden is essential.

Equally, it is both senseless and dangerous to competently sterilise, applying a validated process to a low bioburden product, and then allow it to become recontaminated. This can perhaps most readily happen when a product is aseptically filled and/or packaged after bulk sterilisation. It can also happen when an autoclave load is spray-cooled, or air is admitted to a sterilisation chamber, if there is a failure of container seals, or if there are cracks, pinholes or tears in the containers. Much therefore needs to be known about container quality and integrity, and about the microbial quality of the cooling water and the admitted air. There is also the possibility of what might be termed 'macro-contamination' – a mix-up between sterilised and non-sterilised items as a consequence of inadequate segregation between lots leaving a steriliser, and those waiting to be loaded into it. It has happened.

Chapter 4 of this book set out the various factors which need to be considered before a product is released for sale or supply, as laid down in the Joint UK Professional Bodies' 'Code of Practice for Qualified Persons' (IoB, RPSGB, RSC, 1998). These considerations apply just as much to sterile as to non-sterile products, but in addition there are a number of further matters to be considered. These may be set down, as a useful starting point for a consideration of the extra requirements for quality assurance in the manufacture of sterile products, as follows:

1. Have the products or materials been handled and processed in premises, and under environmental conditions, appropriate to the manufacture of the type of sterile product concerned?
2. Have the personnel involved (at all levels, including those concerned with cleaning, maintenance, monitoring and testing) been properly and thoroughly trained in the disciplines relevant to sterile products manufacture? This training should include hygienic practices, at least the elements of microbiology, and an inculcation of a thorough awareness of the consequences to patients of failure to do the job properly.
3. Have all persons entering sterile products manufacturing areas been, at all times, appropriately clad in the protective clothing prescribed for the area?
4. Has the product, or material, been subjected to the prescribed validated sterilisation procedure, in precise conformity with all laid-down process parameters, including loading patterns? Is there evidence (including automatic, and any manual, steriliser records) available that this was, in fact, so? For example:
   (a) For autoclaves and hot air ovens, time/temperature (and pressure, if relevant) recorder charts;
   (b) For a radiation sterilisation, evidence that the required radiation dose has been delivered to the load, either by means of examination of the exposed dosimeters themselves, or on the basis of unquestionably authoritative certification by person or persons who have, in turn, examined the exposed dosimeters;

(c)   For an ethylene oxide sterilisation, evidence of the quality of the incoming supply of ethylene oxide, load preconditioning records (time, temperature, relative humidity), sterilisation cycle records (time, temperature, pressure, humidity, gas concentration), biological indicator incubation results, and de-gassing records (time, temperature);

(d)   For a filtration sterilisation and aseptic fill:

— identification of the filter used;
— evidence of sterilisation of filter system before use;
— results of filter integrity test(s);
— prefiltration bioburden data;
— details, and evidence, of sterilisation of product containers and other package components, before filling;
— aseptic filling area environmental monitoring data;
— sterility test results;
— evidence of aseptic filling validation.

Premises and services for sterile products manufacture

Clean rooms

Much of the manufacture and filling of sterile products is carried out in clean rooms, or at least within confined areas which have a defined and controlled level of microbial ('viable') and particulate contamination.

A 'clean room' in this special sense is not merely a room that is clean. It is a room which is classifiable into one or other of several classes, or grades, of 'clean-ness'.

The concept and design of clean rooms was first developed (in the early 1960s) for the microelectronics and aerospace industries. In these industries, it is important to protect microelectronic components against even the finest particles. Viable contaminants, as such, are of no special significance to microcircuits, only in so far as bacteria etc. are themselves particles which cause defects in the sub-micron circuit elements.

Because of this origin in industries where product *sterility* is not the aim, classifications of the various classes of clean room are usually based upon the number and size of the particles (purely as *particles*) permitted per unit volume of the air in the room. Many published clean room standards also have specifications for humidity, temperature, lighting and air pressure. It was only later that the pharmaceutical and related industries adopted the concept, and then added to it certain permissible levels of microbial (or viable) contamination. Even so, a lot of what is said and written on this subject still sounds or reads as if it were based on a premise that it is the inanimate particles that are crucially important. In fact (all other things being equal) the presence or absence of viable contamination in a parenteral product is a quality and patient safety issue which is even more critical than the presence or absence of non-viable contamination. It has to be said, however, that although there has been a lack of convincing demonstration of a direct linear relationship between the numbers of non-viable, and the numbers of viable particles in a given volume of air, it is entirely reasonable to suppose that where there are low levels of non-viable particles there will concomitantly be low levels of micro-organisms. Micro-organisms are not usually found floating freely in air, but most characteristically are to be found associated with particles or droplets.

The unit of measure used to define clean rooms is the micrometre (μm = 0.001 mm), very commonly termed (without the utmost in metrological/terminological rigour) a 'micron'. 'Micron' is now well understood, and is probably justified by common usage. The first official published Standard for Clean Rooms was the US's 'Federal Standard 209: Clean Room and Work Station Requirements, Controlled Environment'. This standard has gone through a number of revisions over the years since the 1960s – 209B, 209C, 209D and 209E – but the basic idea behind the US classification has remained the same. It is also the easiest official clean room standard to grasp and remember. It is based on permitted numbers, per cubic foot of air, of particles of a size 0.5 μm and larger – an interesting, though convenient mix of imperial and metric units.

US Federal Standard 209 (E) clean room standards

There are three classes of US Federal Standard 209 Clean Room which are particularly relevant to sterile products manufacture: Class 100, Class 10 000 and Class 100 000, as given in Table 20.1.

This standard defines a number of other clean room parameters and conditions, such as temperature, humidity, air pressure, operator clothing and behaviour, and the instruments and devices used to measure and count particles in the air, but to date it has made no reference to permitted levels of micro-organisms.

BS 5295 clean room standards

Now thus far it is all quite simple. Unfortunately, things get a little more complicated, although the complication is more apparent than real. Following the lead given by the US Federal Standard 209, a number of national and other bodies have produced standards for clean rooms, in essence very

Table 20.1   US Federal Standard 209E. Maximum permitted number of particles per cubic foot of air in room

Class	Particle size	
	0.5 μm and larger	5.0 μm and larger
Class 100	100	0
Class 10 000	10 000	65
Class 100 000	100 000	700

like the US Standard, but with changes in the nomenclature used for the various Classes, or *Grades*. This tends to make things seem more confused than they really are. Since different speakers and writers on this subject tend to vary in the standard to which they refer, it is worth exploring some of these standards, and attempting to clarify the relationships between them.

In 1976, British Standard 5295 'Environmental cleanliness in enclosed spaces' was published. This defined four main classes of clean room. In sterile products manufacturing areas, normally only the first three of them are of interest or concern, Class 1, Class 2 and Class 3. While at first sight these may look different, they are in fact closely similar to the Federal Standards – Class 100, Class 10 000 and Class 100 000, respectively.

What British Standard 5295 did was to express the permitted number of particles in each class in terms of a cubic metre of air, not per cubic foot as in the US Federal Standard.

The BS 5295 (1976) figures for the three classes are summarised in Table 20.2.

Table 20.2 BS 5295 (1976) Clean Room Standard. Maximum permitted number of particles per cubic metre of air in room

Class	0.5 μm (or larger)	1.0 μm (or larger)	5.0 μm (or larger)	10 μm (or larger)
1	3000	N/A	0	0
2	300 000	N/A	2000	30
3	N/A	100 000	20 000	4000

Now, for example 100 particles per cubic foot is *roughly* equivalent to 3500 per cubic metre, and 10 000 per cubic foot is more or less the same as 350 000 per cubic metre. So, in the end the specifications for the different classes of clean room in BS 5295 (1976) are quite close to the US Standard, i.e. the US Standard was re-calculated in terms of a cubic metre of air, and then rounded-down to make it a little tighter. We can therefore say that *more or less*, and for our purposes, that:

— US Fed. Std. Class 100 approx. = BS Class 1
— US Fed. Std. Class 10 000 approx. = BS Class 2
— US Fed. Std. Class 100 000 approx. = BS Class 3

Clean room standards and GMP guidelines

US FDA guidelines

The US CGMPs for finished pharmaceuticals (US FDA, 1990) make no mention of clean rooms, in the specific sense, and offer no quantitative standards, neither for viable nor non-viable particles. Subpart C (Buildings and facilities) includes, under Section 211.46 (Ventilation, air filtration, air heating and cooling) the following:

(a) Adequate ventilation shall be provided.
(b) Equipment for adequate control over air pressure, micro-organisms, dust, humidity, and temperature shall be provided when appropriate . . .
(c) Air filtration systems, including prefilters and particulate matter air filters, shall be used when appropriate on air supplies to production areas.

The US CGMPs for drug products do not contain any statement on environmental standards any more specific than that. Nor are the US GMPs for medical devices any more explicit. Indeed they are rather less. Under Subpart C (Buildings), Section 820 (Environmental control) they state, in part:

> Where environmental conditions at the manufacturing site could have an adverse effect on a device's fitness for use, these environmental conditions shall be controlled to prevent contamination of the device and to provide proper conditions for each of the operations performed. . . . Conditions to be considered for control are lighting, ventilation, temperature, humidity, air pressure, filtration, airborne contamination, and other contamination. Any environmental control system shall be periodically inspected to verify that the system is properly functioning. Such inspections shall be documented.

One might expect that the FDA's *Guideline on Sterile Drug Products Produced by Aseptic Processing* (US FDA, 1987) would be somewhat more specific, and indeed it is. It does not, however, refer to 'clean rooms' as such, but it does draw a distinction between a 'Critical Area, . . . in which the sterilised dosage form, containers and closures are exposed to the environment', and a 'Controlled Area, where unsterilised product, in-process materials, and container/closures are prepared'.

According to this FDA guideline, air in a 'critical area' 'in the immediate proximity of exposed sterilised containers/closures and filling/closing operations is of acceptable quality when it has a per-cubic-foot particle count of no more than 100 in a size range of 0.5 micron and larger (Class 100) when measured not more than one foot away from the work site, and upstream of the air flow.' In a 'critical area' the air 'should also be of a high microbial quality. A incidence of no more than one colony-forming unit per 10 cubic feet is considered as attainable and desirable.'

This FDA guideline considers that, in a 'controlled area', the air:

> . . . is generally of acceptable particulate quality if it has a per-cubic-foot particle count of not more than 100,000 in a size range of 0.5 micron and larger (Class 100,000) when measured in the vicinity of the exposed articles during periods of activity. With regard to microbial quality, an incidence of no more than 25 colony forming units per 10 cubic feet is acceptable.'

At the time of writing it is understood that a revised version of this FDA guideline is in an advanced stage of preparation.

UK guidelines

The 3rd edition of the UK Orange Guide (1983) set out, probably for the first time in any official GMP guideline, its own 'Basic environmental standards for the manufacture of sterile products'. These were based on the

British Standard 5295 (1976), but with the addition of a series of maximum permitted levels of viable organisms per cubic metre of air.

These standards were summarised in a table, the main features of which are shown in Table 20.3. In addition to giving levels for particles generally, which are similar to those of BS 5295 (1976), this table also gives figures for:

- Air filter efficiency.
- Air changes (per hour) in the room.
- Viable organisms per cubic metre.

There is also a cross-reference to other classifications, including BS 5295 and US Fed. 209 and a note that air pressures should 'always be highest in the area of greatest risk', and that 'air pressure differentials between rooms of successively higher to lower risk should be at least 1.5 mm (0.06 inch) water gauge' (i.e. approximately equivalent to a 15 Pa air pressure differential). This exemplifies the concept of the air pressure 'cascade'. Air pressure in sterile manufacturing areas should generally be higher than in the 'world', or factory, outside. Furthermore, the pressure should be highest where a sterile product is, or is liable to be, exposed (i.e. is at greatest risk from contamination – cf. the FDA 'critical area'), with the pressure becoming successively lower in the various interconnecting rooms, as the risk decreases. The intention is that sterile manufacturing areas should always be flushed by filtered air in a way that will most efficiently sweep contamination *away* from the more to the less critical zones.

Note that the UK GMP classification drops the term 'Class' and uses 'Grade'. There are also Grades 1/A and 1/B. Grade 1/A refers to required conditions where product is manipulated at, or under, a special unidirectional airflow (laminar airflow, or LAF) workstation, and Grade 1/B to high standard general room conditions, in which for example such a LAF workstation would be sited. This standard also made it clear that, except for 1/A, it is intended that the various specified *particle* levels should be achieved when the room is unmanned and no work is in progress, but should be recoverable within a short period after personnel have left. The assumption was that it is not possible to retain these conditions generally when people are working in the room, and also that the filtered air supply is running continuously, and thus rapidly flushes out the contamination caused by people. However, as is made very clear, it is vital that the specified conditions should be maintained at all times 'in the zone immediately surrounding the product whenever the product is exposed'. That is another important concept in sterile products manufacture – the provision of a general high standard clean room environment with additional localised protection where product is, or could be, exposed.

EC guidelines

There are a number of other published clean room classifications. They all tend to be similar, but use different 'labels' for the different classes. For

Table 20.3 Basic environmental standards for the manufacture of sterile products (UK Orange Guide (Sharp, 1983))

Grade	Final filter efficiency (as determined by BS 3928)	Recommended minimum air changes per hour	Max. permitted number of particles per cubic metre equal to or above:		Max. permitted number of viable organisms per cubic metre*	Nearest equivalent standard classification	
			0.5 μm	5 μm		BS 5295	US Fed Std. 209B
1/A (unidirectional airflow work-station)	99.997%	flow of 0.3m/s (vertical) or 0.45 m/s (horizontal)	3000	0	<1	1	100
1/B	99.995%	20	3000	0	5	1	100
2	99.95%	20	300 000	2000	100	2	10 000
3	95.0%	20	3 500 000	20 000	500	3	100 000

Air pressure should always be highest in the area of greatest risk to product. The air pressure differentials between rooms of successively higher to lower risk should be at least 1.5 mm (0.06 inch) water gauge.

*This condition should be achieved throughout the room when unmanned, and recovered with a short clean-up period after personnel have left. The condition should be maintained in the zone immediately surrounding the product whenever the product is exposed. (Note: It is accepted that it may not always be possible to demonstrate conformity with particulate standards at the point of fill, with filling in progress, due to generation of particles or droplets from the product itself.)

Modified from the UK Orange Guide (Sharp, 1983).

Table 20.4   EC GMP Guide (1992) air quality classifications

Grade	Max. permitted number of particles per m³ equal to or above:		Max. permitted number of viable micro-organisms per m³
	0.5 μm	5 μm	
A (LAF workstation)	3500	none	<1*
B	3500	none	5*
C	350 000	2000	100
D	3500 000	20 000	500

*Reliable only when a 'large number' of air samples are taken.
Modified from the EC GMP Guide (EC, 1992).

example, a later, revised edition of BS 5295 dropped the numbers and used letters for its different *Classes*. The EC GMP Guide (1992) refers to *Grades* A, B, C and D – and this is really the terminology which all members of the European Community (or Union) should be using. Regrettably, there remains widespread and confusing variation in usage, hence this attempt to clarify things and draw comparisons.

The EC GMP Guide's 'Air classification system for the manufacture of sterile products' is summarised in Table 20.4.

Notes appended to this EC table read:

— Laminar air flow systems should provide an homogeneous air speed of 0.30 m/s for vertical flow and 0.45 m/s for horizontal flow.
— In order to reach the B, C and D air grades the number of air changes should generally be higher than 20 per hour in a room with good air flow pattern and appropriate HEPA filters.
— Low values involved here* are only reliable when a large number of air samples are taken.
— The guidance given for the maximum permitted number of particles corresponds approximately to the US Federal Standard 209C as follows: Class 100 (grades A and B), Class 10,000 (grade C) and Class 100,000 (Grade D).
— It is accepted that it may not always be possible to demonstrate conformity with particulate standards at the point of fill when filling is in progress, due to generation of particles or droplets from the product itself.

The EC GMP Guide offers no suggestions on air pressure differentials, nor does it define 'good airflow pattern'.

Air quality standards compared

Table 20.5 shows how the standards so far discussed, plus some others, relate more or less, to one another.

Table 20.5 Air quality standards compared (approximate comparisons)

Federal Standard 209	Class 100	Class 10 000	Class 100 000
Federal Standard 209 E	Class M 3.5	Class M 5.5	Class M 6.5
BS 5295 (1976)	Class 1	Class 2	Class 3
PIC (1981)	Grade A/B	Grade C	Grade D
UK Orange Guide (1983)	Grade 1(A/B)	Grade 2	Grade 3
EC Guide (1989/92)	Grade A/B	Grade C	Grade D
BS 5295 (1989)	Class E/F	Class J	Class K

Note: In Table 20.5, from issue 'E' onwards, the US Federal Standard 209 introduced (in addition to, and NOT in replacement of, the original classification based on particles per cubic foot) a parallel series based on particles per cubic metre. These all have the prefix 'M'. It is necessary to point out that this 'M' should be taken to stand for 'Metric', and to warn against the confusion which has arisen in some quarters by an erroneous assumption that this 'M' stands for 'Microbial'. It does not.

The 1996 EC annex

Unfortunately, the matter may not be left to rest here for, in 1996, a revised version of Annex 1 to the EC GMP Guide ('Manufacture of Sterile Medicinal Products') was issued (EC, 1996), which some have felt serves to cloud rather than to clarify the issue. This revised EC annex offers a new tabular classification for airborne particle levels (see Table 20.6). It is noteworthy that this table differs from its British and EC antecedents in, as it were, 'divorcing' inanimate particulate requirements from microbial limits. Hitherto, for example, 'Grade B' meant: in one cubic metre of air, no more than 3500 particles at the 0.5 μm level, none at 5 μm, *and* no more than five micro-organisms. Now, in this newer classification, a given Grade (A, B, C or D) refers *only* to the permitted inanimate particle levels. Furthermore, two sets of figures (different except, obviously, for Grade A) are given. One for the 'at rest' state, and one for the 'in operation' state.

Table 20.6 The EC GMP Guide, Annex 1 (revised July 1996) 'Airborne particulate classification'

Grade	Maximum permitted number of particles/m³, equal to or above:			
	At rest (b)		In operation	
	0.5 μm	5 μm	0.5 μm	5 μm
A	3500	0	3500	0
B(a)	3500	0	350 000	2000
C(a)	350 000	2000	3500 000	20 000
D(a)	3500 000	20 000	not defined (c)	not defined (c)

See the text for explanation of notes.

Textual comment, printed in this EC annex in relation to this table reads as follows:

> For the manufacture of sterile medicinal products normally 4 grades can be distinguished.
>
> - Grade A: The local zone for high risk operations, e.g. filling zone, stopper bowls, open ampoules and vials, making aseptic connections. Normally such conditions are provided by a laminar air flow work-station. Laminar air flow systems should provide an homogenous air speed of 0.45 m/s ± 20% (guidance value) at the working position.
> - Grade B: In the case of aseptic preparation and filling, the background environment for Grade A zone.
> - Grade C and D: Clean areas for carrying out less critical stages in the manufacture of sterile products.

Notes (a), (b), and (c) appended to Table 20.6 read:

> (a) In order to reach the B, C and D air grades, the number of air changes should be related to the size of the room and the equipment and personnel present in the room. The air system should be provided with appropriate filters such as HEPA for grades A, B, and C.
> (b) The guidance given for the maximum permitted number of particles in the 'at rest' condition corresponds approximately to the US Federal Standard 209E and the ISO classifications as follows: grades A and B correspond with class 100, M 3.5, ISO 5; grade C with class 10,000, M5.5, ISO 7 and grade D with class 100,000, M6.5, ISO 8.
> (c) The requirement and limit for this area will depend on the nature of the operations carried out.

Thus, no mention is made of differential room air pressures, and required air changes are not quantified.

Three further tables are also provided in this EC annex. Two give 'examples of operations to be carried out in the various grades', in relation to terminally sterilised products, and to aseptic preparation.

Summary of EC table of 'examples of operations for terminally sterilised products':

— Grade A: Filling of products, when unusually at risk.
— Grade C: Preparation of solutions, when unusually at risk; filling of products.
— Grade D: Preparation of solutions and components for subsequent filling.

Summary of EC table of 'examples of operations for aseptic preparations':

— Grade A: Aseptic preparation and filling.
— Grade C: Preparation of solutions to be filtered.
— Grade D: Handling of components after washing.

The textual matter relating to these summaries may provide some clarification. It reads:

The particulate conditions given in the table for the 'at rest' state should be achieved in the unmanned state after a short 'clean-up' period of 15–20 minutes (guidance value) after completion of operations. The particulate conditions for grade A in operation given in the table should be maintained in the zone immediately surrounding the product whenever the product or open container is exposed to the environment. It is accepted that it may not always be possible to demonstrate conformity with particulate standards at the point of fill when filling is in progress, due to the generation of particles or droplets from the product itself.

Further comment on the application of the various grades appears, in the revised EC annex, in the sub-sections on 'Terminally sterilised products' and on 'Aseptic preparation', thus:

Terminally sterilised products:

Preparation of components and most products should be done in at least a grade D environment in order to give low risk of microbial and particulate contamination, suitable for filtration and sterilisation. Where there is unusual risk to the product because of microbial contamination, for example, because the product actively supports microbial growth or must be held for long periods before sterilisation or is necessarily processed not mainly in closed vessels, preparation should be done in a grade C environment.

   Filling of products for terminal sterilisation should be done in at least a grade C environment. Where the product is at unusual risk of contamination from the environment, for example because the filling operation is slow or the containers are wide-necked or are necessarily exposed for more than a few seconds before sealing, the filling should be done in a grade A zone with at least a grade C background. Preparation and filling of ointments, creams, suspensions and emulsions should generally be done in a grade C environment before terminal sterilisation.

Aseptic preparation:

Components after washing should be handled in at least a grade D environment. Handling of sterile starting materials and components, unless subjected to sterilisation or filtration through a microorganism-retaining filter later in the process, should be done in a grade A environment with grade B background.

   Preparations of solutions which are to be sterile filtered during the process should be done in a grade C environment; if not filtered the preparation of materials and products should be done in a grade A environment with a grade B background.

   Handling and filling of aseptically prepared products should be done in a grade A environment with a grade B background.

   Transfer of partially closed containers, as used in freeze drying should, prior to the completion of stoppering, be done either in a grade A environment, or in sealed transfer trays in a grade B environment.

   Preparation and filling of sterile ointments, creams, suspensions and emulsions should be done in a grade A environment, with a grade B background, when the product is exposed and is not subsequently filtered.

Table 20.7   Recommended limits for microbial contamination (average values)

Grade	Air sample cfu/m³	Settle plates (diam. 90 mm) cfu/4 hours*	Contact plates (diam. 55 mm) cfu/plate	Glove print 5 fingers cfu/glove
A	<1	<1	<1	<1
B	10	5	5	5
C	100	50	25	–
D	200	100	50	–

*Individual settle plates may be exposed for less than 4 hours.
Data from the revised (1996) EC 'Sterile Products Annex'.

There remains to be considered the revised EC annex view of what we have termed the 'divorced' environmental microbial standards. Paragraph 5 of the 1996 annex reads:

> 5.   In order to control the microbiological cleanliness of the various grades in operation, the areas should be monitored. . . . Recommended limits for microbiological monitoring of clean areas in operation . . . [are given in Table 20.7].

(For a cogent analysis of this revised EC annex, see Walker, 1997.)

The sterile products manufacturing area or 'suite'

Before we turn to the layout of a sterile suite there is the *absolutely fundamental* point which cannot be stressed too often (UK GMP Guide, 1983):

> *All sterile products must be manufactured under carefully controlled and monitored conditions, and sole reliance should NOT be placed on any terminal process or test for assurance of the microbial and particulate quality of the end-product.*

In other words, great care must be taken to protect the product from contamination *throughout the entire manufacturing process*, and it is not sufficient merely to rely on a final filtration and/or sterilisation to 'clean things up'. It certainly cannot be hoped that if it fails to do so, then end-product testing particularly by the notably fallible sterility test will detect any problems. That is why sterile products are manufactured in specially designed sterile manufacturing areas or 'suites' of one or more clean rooms.

A clean room, as originally conceived, may be defined thus:

> A clean room is an enclosed space with quantitatively specified control of: particles, temperature, pressure and humidity, constructed with non-porous surfaces which are easy to clean and maintain, with controlled access via airlocks, and operated in accordance with procedures designed to keep contamination below a defined low level.

It needs to be noted that:

1.   Although it is customary to classify clean rooms on the basis of a single parameter – the room air particulate level – the term 'clean room' implies a number of other important factors.
2.   The definition, as given, does indeed refer to a clean room 'as originally conceived'. It was only when this engineering concept was applied to the manufacture of pharmaceuticals, medical devices and other healthcare products that standards for permitted microbial levels were grafted on to it.

There are a few other expressions which also need to be defined:

- *Airlock*. This is an enclosed space with a door at each end, which is placed between rooms (for example, two different grades or classes of clean room) in order to control the airflow between the rooms when they need to be entered. It is usual to arrange, by mechanical, electromagnetic, or electronic devices (or, less desirably, by visible or audible warning systems) that both doors are not open at the same time. (That would defeat the whole object of the airlock.) Airlocks may be intended either for the passage of people or of materials.
- *Pass-through hatch*. This is a sort of mini-airlock, inserted in a wall between two different rooms, usually at bench height. It serves the same purpose as an airlock, and is usually used for the passage of materials or smaller items of equipment. Again, the two doors should not be opened (or openable) at the same time.
- *Double-ended steriliser*. This is a steriliser that has a door at each end. When inserted through a wall to a clean room it means that items can be loaded into the steriliser on one side of the wall, and (following sterilisation) can be taken out on the other. There are two main advantages. Use of a double-ended steriliser guards against the contamination of a clean room which could happen if goods were transported in or out by other means, and it also helps to prevent mix-ups between sterilised and unsterilised materials.
- *Sterilising tunnel*. This is an enclosed conveyor system on which, for example, ampoules and vials can be conveyed into a filling room whilst (during their journey through the tunnel) they are subjected to sufficient heat to sterilise them, and usually also to destroy pyrogens.

Layout of a sterile products suite

A basic problem which confronts a writer on this topic is that of what system (or nomenclature) to use to denote the different air classes, grades or levels. What system will be most readily comprehensible to the widest range of readers? As a member of the European Union, the author realises that he *ought* to employ the classification and terminology of the 1996 'Sterile products' annex to the EC GMP Guide. However, in the light of this particular annex's ambiguities and imprecisions, and in the full recognition that it represents a 'movement towards a common lower standard' (Walker, 1997), he is reluctant to do so. In the discussions which follow therefore, such terms as 'Grade' and 'Class' have been abandoned and the different levels of air quality have simply been designated as Levels A, B, C and D, with Level A referring to the conditions at or under an operational laminar airflow workstation, and the others corresponding respectively to the grades of the original version of the European 'Annex 1 – Manufacture of Sterile Medicinal Products'.

For ease of reference, the relationships between this terminology, adopted for the purposes of this chapter, and the US Federal Standard are as follows:

- Level B – approx. equivalent to Class 100 with the additional requirement of not more than 5 cfu/m³
- Level C – approx. equivalent to Class 10 000 with the additional requirement of not more than 100 cfu/m³
- Level D – approx. equivalent to Class 100 000 with the additional requirement of not more than 500 cfu/m³

Figure 20.1 illustrates a basic sterile products suite. It is like no sterile products area ever built, or ever likely to be built. The drawing is not to any scale, it does not indicate true relative sizes, and a number of things (e.g. doors) are omitted. It is merely intended to indicate the relationships between different areas and activities, and how they all fit together.

Points to note concerning Fig. 20.1:

1. The sterile manufacturing suite should be separate and apart from other manufacturing areas – either a separate building, or a discrete, walled off part of a more general manufacturing site. Entry should only be permitted to authorised personnel via controlled, preferably airlocked, entry doors.
2. The environmental air quality within the general area (that is, the area outside the clean rooms but within the overall suite) need not necessarily conform to the higher standards, although this will depend on the type of work that is carried out. Nevertheless, the air and all surfaces should at least be 'very clean' by any normal (or 'domestic') standards – Level D would normally be appropriate.
3. The essential heart of the suite is the set of clean rooms. Three are shown in the example:

   - A solution preparation room – Level C.
   - A filling room for terminally sterilised products ('fill (T)') – Level C.
   - A room for aseptic filling and any other aseptic manipulations – Level B, with local LAF protection Level A.

The material and workflow is as follows:

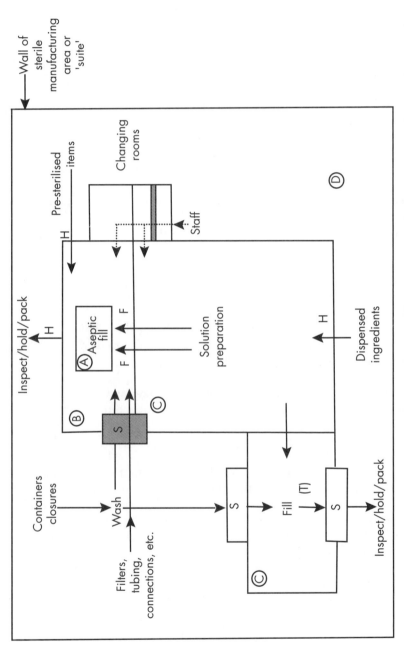

Figure 20.1 Conceptual/schematic diagram of a sterile manufacturing suite. F, filter; H, pass-through hatch; S, steriliser. Levels of air quality indicated by A, B, C, D (see text). —→ Material/work flows. ······▸ Personnel entry.

- Dispensed ingredients, for the manufacture of bulk solutions and suspensions, etc., are passed via a pass-through hatch, or an airlock, into the solution preparation room.
- When manufactured, bulk solutions *intended for aseptic filling* can be pumped, via sterilising grade filters, to the aseptic fill room (filters on the aseptic side; other methods are possible).
- In the aseptic fill room the sterile filtered solution is filled into containers which have previously been washed, rinsed, and passed into the aseptic filling room through a double-ended steriliser, or through a sterilising tunnel. Following filling, the filled sterile product then passes out from the filling room via a hatch, for inspection, labelling and further packaging.

It is essential in this type of aseptic filling process that the containers are clean and sterile at the time they are filled. There is the alternative form of ampoule which is completely sealed as purchased. In use, it is usually assumed that the inside of the ampoule is clean and sterile, and therefore does not need washing, etc. (Indeed, the inside cannot be washed!) Nevertheless, the outsides of these ampoules must be clean and sterile before they pass into the aseptic filling room.

The route for bulk solutions which are intended to be filled and then terminally sterilised is as follows. The bulk manufactured solution is passed to filling room (T) – either by pump, or by use of a mobile sealed mixing vessel wheeled through the door (not shown) – to be filled into clean, washed rinsed and dried, and preferably, but not necessarily, sterilised, containers. The filled containers then pass out of filling room (T) through a double-ended steriliser, in which the product, sealed in its containers, is terminally sterilised.

As the diagram shows, once a bulk solution has been prepared, there are two alternative ways (depending on the nature of the product) by which it can be further processed, and these illustrate the two main, and different, approaches to making sterile products:

1. Filling and sealing the product into its final container and then sterilising it (terminal sterilisation).
2. Sterilising a product at some earlier, bulk stage and then carrying out further processing, filling and sealing into sterile containers, using aseptic techniques and taking aseptic precautions.

Room standards for different operations

The aseptic fill room should be Level B, and both the solution preparation room and the filling room (T) should be Level C. In addition, in the Aseptic fill room, there should certainly be additional localised high-quality filtered air, provided by LAF units (Level A) protecting the point of fill, and wherever else the product is exposed. It is also at least desirable that there should be additional localised filtered air protection at the place(s) where product is filled in the filling room (T).

It is not usually considered necessary to have Levels A, B or C conditions in rooms or areas used for the *initial* preparation of containers, caps/closures, items of equipment, components, etc. prior to washing and sterilisation, always provided that precautions are taken to prevent re-contamination once such items have been cleaned and/or sterilised.

However, even the 'general areas' within a sterile products suite should at least be *very clean* by everyday standards and, some sterile product manufacturers do in fact specify, at least Level D for their more general areas.

Where any sterilised product, or container, is exposed (or could become exposed) in the room, then the room environment ('background') should be Level B when the room is unmanned, and with Level A conditions maintained at critical points (critical for the product, that is) when the room is manned and operational. This applies not only to aseptic filling of previously sterilised liquids, but also to activities such as:

- Mixing different previously sterilised ingredients to form a bulk product which will not (or cannot) then be sterilised. An example would be the incorporation of a sterile powder into a sterile ointment base to form an eye ointment.
- Capping of vials of freeze-dried material.

For the preparation of bulk solutions and other products which are subject to later sterilisation, and for the final cleaning (before sterilisation) of some components and items of equipment, Level C conditions are required.

Other features of a sterile manufacturing area

Other important quality-influencing factors bearing upon the way a sterile products manufacturing suite is designed, constructed, finished and used include the following:

Changing rooms

The possible ways of passing things in and out of these clean rooms include passage via:

- Airlocks
- Pass-through hatches
- Double-ended sterilisers
- Sterilising tunnels.

The method adopted will depend on the nature of the product or material, and the nature of the process.

The other important articles which have to be got in and out of clean rooms are the people who work in them. And when it is recalled that it is people who are the most likely source of contamination, it becomes clear why special arrangements have to be made for their entry to and exit from clean rooms.

This is done through special changing rooms. The schematic diagram (Fig. 20.1) shows one possible arrangement in the form of a single, three-stage changing room. The idea here is that staff enter through a door from the 'general' area already clad in some form of clean protective clothing. This first stage is separated from the second by what is usually called a 'step-over barrier'. In fact it would be more correct to call it a 'sit-over barrier', for it is usually more like a solid bench, about seat height, extending from the floor (no gaps underneath) and completely crossing the room. Staff entering the room sit on this bench while changing their footwear, one shoe at a time. As the first foot is changed it is swung over the bench, to be followed by the other when that shoe has been changed. The object is to make sure that the dirty shoes do not touch the floor in the second stage, and that the new clean footwear does not touch the dirtier floor in the first stage.

In the second stage, a first scrub-up and a further change takes place, into special clean (but not necessarily sterile) protective garments, and then staff can enter the solution preparation and other Level C rooms.

However, before entry into an aseptic fill room, a third stage is necessary, with a change into more thoroughly protective *sterile* garments (protective of the product against contamination from the wearer, that is).

Notice that, since there are doors on the first entry to the changing room, between the second stage and solution preparation, between the second and third stages, and between the third stage and aseptic fill, changing rooms also act as airlocks for the passage of people. (And the same considerations regarding interlocking of doors apply.)

There are many possible variations on this simple arrangement. For example:

- Some arrangements have separate rooms, or routes, for entrance and for exit, and this (laudably) is becoming an increasing trend.
- Some have an entirely separate changing room for just an aseptic room.
- Some have separate male and female changing rooms, and others, by careful timing, manage to operate a 'unisex' system.

Air supply

As already discussed, the air supplied to various rooms must be of quantitatively specified quality. Air from the outside world, or from the rest of the factory is neither suitable or acceptable.

Hence, no windows (or certainly no *openable* windows) to the outside are permissible. It follows that the air to the various rooms must be a forced supply, delivered via ventilation trunking, through filters designed and tested to ensure that air which has passed through them is of the required quality (that is, contains no more than the specified number of particles, and organisms, per cubic foot or cubic metre).

While it is common for coarser pre-filters to be used, in order to reduce the clogging of the final filters, it is important that the final air filters should be fitted at, or as close as possible to, the point of entry of the air into a room. This is usually at various places in the ceiling. It is also usual to design clean rooms so that it is possible to change these filters, as and when necessary, without having to do so from within the room itself (that is, for example, by making the change from above a 'false' or suspended ceiling). This is to avoid contaminating the room with particles from the 'dirty' side of the filter, and to avoid more personnel than absolutely necessary having to enter the room.

Another important feature is that this filtered air should be supplied under pressure, so as to make the whole area at a positive pressure in relation to surrounding areas, and as necessary give a pressure differential *between* different rooms within the suite. As we have seen, the whole idea is that there should be a 'flushing-out' of the suite, from the more to the less critical areas, and thence to the outside.

It is generally considered that there should be a pressure differential between rooms of successively higher to lower risk of at least 15 Pa (approx. 1.5 mm water gauge = 0.06 inches water gauge), although some authorities (see e.g. BS 5295) consider that a pressure differential of 10 Pa between one classified area and another adjacent one of lower classification is acceptable, provided that the differential between the classified areas and adjacent unclassified areas is at least 15 Pa. Thus, the air pressure in the aseptic fill room should be higher than in solution preparation, and the pressure in both should be higher than in the changing rooms, which should in turn be at least 15 Pa higher than in the general unclassified area. To give an indication of this our simple diagram of a sterile suite can be redrawn to show just the airflow patterns (see Fig. 20.2).

Air can flow from one room to another through airlocks, hatches, ports for conveyors or tubing, or through low-level grilles specially installed to aid the overall air balance.

Pressure-sensing devices (water gauges, manometers) must be installed to show the pressure differentials between rooms, and there should be audible or visible warning systems which sound or display alarm signals if the air supply fails and the required pressure drops.

Designing and installing air supply systems is a highly specialised business, as is the balancing of air pressures to achieve the correct differentials and flows. Most commonly, clean rooms are constructed and installed, under contract, by specialists in this field. Careful selection of an appropriate specialist is crucial to success. (Not to put too fine a point on it, some are better than others.) Just as important is a clear, precise definition of just exactly what is wanted, and close and careful monitoring of the project, as the contract proceeds. When the installation has been completed and commissioned, it should be 'handed-over', complete with a certificate of conformity to specification. This should contain certification of at least:

1. *Air filter integrity* – all air inlet filters tested to confirm filter and seal integrity, and conformity to the specified standard. (Filter efficiency can be tested by introducing particulate contamination upstream of the filter, and measuring the contamination level downstream. Percent efficiency is then expressed as the difference between particle concentration upstream (PCU) and particle concentration downstream (PCD) as a percentage of PCU, i.e. (PCU – PCD)/(PCU) × 100%.
2. *Air velocity* – measured by anemometer to determine air velocity (m/s) at the internal filter face of each air inlet.
3. *Air change rate* – calculated for each clean room from the air velocity, and the internal volume of the room.
4. *Air particle counts* – as measured in each clean room, in terms of the number of particles (of specified size) per cubic metre, or cubic foot, at the positions and heights specified in the standard against which the clean rooms were constructed and commissioned.

In addition, reports should be provided of checks on airflow patterns, room pressure differentials, lighting levels, heating and humidity.

Once the system has been installed and the suite is operational it is necessary to continue to check and monitor air filter (and seal) integrity and efficiency and that the air pressures and flows remain as required and as specified. It is also necessary to check airflow rates at filter faces, and room air change rates (which should be at least 20 air changes per hour).

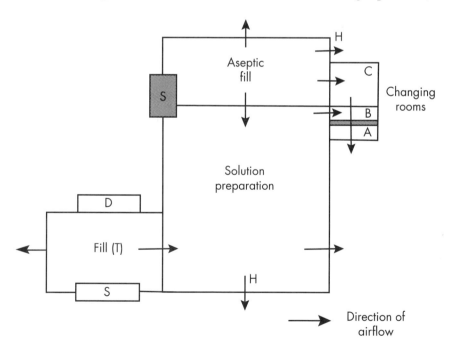

Figure 20.2 Direction of airflow in a typical sterile suite. (For key, see Fig. 20.1.)

Air quality monitoring

The quality of the air, and surfaces, within the rooms must also be regularly monitored by:

- Total particle counters;
- Air samples (for viable organisms);
- 'Settle plates' to check microbial deposition on surfaces;
- Surface swabs and contact plates;
- 'Finger dabs'.

There will, of course, be people working in these clean rooms. There therefore needs to be heating or cooling of all this high quality air to ensure the right level of comfort, particularly for operators clothed in the special clean room garments, which can make them uncomfortably hot. It is important that operators do not get too warm, since the more they sweat, the more particles and organisms they will shed.

Total particles per unit volume of air may be determined by drawing a sample of air (of known volume) through a gridded filter membrane (capable of retaining particles of at least the size under investigation, e.g. of at least 0.5 μm), and then examining the membrane under a microscope for the size and numbers of particles. This is the reference method for demonstrating compliance with BS 5295. However, more often used are the various commercial brands of optical particle counters. In these the air sample is passed through a light beam, with a light scattering detection device, with the resulting signal being electronically processed to display and/or print out particle counts at different size ranges. To detect the finest particles, some models use laser beams.

Microbial levels in a clean room may be determined by use of:

- Settle plates
- Air samplers
- Surface sampling
- 'Finger dabs'.

Settle plates are Petri dishes containing sterile nutrient agar. The plates are most usually 90 mm diameter (surface area approx. 0.006 m^2), although plates of 140 mm diameter (approx. 0.015 m^2 surface area) have been used. It is thus necessary when reporting settle plate results (and when establishing standards for settle plate counts) to state both the size of the plate(s) and the time of exposure. For valid comparisons to be made between results obtained using different plate sizes, the results should be expressed as cfus/100 cm^2/hour.

The most commonly used growth medium is Tryptone Soya, but others such as Rose Bengal and Sabouraud's medium have been used for specialised purposes. The plates are exposed in the room for a predefined (and subsequently recorded) time, and then incubated for a specified time at a specified temperature, and then examined. The number of colony-forming units (cfu) and the types (or species) of micro-organisms found are recorded.

It has been argued that settle plates do not give a measure of the concentration of micro-organisms in the air in a room. This is true, but it may equally be argued that, in providing a direct measure of the organisms which are depositing from the air and on to surfaces (or into containers), they do provide an indication of what the sterile product manufacturer really requires to know – the likely microbial contamination entering into, or on to, products (Whyte, 1996).

At one time it was considered that settle plates were only suitable for exposure for relatively short periods (0.5 to 1 hour), on the grounds that longer exposure times cause the agar to dry out, and thus fail to culture the organisms which deposit on it. This view is no longer generally held, given that the agar has not been poured too thinly. If the agar layer fills at least half the Petri dish, plates may be exposed to good effect for several hours (Whyte & Niven, 1986; Russell *et al.*, 1984).

Air samplers are commercially available in a number of different types:

- *Cascade samplers.* Here the air being sampled is drawn through perforations onto a stack of agar plates, separated one from the other by perforated plates, the perforations in a plate decreasing in diameter from top to bottom of the stack. Organisms attached to the larger particles in the air sample are deposited on the top agar plate. Those attached to the smaller particles cascade down through the perforations until they impact on an agar plate lower down. After the specified time the agar plates are incubated and examined, as for settle plates.
- *Slit to agar sampler.* Here the air sample is drawn through slits and impinges on a rotating agar plate. The dimensions of the slits, their distance from the agar surface and the airflow rate are adjusted to give optimum capture of the contaminants in the air. The agar plate is incubated and examined as before.
- *Single sieve to agar sampler.* Here the air is drawn through a perforated disc so as to impinge on an agar plate, which is then incubated and examined as in the other methods.
- *Centrifugal sampler.* Here air is drawn into the sampling head by the blades of a rotating fan-like impeller. This directs the air onto an agar strip fitted around the inner circumference of the sampling head. After a pre-set sampling time the agar strip is incubated and examined.
- *Filtration.* Here air is drawn, at a controlled rate for a specified time, through a micro-organism retaining membrane filter, which is then placed on an agar plate, incubated and examined for organism growth.
- *Liquid impingement.* Here the air is drawn through an aqueous

medium contained in an aspirator bottle, for a specified time. The liquid is then filtered through a membrane, which is then placed on an agar plate and incubated.

In all these air sampling methods, knowledge of the sampling rate, the time period over which the sample was taken, and of the number of cfu's counted after incubation will enable the determination of the number of viable organisms present in unit volume (1 cubic metre or 1 cubic foot) of air in the room.

Surface sampling   Surfaces of walls, floors, work and equipment surfaces can be sampled using moistened sterile cotton swabs, which are then 'streaked-out' on an agar plate, which is then incubated. Alternatively, and more conveniently except for less accessible surfaces, contact (or 'Rodac') plates can be pressed lightly onto flat surfaces and incubated. The colonies can then be counted to derive a quantitative estimate of surface contamination levels. Following the application of a swab, or a contact plate, the relevant surface area should be wiped with a disinfectant wipe.

Finger dabs   Although 'finger dabs' do not directly measure the microbial contamination of the air in a clean room, they do give an indication of the contamination picked up by operators from surfaces in the room.

After, or as, they leave the room, operators touch the tips of all digits of both gloved hands onto an agar plate, which is then incubated. (It should go without saying that the gloves should be discarded and fresh ones put on before an operator continues to work.)

A similar technique can be employed as a training exercise, outside the sterile area, by applying operators' ungloved fingers (and indeed noses, ears or whatever) to an agar plate to provide them with a graphic illustration of the organisms present on the human body surface.

Frequency of monitoring/checking of clean room parameters

Physical

(a) *Room pressure differentials.* There should be a continuous automatic manometric measurement, linked to unmistakable visual and/or audible warning signals which are triggered whenever pressure drops below the specified level. The manometer gauges should also be visually checked hourly, and the reading recorded at least once per day (or per shift). It is essential that the manometers are regularly calibrated.

(b) *Air velocity and room air change-rates.* Perform and record every six months.

(c) *Air particle counts.* Perform daily (or batch-wise) in the more critical areas, and weekly in the less.

(d) *Air filter integrity and efficiency test.* Carry out once or twice a year, unless results of in-process physical and microbial monitoring indicate a more urgent need.

Airflow directions and patterns should also be occasionally checked, as convenient. (Clearly, it is not possible to check this by smoke tests when the rooms are in operation. It is usually possible to check quite simply the direction in which air is passing through a grille. But beware – air moving rapidly away from the surface of a hand can produce a sense of cooling which can be (and indeed has been) misinterpreted as if air were blowing on the skin surface.)

It is quite common for sterile products manufacturers to have the more crucial physical parameters examined and independently certified, say once or twice a year, by an external contract specialist. While there is no absolute necessity to do this, it can be said, with good reason, that in such a critical area of manufacturing, where lives could be at stake, it does add a significant extra layer of assurance.

Microbial

While there is something like general agreement on the frequency of monitoring of physical clean room parameters (for example, frequency rates similar to those set out above are to be found in BS 5295), no such official or general agreement exists in regard to frequency of microbial monitoring. Both the EC GMP Guide and the US CGMPs remain silent on this important point. Nor is the FDA's *Guideline on Sterile Drug Products Produced by Aseptic Processing* (US FDA, 1987) prepared to commit itself any further than to say, in this context, 'the written monitoring program should have a scientifically sound sampling schedule, including sampling locations and frequency'.

In the circumstances, the following seems to be a reasonable schedule for the different levels of clean room:

- In clean rooms at Level A – daily or batch-wise.
- In clean rooms at Level B – daily.
- In clean rooms at Level C – weekly.
- In clean rooms at Level D – weekly, without all microbial monitoring necessarily being carried out on each occasion.

Standards for clean room monitoring tests

The standards against which the results of *physical* monitoring tests are to be assessed present no problem. They are as discussed above, and related to the specification against which the room (or suite) was constructed. As before however, there still seems to remain areas for discussion in regard to *microbial* monitoring. The 'recommended limits for microbiological monitoring' of the revised (1996) EC Annex 1 on the 'Manufacture of sterile products' are as given in Table 20.7.

For more detailed information, see Technical Monograph No. 2 of the Parenteral Society (1989).)

The sterile manufacturing area – construction, materials and finishes

The surfaces of all floors, walls and ceilings should be hard, smooth, impervious and unbroken (i.e. no cracks, holes or other damage). There are three good reasons for this:

1.   To prevent the shedding of particles from damaged, or poorly finished, brick, building block, plaster, etc.
2.   To prevent the accumulation of dust, dirt and micro-organisms on, or in, rough or broken surfaces.
3.   To permit easy and repeated cleaning and disinfection.

Various materials have been used for floors, including welded sheet vinyl, terrazzo and various 'poured' resin floors. A variety of basic structural materials is used for walls – bricks, blocks, plastic coated metal panels, glass reinforced plastics. All are acceptable, provided that the final finish provides a *smooth, impervious, unbroken* surface. Thus if a wall is constructed of brick or structural block, it must be plastered smooth and then coated with a hard-setting finish (polyurethane, epoxy, etc.), sprayed or painted on.

Welded sheet vinyl is also used as a wall finish, often as a continuation of the same material when it has also been used as a floor surface.

Where windows are installed they should not be openable. They should be flush-fitted on the controlled (or classified) area side. Where windows are fitted in a dividing wall between two classified areas or rooms, they should be double glazed so as to present a flush, ledgeless fit on both sides. If communication is necessary between adjacent clean rooms, this should be via 'speech panels' (polymeric membranes which transmit sound while maintaining an air-tight seal). They can be used back-to-back in double glazed windows. When installed in the more critical clean rooms the usual protective grilles should be removed as they are difficult to clean. Telephone and intercom installations should generally be avoided, certainly in aseptic processing rooms. If they are deemed essential, in for example a solution preparation room, they should be purpose-designed, flush mounted and with easily wipeable touch-sensitive controls.

Ceilings in sterile areas are often 'false' or suspended, to allow for the installation of air supply ducting, and other services. It is important that any suspended ceiling is effectively sealed from the room below, to prevent any possible contamination from the space between the false and the 'real' ceiling.

Where floors meet walls, and walls meet ceilings, the joins should be coved, so as to avoid sharp corners which are difficult to clean and would harbour dust, dirt and micro-organisms. It is also important that any such coving should be flush to both floor and wall (or wall and ceiling) (Fig. 20.3).

All too often coving is so badly installed that it creates two dirt- and bacteria-collecting corners where previously there was only one.

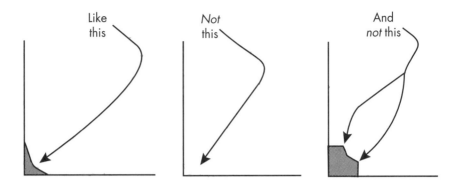

Figure 20.3   Coving design for clean rooms.

It is also important that all potential dust-collecting surfaces should be kept to a minimum. All lights, doors, windows, air supplies and exit grilles and the like should be flush-fitting with no, or a minimum of, ledges or ridges. Light fittings should be flush-fitted, permanently sealed-in units, with access for lamp replacement from a service void above the false, or suspended ceiling. Because of the difficulties of cleaning the sliding gear, sliding doors should be avoided. Doors should normally open inward to the higher standard, or more critical room, so that operators can back in, without having to touch the 'dirtier' side with their gloved hands. Doors into, within, and from changing rooms should be fitted with warning systems or interlocks to prevent more than one door being opened simultaneously, thus causing a drop in overall pressure levels. Electromechanical interlocks are perhaps more effective from this point of view, but are a potentially serious hazard to operators in the event of fire. Unless the safety of workers can be assured by other means (e.g. by the installation of sealed 'burst panels' in clean room walls) interlocking bolt systems are probably best avoided. Given well trained and disciplined operators (which all workers in sterile products manufacturing areas should unquestionably be) clear warning light systems, actuated by door-mounted microswitches should be more than adequate.

There will, inevitably, be bench and work surfaces but these must be constructed (with hard, smooth, impervious and unbroken surfaces) so that it is always possible to clean everything thoroughly on, in, under, and around them. There should be easy access around, and under, all furniture and equipment within a clean room. On the whole, wood, and certainly bare wood, should not be used as a material of construction within a clean room.

Any pipework, ducting or conduit supplying air, water, electricity or gas to a clean room should be supplied via the void above a false ceiling, and/or sealed within the walls. If pipework or ducting passes through a wall, it should be completely sealed within the wall through which it passes. There should be no pipes set so close to walls as to create difficult-to-clean dirt traps.

Sinks and drains should be excluded from manufacturing areas wherever possible, and avoided entirely in clean rooms in which aseptic operations are carried out. Where drains must be installed, they should be fitted with effective, easily cleanable traps and air breaks to prevent back-flow. They must be easy to clean and disinfect – and, of course, they must *be* clean and disinfected.

Where sinks are installed (for example in changing rooms and in bulk solution preparation areas) they should preferably be made of stainless steel, and be designed, installed and maintained so as to minimise risks of microbial growth and contamination. In changing rooms, foot controls for the supply of water and antibacterial liquid soap for washing hands, and automatic warm-air hand dryers are much to be preferred. Sinks and hand washbasins, and the drains from them, should be regularly disinfected.

Wherever possible, major items of equipment should either be movable, for the purposes of cleaning and disinfecting both the equipment and the floor or wall area under or adjacent to it, or built into the fabric of the room so as to present only smooth, cleanable surfaces, and no inaccessible gaps and recesses. Where built-in work benches join walls, flexing of the working surface can cause stress and consequent cracking at the junction. The joint can be sealed with a well and smoothly applied flexible sealant, silicone or urethane, but probably the better alternative is the use of free-standing, movable stainless steel tables rather than fixed bench-work. In general, it can bear being repeated that all surfaces should be smooth, impervious and unbroken, that there should be NO uncleanable gaps, cracks, spaces, holes or recesses and that there should be a minimum of ledges, shelves, cupboards and equipment.

Unidirectional airflow workstations

'Laminar airflow' (LAF) is the term applied to a supply of sterile air forced through high efficiency particulate air (HEPA) filters so that it flows, non-turbulently, in just one direction, over the material or product which is in need of special protection. The object is to sweep away (and keep away) any potential microbial or other particulate contamination. The actual filter faces from which the air emerges are usually fitted with side screens, curtains or shields which surround, or partially surround, the product, material or equipment which needs to be protected. Alternatively, they may be obtained already purpose-built into laminar flow cabinets. Unidirectional, or laminar, airflow may be either vertical or horizontal.

Sometimes seen are entire laminar airflow rooms, that is, rooms in which one whole wall is made up of HEPA filters. The idea is that the whole room is 'swept clean' with the flow of unidirectional filtered air. Such rooms are, however, not commonly installed in sterile pharmaceutical manufacturing units, where it is much more usual to see laminar airflow cabinets ('contained workstations' or 'unidirectional airflow cabinets') installed where extra protection against contamination is required,

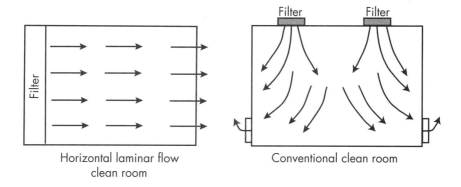

Figure 20.4   Two airflow systems for clean rooms (elevation view).

within a standard (or 'conventional') clean room. A conventional clean room is a clean room which is not a totally laminar flow room, but a room where normally the air enters through filters installed in the ceiling, and exits through grilles placed low in the walls, and/or under doors, etc. (see Fig. 20.4).

Isolation and BFS technology

Isolation technology is concerned with the containment and close control of the environment immediately surrounding the work in process. It has two possible main objectives – protecting the product from contamination from the operator(s), and protecting operator(s) from any hazardous products or materials. A well designed, constructed and operated isolator, avoiding as it can any direct contact between human operators and the immediate product environment, can significantly reduce the risk of microbiological contamination of products and materials processed within them. Problems to be guarded against are the possibility of puncturing of the fabric of an isolator, and of leakage, particularly around any transfer devices or ports. The revised EC annex on sterile procedure considers that when used for aseptic processing, isolators should be sited in at least a Grade D background operating environment.

Isolator processes should be validated, with particular regard for the quality of the air both inside and outside of the isolator, cleaning and disinfection of the isolator, and the integrity of the isolator and any transfer mechanisms. They should be physically and microbiologically monitored, as for any other aseptic process, with attention being given to leak testing of the isolator and any glove or sleeve system.

Blow-fill-seal (BFS) machines are specialist purpose-built pieces of equipment in which, in one continuous operation, containers are formed from a thermoplastic granulate, filled and then sealed, all in a continuous automated operation. Originally developed for other purposes, they have

for some years been available adapted for use in the manufacture of pharmaceutical, device and other healthcare products, specifically sterile pharmaceutical products.

In this process, bulk solution prepared under microbiologically clean
or sterile conditions (as appropriate) is delivered to the machine via a bacteria-retaining filter; pipework, filter housings and machine parts in contact
with the product having been previously steam sterilised in place. Filtered
compressed air and granules of a plastics material conforming to a predetermined specification and known to be compatible with the product to be
filled (usually polyethylene, polypropylene or polyethylene/polypropylene
co-polymers) are also supplied to the machine.

Within the machine, the plastics granules are extruded downwards
under pressure (up to 350 Bar) as a hot hollow mouldable plastics tube
(termed in the trade a 'parison') or tubes. As a result of the high pressure
extrusion process, the parison reaches a temperature of 170° to 230°C.
The configuration and internal integrity of the parison is maintained by an
internal downward flow of filtered air under pressure. The two halves of
a mould close around the parison and seal the base. Simultaneously, the
top of the parison is cut free by a hot knife. The plastics material is now
formed into a container (or containers, as determined by the design of the
mould) by vacuum and/or sterile air pressure. The container(s), having
been transferred to the filling position (still within the mould) is/are
immediately filled with a carefully metered volume of the solution, dis-
placing the sterile air. Both the air and the solution are filtered through
micro-organism retaining filters immediately before entry into the forming,
or formed, container(s).

When the required volume is filled into the container(s) the filling unit
is raised and the containers are sealed automatically. The mould then opens,
releasing a package formed, filled and sealed all in the one continuous, automatic cycle which takes a matter of seconds (usually around 10–25 seconds,
depending on the volume filled). Meanwhile, parison-extrusion continues,
and the cycle repeats. The filled and sealed units will usually require crop-
ping or deflashing of excess plastic.

In versions of these machines adapted for aseptic manufacture, the
filling cycle occurs in an internal sterile filtered air-flushed environment (the
so-called 'air shower'). The machines can also be used to fill suspensions,
ointments, creams and liquids other than aqueous solutions, although with
such products it is not necessarily always possible to employ the final aseptic
product filtration facility.

'Multiblock' versions of these machines permit the formation of a
number (or set) of containers at each pass, from one parison in one mould.

As mentioned in Chapter 19, some impressive claims have been made
for the advantages of blow/fill/seal technology in providing greater confidence of sterility in aseptic processing. The evidence presented would appear
to suggest that these claims have not been made without justice. However,
regulatory bodies have largely viewed the technology, up until now, with
greater scepticism.

Services for sterile products areas

Services for manufacturing departments generally have already been covered in Chapter 9, where the various grades of water, and the systems for supplying them were discussed. The special requirements for air supply have been covered in this present chapter. It is especially important that all services to sterile products areas should be supplied and/or installed so as not to represent risks of contaminating the product or the manufacturing environment. The US FDA's *Guideline on Sterile Drugs Produced by Aseptic Processing* (US FDA 1987) also notes that 'gases other than ambient air may also be used in controlled areas. Such gases should, if vented to the area, be of the same quality as the ambient air. Compressed air should be free from demonstrable oil vapour.'

For comprehensive information on the design, layout, construction and servicing of sterile products suite, see the *Baseline Pharmaceutical Engineering Guide, Vol. 3: Sterile manufacturing facilities* (ISPE, 1999).

Validation of sterilisation processes

All sterilisation processes must be validated. See Chapter 23, 'Validation: applications'.

Personnel

Even more than in relation to other types of manufacture, the people involved in sterile manufacturing are the single most important factor. The person, or persons, who manage sterile products departments should have a full understanding of, and experience in, the special techniques, technologies and disciplines required – and of the underlying physical, chemical, microbiological and clinical principles. They should be able to impart their knowledge and understanding to their staff, who should also be selected with care. Workers in sterile product areas should be mature (and that does not necessarily mean old) intelligent people who can fully understand not only what they have do, but also the reasons for so doing it. They must have innately high standards of personal hygiene, and be readily able to abide by the special disciplines involved. They should also be free from any disease or condition which could represent an abnormal microbiological hazard to the clean room environment, and hence to the product. These conditions include, in addition to chronic gastrointestinal and respiratory tract diseases, short-term conditions such as colds, acute diarrhoea, skin rashes, boils, open superficial injuries and peeling sunburn. Operators should be required to report any such conditions, and supervisory staff should be on the look-out for them. There should be periodic health checks.

In addition to those who have chronic skin, respiratory or gut diseases, persons who have allergies to the synthetic fabrics used in clean room clothing, who are abnormally high shedders of skin flakes or dandruff, have nervous conditions resulting in excessive itching, scratching etc. or who suffer from any degree of claustrophobia are really not fitted to work in clean rooms.

No person who reports that they have a condition which would preclude their working in a clean area should suffer any penalty for so doing. The thought of loss of earnings might well persuade even the most exemplary worker to keep quiet about an adverse health condition.

A certain calm resoluteness of character is also most desirable. To be alone, or perhaps be just one of two or three, in a clean room, in a full sterile suit with gloves, hood, mask and possibly goggles can prove a lonely, depressing, demotivating experience for some temperaments. Conversely, while a casual, 'whistle-as-you-work' attitude may well be salutary in some areas of human activity, it is entirely inappropriate in a clean room.

To minimise the contamination inevitably caused by the presence of people, the numbers entering and working in clean rooms should be kept to the minimum necessary for effective working. All activities, such as in-process testing and control, visual inspection and the like which do not need to be conducted in a clean room should be performed outside it.

All personnel, and that includes cleaning staff and maintenance engineers, required to work in, or otherwise enter a clean area, should be trained in the techniques and disciplines relevant to the safe and effective manufacture of sterile products. This training, which should not be a 'one-off' exercise but must be regularly reinforced with refresher training, should include coverage of personal hygiene, the essential elements of microbiology and the purpose and correct wearing of protective clothing. Operators should be taught to 'know the enemy', and practical demonstrations of growing cultures, finger dabs and the like will help to get the message home. Training should also include a strong motivational element, stressing responsibilities to patients' health and life, which are, quite literally 'in your hands'.

Any outside persons, such as building or maintenance contractors, who have not received the training and who need to enter clean areas should only do so under close supervision, and when wearing protective clothing appropriate to the area.

Clothing and changing

Personnel should only enter a clean area via changing rooms, where washing and changing should proceed in strict accordance with a written procedure. The operators should have been trained to follow this procedure, and a copy of it clearly displayed on the changing room wall. The procedure should be designed to minimise contamination of the protective clothing, through, for example, contact with the floor on the 'dirtier side', or with operators' shoes. Outdoor clothing should not be taken into clean room changing rooms. The assumption should be that outdoor garments have already been removed elsewhere, and that personnel are already clad in the standard 'general factory' protective clothing. Wristwatches and jewellery should be removed as part of the changing process. Plain, simple wedding rings are generally considered to be an exception which is both reasonable, sympathetic and expedient, many people finding it impossible (physically or emotionally) to remove their wedding rings. However, the FDA are said not to agree on this point. Cosmetics, other than perhaps simple particle-free non-shedding creams should not be worn.

Protective garments, which should include head- and footwear, should be made from textiles specially manufactured so as to shed virtually no fibres or particles, and to retain any particles shed by a human body within. They should be comfortable to wear, and loose fitting to reduce abrasion. Fabric edges should be sealed and seams all-enveloping. Unnecessary tucks and belts should be avoided, and there should be no external pockets. The garments should be worn only in the clean areas. A fresh set of clean (and if necessary sterilised) protective garments should be provided each time a person enters, or re-enters a clean room. This should rigorously be enforced where aseptic processing is in operation. In other, less critical, clean rooms, it may be possible to relax this requirement and provide fresh garments once per day, if this can be justified on the basis of monitoring results and other control measures. Even so, fresh head- and footwear, and gloves should be provided for each working session.

Protective clothing, following use, should be washed or cleaned (and as necessary sterilised), and thereafter handled in such a way as to prevent it gathering contaminants, and to minimise attrition of the fabric. It needs to be recognised that repeated wearing and laundering/cleaning (and sterilisation) can cumulatively damage the fabric so that it becomes no longer suitable for use. This is clearly something which needs to be monitored and controlled, and some methods and standards have been published (see, for example, ASTM, 1968; AS 2013, 1977; AS 2014, 1977; BS 3211, 1986).

In Levels C and D standard clean rooms, one- or two-piece trouser suits should be worn, close fitting at the neck, wrists and ankles, with high necks. Hair, including any facial hair (beard or moustache) should be covered. Trouser-bottoms should be tucked into overshoes or boots, and sleeves into gloves.

In Level B rooms, and/or when working at Level A workstations, sterilised non-shedding cover-all trouser suits (preferably one-piece) should be worn. Headwear should be of the helmet or cowl type, and totally enclose the hair and any beard/moustache. It should be completely tucked into the neck of the suit. Footwear should be of the boot, or 'bootie' type, totally enclosing the feet. Trouser bottoms should be completely tucked into the footwear. Powder-free rubber or plastic gloves should be worn with the garment sleeves neatly and completely tucked inside the gloves. Gloves should be regularly disinfected (e.g. with a sterile alcoholic spray or foam) during extended operations. Disposable face masks, covering both the nose and mouth should be worn, and should be discarded at least each time the wearers leave the clean room, and whenever they become 'soggy'. In the latter circumstances, it is of course necessary to leave the clean room to change the mask. Operators should be trained not to touch masks, or any other part of their face, with their hands when in a clean room.

There is a school of thought which holds that, when working in an aseptic processing area, operators should wear close-fitting goggles. Indeed, the US FDA have been known to insist upon it. There are, however, those who would argue that any benefit, in terms of reduction in contamination hazard, is out-weighed by the risks introduced by the additional operator discomfort and the misting of the goggle lenses.

When working at contained LAF workstations, operators should always work down-stream of the filter face and of any product, material or equipment which is being processed or manipulated at the workstation. In other words, work should be conducted so that any operator-derived contamination is swept in a direction away from the work in hand. Hands or arms should not be interposed between the filter face and the product, as this would cause the air stream to sweep contamination from the operator onto the work – the very reverse of what is required.

Instructions to operators on entering and working in clean rooms

To conclude this passage on the personnel aspects of sterile product manufacture, the following instructions to operators will serve as a checklist, and perhaps as the basis for an SOP, or a training hand-out.

○ Keep body, hair, face, hands and fingernails clean.

○ Report any illnesses, cuts, grazes, or respiratory, gut, or skin problems.

○ Follow the written changing and wash-up procedure EXACTLY.

○ Check that your protective clothing is worn properly.

○ Do not wear cosmetics, jewellery or wristwatches.

○ Leave all personal items (wallets, coins, keys, watches, tissues, combs, etc.) in the changing room.

○ Do not take papers, documents or paper materials into clean rooms, unless these have been specifically approved. (Paper, cardboard and similar materials are great shedders of particles and fibres.)

○ No eating, chewing, drinking.

○ Always move gently and steadily.

○ Do *not* move vigorously. No frivolous activity, singing or whistling.

○ Avoid talking unless absolutely necessary.

○ Avoid coughing or sneezing. If these are unavoidable, leave the clean room. (We spray a lot of fine drops and microbes about when we talk, sing, whistle, cough, sneeze or splutter.)

○ Do not touch other operators.

○ Avoid scratching, touching nose and mouth and rubbing hands.

○ Where gloves are worn, regularly disinfect them, as instructed.

○ Always check for worn or damaged garments and torn gloves, and change them as necessary. (Even a pin-hole in a glove could have disastrous consequences for a patient.)

○ Keep garments fully fastened up. Do not unfasten or loosen them.

○ Unless there is a special hazard involved, do not pick up dropped items from the floor.

○ When working at a laminar flow workstation it is important to ensure that:

   • Nothing is placed between the air filter face and the object, material or product which is being handled and which needs to be protected. (This would disturb the smoothly sweeping flow of unidirectional air which is keeping the vital areas clean.)

   • Always work downstream from the air filter face, and do not let your hands or arms come between the item which is being protected and the air filter face. Blowing contamination from you onto a product defeats the whole object, and could be a danger to patients.

In-process control of sterilisation processes

It is a statement of the obvious, but it cannot be over-stressed that for a sterilisation process to be effective, all of the material, product, batch, lot or load must be subjected to the required treatment. For example, 121°C for 15 minutes is generally considered to be an effective time/temperature cycle for steam sterilisation. This does not mean that it is OK if some part or parts of the autoclave load reach and maintain a temperature of 121°C for 15 minutes. It means that the coldest part, of the coldest item or unit, in the coldest area within the chamber, must reach a temperature of at least 121°C, and be held at that temperature for at least 15 minutes. If it is necessary, in order to achieve such conditions, for some other parts of the load to reach much higher temperatures for significantly longer times, thus risking product degradation, then something is wrong with either the design of the autoclave, or the loading pattern, or both. When a heat sterilisation cycle is validated, it must be regarded only as the validation of a specified cycle, in a particular chamber, containing a specific product or material, loaded into the chamber in a specified pattern. If the loading pattern is changed, the process can no longer be considered to be validated.

Materials and products to be sterilised should not carry a high level of microbial contamination ('bioburden'). Limits should be set on the pre-sterilisation bioburden, and lots intended for sterilisation should be tested for microbial levels before being subjected to the sterilisation process. This does not necessarily mean that sterilisation may not proceed until these test results are available. They should, however, be recorded and form part of the data to be considered when the final release/reject decision is made. The whole object is to present the lowest possible microbial challenge to the sterilisation process. To this end, it is sound quality practice to pass solutions, particularly large volume parenterals (LVPs) through a bacteria-retaining filter before filling and terminal sterilisation.

Various forms of biological and chemical indicators are available for use in connection with sterilisation processes. They can show when a sterilisation has failed, but cannot necessarily demonstrate that the process has been an overall success. Thus, if used alone they are not acceptable as proof that a sterilisation process has been effective. They may be considered as providing no more than back-up to the other evidence which must be available.

Biological indicators (preparations of bacterial cultures, usually spores, of strains known to be resistant to the type of sterilisation process under consideration) are less reliable than physical monitoring and control methods, except in the case of ethylene oxide sterilisation. If used, strict precautions must be taken to avoid releasing the resistant contamination into clean rooms, and into or onto products.

Chemical indicators are commercially available for heat, ethylene oxide and radiation sterilisation. They can take the form of adhesive tapes or patches, colour spot cards, small sealed tubes or sachets. They change colour as a result of chemical reactions activated by exposure to the sterilisation process, but it is possible for the change to take place before the sterilisation time has been completed, and hence (with the exception of the plastic dosimeters used in radiation sterilisation) their inadequacy as proof of sterilisation. The same applies to the preparations of substances which melt at a sterilising temperature. They can show that a temperature has been reached, but not that it has been held, or for how long. Radiation-sensitive coloured discs (not to be confused with plastic dosimeters) that change colour when exposed to radiation serve to distinguish between items which have been exposed to radiation, and those which have not, but do not give a reliable indication of successful sterilisation.

It is vital that there should be a clear and foolproof method of distinguishing between goods which have been sterilised and those which have not. Double-end, through-wall, sterilisers are a notable aid in preventing this potentially lethal form of mix-up. In any event, each basket, tray or other carrier of material or product should be clearly labelled with the material name, its lot number and an unequivocal indication of whether or not it has been sterilised. Autoclave tape is a useful indicator, as long as it is understood that it can only indicate that a lot has been through an autoclave cycle, not that it has been sterilised.

Each *heat sterilisation* cycle should be automatically recorded on a temperature/time chart, or by other suitable automatic means, such as a digital printout. The chart scale should be large enough to permit accurate reading of both the time and temperature. The chart, or printout should form part of the permanent batch record, and thus form part of the data evaluated when making the release/reject decision. The temperature thus recorded should be sensed from a probe placed in the coolest part of the loaded chamber, this point having been determined for each type of load processed. Where control of the cycle is automatic the heat-sensing *control* probe should be independent of the *recorder* probe. (If the same probe were used for both purposes and it was defective, it could actuate an inadequate cycle, yet still signal an apparently satisfactory one.)

In a *steam sterilisation* process it is important to ensure that the steam used is of a suitable quality ('clean steam') and does not contain additives, or other substances, which could cause chemical contamination of the product, material or equipment being sterilised.

After the high temperature (sterilising) phase of a heat sterilisation cycle has finished, there is a risk that as the load cools, air entering the chamber, and particularly any water used in spray cooling, could be drawn into, for example, inadequately sealed vials. Air admitted before the chamber doors are opened should be filtered, and water used for spray cooling should be water for injection quality.

In *ethylene oxide* sterilisation, direct contact between the gas and the microbial cells is essential for effective sterilisation. Organisms occluded in crystals, or coated with other material, such as dried protein, may well not be killed. The nature and quantity of any packaging material can also markedly affect the efficacy of the process. Before exposure to the gas, the materials should be brought into equilibrium with the required temperature and humidity. Throughout the cycle, records should be made of the cycle time, temperature, pressure, humidity, gas concentration and total amount of gas used. These records should form part of the batch record, and be used in the final evaluation of the batch for release/reject. Ethylene oxide sterilisation is an instance where use of biological indicators should be considered mandatory, rather than merely a possible useful adjunct. The generally recommended organism is *Bacillus subtilis* var. *niger,* deposited on a suitable carrier. The positioning of these indicators should be selected following validation studies to determine those parts of the load most difficult to sterilise. Views vary as to the number of biological indicators to be used per load. The UK Department of Heath recommends a minimum of ten indicators for sterilisers with a capacity of up to 500 litres (Department of Health 1981, 1990). The information derived from the use of these biological indicators should form part of the batch manufacturing record, as evaluated when making the final release/reject decision.

During *gamma irradiation sterilisation,* the dose received should be monitored throughout the process by the use of plastic dosimeters inserted in the load in sufficient numbers, and inserted in packs sufficiently close together so as to ensure that in a continuous process there are always at least two dosimeters in the load, exposed to the source. The standard red Perspex dosimeters, as for example prepared by the UK Atomic Energy Authority at Harwell, UK, give a reproducible, quantitative, dose-related change in absorbance which should be read as soon as possible after exposure to the radiation. *Electron beam sterilisation* is rather more difficult to control. The dosimeters used are usually in the form of PVC films. In both cases the dosimetry results should form part of the batch record. Biological indictors can be used, but NOT as a proof of sterilisation. Radiation-sensitive ad-hesive coloured discs are used, but only as a means of indicating that a package has been exposed to radiation and not as proof of sterilisation.

In *filtration sterilisation,* which should only be used when it is not possible or practicable to sterilise by other more secure means, non-fibre shedding filters, which are demonstrably capable of removing micro-organisms, without removing ingredients from the solution or releasing substances into it, should be used. It is often advisable to use a (possibly coarser grade) pre-filter to first remove larger particles and thus reduce the load on the sterilising filter. The once widely-used asbestos filters must not be used unless there is some absolute necessity, and when there is complete assurance that any released asbestos fibres will be removed downstream. Because of the potential additional risk of filtration as compared with other sterilisation methods, it is sound practice to follow the first sterilisation grade filter with a second in series, downstream. This has on occasions been decried as pointless 'belt and braces', but it is impossible to be too careful when lives may be at stake, and no good arguments have been mounted against such a double filtration system.

The integrity of the sterilising (and sterilised) filter assembly, *in situ* (not just the filter in isolation) should be confirmed before use, and rechecked after use by such methods as the so-called bubble-point, pressure-hold or forward-flow tests. Most major filter manufacturers supply automatic integrity-testing equipment, applicable to their own filters and filter housings, and will assist in the selection and operation of integrity test procedures appropriate to specific filters, products and applications. The time during which a sterile filtered bulk solution is held, pending filling and sealing in its final container, should be kept to a defined minimum, appropriate to the conditions under which the bulk filtered solution is stored. Any one filter should not normally be used for more than one working day, unless a longer period of use can be justified by sound validation studies.

After sterilisation

Of major importance is the need to avoid recontamination of a sterilised product or material, and the mix-up of sterilised with non-sterilised items. Ethylene oxide sterilisation is a special case where it is necessary to hold sterilised material under controlled ventilated conditions to allow any residual ethylene oxide and its reaction products to diffuse away. This presents additional problems in the prevention of recontamination and mix-up.

As well as the chemical analytical testing to confirm compliance with specification, sterile products also require to be subjected to further testing which is specific to this type of product. This includes:

- Examination for particles,
- Sterility testing,
- Leak detection testing, and possibly
- Pyrogen (or endotoxin) testing.

Examination for particulate contamination

The EC GMP Guide's revised (1996) Annex 1 'Manufacture of sterile medicinal products', requires that 'filled containers of parenteral products should be inspected individually for extraneous contamination or other defects', and adds that when this is a visual inspection 'it should be done under suitable and controlled conditions of illumination and background'. It adds that operators engaged in this work should pass regular eyesight tests, with spectacles if normally worn, and be given frequent breaks from inspection (an acknowledgement of the very real problem of the decline in the efficiency of the human inspecting machine as a result of eye and general fatigue). Pharmacopoeias (e.g. British, European and United States) have also variously set down requirements for the examination of filled parenterals for visible and sub-visible particles, albeit not necessarily for the 100% inspection that is, perhaps, implied by the EC GMP Guide's use of the term 'individually'. The question thus arises as to why it is considered necessary, or at least desirable, for parenteral products to be free of visible, and in the case of large volume parenterals (LVPs) sub-visible particulate contamination. Although the evidence for adverse clinical effects following injection of particles is equivocal, even conflicting (Barnett, 1994; Sharp, 1991), there is nevertheless a general (understandable, and probably justifiable) perception that particles in injections do represent a significant health hazard. At the very least, it can be said that a lack of particles conveys a highly desirable image of a clean, 'quality' product, indicative of high manufacturing standards. It is also worth recalling that environmental organisms are most commonly not to be found floating freely in the air, but are usually to be found associated with (or 'rafting on') inanimate particles. It is thus not unreasonable to postulate that the presence of particles implies the potential presence of micro-organisms.

Visual inspection is a fallible process, relying as it must on subjective, hardly quantifiable judgements under conditions which are difficult to standardise. Not only is it of doubtful value, it is also a dreary, time-consuming job that most workers would wish to avoid. It is not surprising, therefore, that various automated electronic methods have been developed.

For a comparative review of the techniques and equipment available, see Akers (1985).

Sterility testing

The severe statistical limitations of the compendial sterility test have been discussed in the preceding chapter. There are also microbiological limitations, in particular the fact that there is no 'universal' growth medium upon or in which all forms of micro-organisms may be expected cheerfully to grow. As generally practised, sterility tests will not detect viruses, protozoa, exacting parasitic bacteria or many thermophilic and psychrophilic bacteria. Furthermore, organisms which have been damaged but not killed by exposure to sub-lethal levels of 'sterilisation', may not show up in the standard sterility test, as they may require conditions for growth, in terms of nutrients, temperature and time which the test does not provide.

Despite these acknowledged limitations, the test continues to be performed, even by those who would accept that it has little real significance in terms of the quality of the product. This would appear to be due largely to regulatory requirements, and to a nervous perception of potential legal implications. GMP guidelines appear to accept the limitations by declaring, for example, that 'The sterility test applied to the finished product should only be regarded as the last in a series of control measures by which sterility is assured'. The UK Orange Guide amplifies this very point by adding 'Compliance with the test does not guarantee sterility of the whole batch, since sampling may fail to select non-sterile containers, and the culture methods used have limits to their sensitivity.' The EC 'Sterile Annex' (revised 1996) considers that samples taken for sterility testing should be 'representative of the whole batch, but should in particular include samples taken from parts of the batch considered to be most at risk of contamination'. Examples given are of (a) samples taken from the beginning and the end of an aseptic run, and 'after any significant intervention' and (b) samples from the 'potentially coolest part of the load' in a heat sterilisation.

There will be those who would consider that it would be difficult to encompass these requirements within the limitations of the 20-unit sample that is usually taken, and they would be right. Akers (1985) has considered alternative statistical sampling methods.

Leaks and leak testing

In the context of this chapter, a leak may be defined as:

> Any break or interruption in the physical structure of a container and/or its seal that would permit the egress of its contents or the ingress of any substance, article or material or contaminant, living or non-living.

The Parenteral Society's Technical Monograph No. 3, 'The prevention and detection of leaks in ampoules, vials and other parenteral containers' (Parenteral Society, 1992) rightly lays stress on the primary importance of *preventing* the formation of leaks.

The two main causes of leaks in ampoules are cracks in the glass and faulty sealing. Mechanical cracks can be caused by collision or abrasion of ampoules, one with another, or with or against other objects, during or after filling. In addition, thermal cracks can be caused in the glass through rapid cooling from higher temperatures, for example by contact of hot glass with cold machine parts. Such thermal cracks may develop immediately, or regions of stress may be induced which develop into cracks later. Crack-inducing stresses can be caused during the original ampoule forming operation, or during sterile product manufacture, when heat sealing, ceramic printing and heat sterilising. Faulty ampoule seals can arise from maladjustment or faulty setting of ampoule filling and sealing machines.

Methods aiding prevention are obvious: at all stages from the original forming of the ampoules to the dispatch of the finished product, careful steps should be taken to prevent impact and attrition of glass against glass, or with or against any other objects. Empty and filled ampoules awaiting further processing should be assembled neatly on their bases, and not loaded haphazardly in basket-loads. To prevent thermal stress cracks, contact must be avoided between hot glass and cold metal. Careful attention is necessary to machine adjustment, including flame settings, to avoid faulty sealing. With proper setting, draw sealing is less likely to give rise to faulty seals than tip sealing.

There are a number of 'traditional' methods for leak testing ampoules. They include various pressure/vacuum tests such as the common dye intrusion (or 'dye bath') test, liquid loss and 'blotting paper' tests. These, and other techniques have been (and are) used, and they all have their limitations, even hazards; for example that of dye solution entering an ampoule through a leak and then escaping subsequent detection.

Although not entirely free of problems and limitations, automated high voltage detection methods are more sensitive, and are not subject to the limitation of 'traditional' methods such as fallibility of human inspectors and hazards of undetected dye intrusion. They also have the further advantage that they can detect points of weakness, such as areas of thin glass, which at the time of testing are potential, if not actual, leaks.

With glass vials, again, the major stress should be upon prevention, not merely detection of leaks. Measures to prevent mechanical and thermal stresses and cracks are the same as for ampoules. To minimise leaks arising from dimensional, physical and chemical inadequacies or incompatibilities, it is crucial that detailed and comprehensive specifications are agreed with suppliers of both vials and closures, and that compliance with specification is checked on all incoming deliveries.

In contrast with a fairly general acceptance of the need for 100% leak testing of glass ampoule products, a brief survey carried out in 1991/2 indicated that 100% leak testing of glass vial products was the exception, rather than the rule. This is clearly unsatisfactory from a patient safety point of view, unless it can be shown that there is little if any possibility of leaks in filled and sealed glass vials, which does not appear to be the case. Pressure/vacuum tests can be applied to glass vial products, with the same limitations and problems as for ampoules. However, based on the experience of the relatively few manufacturers of glass vial products who have tried the technique, it seems that automated high voltage detection is applicable to glass vial products. Such trials that have been conducted have shown that leaks do occur in production batches of filled glass vials, both in the vial body and in the closure system.

Leaks in large volume parenteral (LVP) plastics containers can be caused by:

- Faults in the welding or sealing of the container when it is fabricated from the plastics sheet.
- Inadequate 'fit', or sealing, of components (tubes, closures, ports) attached to the bag.
- Mechanical damage caused by contact with sharp or abrasive surfaces during filling, sterilisation and subsequent handling.
- Pinholes or splits occurring during bag printing.

The standard method of checking for leaks in LVPs is 100% visual inspection, perhaps with a gentle manual squeeze, after sterilisation, to check for abnormal quantities of liquid between the bag and its outer overwrap. Some manufacturers apply a light, controlled mechanical pressure via a bar or plate, immediately before the units are examined. As ever, there are limitations in the efficacy of the human visual checking machine.

Leaks in plastics blow-fill-seal (BFS) containers are most commonly caused by:

- Imperfect heat seals.
- Damage inflicted by the scrap (or flash) removing cropper.
- Careless handling.

Leak test methods which can be used include dye bath pressure/vacuum tests, vacuum/'blotting paper' test, and mechanical pressure plus visual examination. Such work that has been carried out to date suggests that automated high voltage detection methods are applicable to filled BFS containers, and appear to be more sensitive than the traditional methods.

Pre-filled syringes and cartridges would clearly seem to represent a serious patient hazard if they have leaks. Somewhat disturbingly, however, it does appear there is virtually no information available on the incidence and causes of leaks, nor on suitable methods of leak detection. This is clearly an area in need of serious attention.

Pyrogen, or endotoxin, testing

A literal translation of the term 'pyrogen' (derived from the Greek) is 'fire generating'. However, the reaction in humans to injection of pyrogens can include chill, shivering, vasoconstriction, dilation of pupils, respiratory depression, hypertension, nausea and pains in joints and head, in addition to (or as a result of) the 'fire', or rapid increase in body temperature, which the term suggests. It is reasonable to assume that a patient receiving an injection is, in most cases, already ill. This additional stress to the system cannot be considered as anything less than highly undesirable.

Some substances, including some active drug substances (or APIs, e.g. some steroids) and some viruses are pyrogenic *per se*, but in terms of sterile products manufacturing on an industrial scale, the most significant pyrogen is the bacterial endotoxin which is derived from the outer cell wall of certain Gram-negative bacteria. This substance is a complex, high molecular weight lipopolysaccharide, soluble in water and relatively heat-stable. It can withstand autoclaving, and can pass through the 0.2 μm pores in the filters commonly used for sterilisation by filtration. Destruction, or removal, of micro-organisms will not necessarily destroy pyrogenic endotoxin. There is thus another very good reason for keeping bacterial contamination at the lowest possible level at all stages in the manufacturing process, in addition to ensuring the lowest possible challenge to the sterilisation procedure. It is to reduce the chance of the presence of endotoxins. Prevention is, as ever, far better than later detection.

Pyrogenic contamination can arise at any stage in the manufacturing process. It may be present in starting materials, most notably in the water used to make solutions, hence the importance of good quality water, produced by well designed and monitored systems. It can be present on the surfaces of containers. It is unlikely to be present on glass containers, as manufactured, in view of the temperatures at which glass is blown or moulded, but it can be introduced by washing and rinsing glass containers with water which is not pyrogen-free. It can be removed from glass containers by exposure to temperatures of 250°C or above, in for example a sterilising and depyrogenating tunnel. Once present in a solution, it is difficult if not impossible to remove. The answer is to not let it develop in the first place.

The traditional test for the detection of pyrogenic substances relies on the fact that the febrile response of rabbits resembles that of humans. The solution under test is injected into rabbits, and the rise, if any, in their rectal temperatures measured over the period of the test. The rabbit test has a number of disadvantages: it is a limit, rather than a quantitative test, it is time-consuming and subject to the variability and vagaries inherent in all biological test methods, and it cannot be used for solutions of substances which themselves prompt or inhibit a pyrogenic response.

A method which overcomes these problems, which can be used for quantitative determinations, and is more sensitive at low endotoxin levels is based on a discovery that a lysate of the amoebocytes from the blood of the so-called horseshoe crab (*Limulus polyphemus*, found mainly along the north-eastern seaboard of the American continent), in contact with bacterial endotoxin shows turbidity, or undergoes clotting (gelation). This is the limulus amoebocyte lysate, or LAL, test. LAL test kits are widely available from commercial suppliers. Although, at its most simple, the turbidity/gelling end-point is determined visually, the method has been refined to permit more precise turbidimetric, calorimetric, or nephelometric determinations (see Akers, 1985).

Parametric release

The concept (or, it would be more correct to say, the terminology) of 'parametric release' is another fairly recent development. 'Release' refers to approving a batch of product for distribution and sale, or for further processing – and surely this is always done (or should be done) after the consideration of a number of relevant parameters? (See 'The Qualified Person: Requirements', in Chapter 11.)

The terminology emerged in the early to mid-80s and originally was related solely to the sterility (or otherwise) of terminally heat-sterilised products. That is, it did not originally bear upon other release criteria, or on the release of any other products, sterile or otherwise.

One of the first (if not *the* first) 'official' publications on this subject is the FDA's 'Compliance Policy Guide' on 'Parametric release – terminally sterilised drug products'. This guide provides a definition as follows:

> Parametric Release is defined as a sterility release procedure based upon effective control, monitoring and documentation of a validated sterilisation process cycle, *in lieu of* [author's emphasis] release based upon end-product sterility testing.

If 'sterility release' may be based on 'effective control . . .' in place of a sterility test result, then the inverse corollary is surely implied that if a sterility test *has* been passed, then 'effective control, monitoring and documentation of validated sterilisation process' is not necessary – which is contrary to all the principles of quality assurance in the manufacture of sterile products, and is thus presumably not what the FDA really meant.

This FDA guideline then goes on to list the actions which must be taken (and documented) as preconditions for parametric release. In brief, they are given as:

1. Validation of the cycle to achieve a reduction of the known microbial bioburden to 10^0 [unity], with a minimum safety factor of an additional six logarithm reduction. (Validation studies to include heat distribution, heat penetration, bioburden, and cycle lethality studies.)
2. Validation of integrity of container/closure.

3.   Pre-sterilisation bioburden testing on each lot, pre-sterilisation, and checking comparative resistance of any spore formers found.
4.   Inclusion of chemical or biological indicators in each truckload.

Some would ask, is this not, with the possible exception of the inclusion of biological indicators in *every* load, a list of things which should be done anyway, whether the lot is to be sterility tested or not?

This form of 'parametric release' provides an indication of the type and range of process parameters which need to be considered before a product may reasonably be released without testing the end product for a specific quality characteristic. In this particular instance a notably unreliable test procedure (the sterility test) may be abandoned, with at least a theoretical possibility of regulatory approval, in favour of a rigorous concentration of effort on actions that will provide a significantly higher level of assurance of sterility. An excellent notion, in this context, and one which has been adopted (with official approval) by a few manufacturers of sterile products. But they are surprisingly few. The reason for this probably lies in a not unfounded fear that, should action be taken for damages in the case of an alleged sterility failure, learned judges will probably consider 'passed pharmacopoeial sterility test' a better defence than technical and statistical arguments that they will not understand.

References

Akers M (1985). Particulate matter testing; Pyrogen testing; Sterility testing. In: *Parenteral Quality Control*. New York: Marcel Dekker.

AS 2013 (1977). *Clean Room Garments*. North Sydney: Standards Association of Australia.

AS 2014 (1977). *Code of Practice for Clean Room Garments*. North Sydney: Standards Association of Australia.

ASTM (1968). *Sizing and counting particulate contamination in and on clean room garments*. ASTM F51–68. American Society for Testing Materials.

Barnett M I (1994). Particulate contamination. In: Lund W (ed.), *The Pharmaceutical Codex: Principles and practice of pharmaceutics,* 12th edn. London: Pharmaceutical Press.

DoH (1981). *Guide to Good Manufacturing Practice for Sterile Medical Devices and Surgical Products*. London: Department of Health. (Available from HMSO.)

DoH (1990). *Guidance on Ethylene oxide sterilisation*. London: Department of Health. (Available from HMSO.)

EC (1992). *The Rules Governing Medicinal Products in the European Community, Vol. IV: Good Manufacturing Practice for Medicinal Products*. Luxembourg: Commission of the European Communities. Available from The Office for Official Publications of the European Communities, Luxembourg. Also available from The Stationery Office (HMSO), London, and The EC Information Service, Washington, USA. Also stated *verbatim* with guidance on the detailed interpretation of these rules in MCA, 1997. (Referred to as the EC GMP Guide.)

EC (1996). *Annex 1, Manufacture of Sterile Medicinal Products*. Revised July 1996. Luxembourg: Commission of the European Communities. Reproduced in MCA (1997).

IoB, RPSGB, RSC (1998). Code of Practice for Qualified Persons (1998). Appendix to *Joint Register of Qualified Persons*. London: Institute of Biology, Royal Pharmaceutical Society of Great Britain, and Royal Society of Chemistry.

ISPE (1999). *Baseline Pharmaceutical Engineering Guide, Vol. 3: Sterile manufacturing facilities*. The Hague: ISPE.

MCA (1997). *Rules and Guidance for Pharmaceutical Manufacturers and Distributors*. London: Medicines Control Agency. Available from The Stationery Office (HMSO), London.

Parenteral Society (1989). *Environmental Contamination Control Practice*. Technical Monograph No.2. Swindon: Parenteral Society.

Parenteral Society (1992). *Prevention and Detection of Leaks in Ampoules, Vials and other Parenteral Containers*. Technical Monograph No.3. Swindon: Parenteral Society.

Russell M P, Goldsmith J A, Phillips I (1984). Some factors affecting the efficiency of settle plates. *J Hosp Infect* 5, 189–199.

Sharp J, ed. (1983). *Guide to Good Pharmaceutical Manufacturing Practice*, 3rd edn. London: HMSO. Also stated *verbatim* with guidance on the detailed interpretation of these rules in MCA, 1997. (Referred to as the UK Orange Guide.)

Sharp J (1991). Particulate contamination of injections. In: Sharp J, *Good Manufacturing Practice – Philosophy and Applications*. Illinois: Interpharm Press.

US FDA (1987). *Guideline on Sterile Drug Products Produced by Aseptic Processing*. Rockville, MD: Center for Drugs and Biologics and Office of Regulatory Affairs, Food and Drug Administration.

US FDA (1990). *Code of Federal Regulations, Vol. 21, Ch. 1, Part 210,* Current good manufacturing practice in manufacturing, processing, packaging or holding of drugs, general; *CFR Vol. 21, Ch. 1, Part 211,* Current good manufacturing practice for finished pharmaceuticals; *CFR Vol. 21, Ch. 1, Part 820,* Good manufacturing practice for medical devices (revised 1995). US Food & Drug Administration. (Collectively referred to as the US CGMPs.)

Walker R (1997). Application of the new sterile products annex – a personal view. *Ind Pharm* Issue 2 (August 1997).

Whyte W (1996). In support of settle plates. *J Pharm Sci Technol* 50 (4), 201.

Whyte W, Niven L (1986). Airborne bacterial sampling: the effect of dehydration and sampling time. *J Parenter Sci Technol* 40, 182.

21

Non-sterile manufacture and packaging

The bourgeoisie in the long run only changed the form of the pack
Leon Trotsky, *History of the Russian Revolution*, Vol. 3, Ch. 1, 1933

The length of the previous chapter on sterile manufacture is a reflection of the range of *additional* quality assurance/good manufacturing practice (QA/GMP) requirements specific to the manufacture of sterile products. In contrast, this chapter covering some other major manufacturing operations, will be relatively short. This is not to suggest that quality considerations are not important in these other areas. It is merely that these issues are largely covered by more general QA/GMP considerations, and because any special or additional requirements are, in comparison with sterile products manufacture, relatively few.

Solid dose manufacture (tablets and capsules)

Contamination

Although any significant level of microbial contamination can be a potential health hazard, reports of serious health hazards as a result of viable organisms in solid dosage forms have been rare, although there have been a few. The main potential contamination hazard is more likely to be cross-contamination by dusts from the products themselves and/or from the materials used in them. Thus, the prevention of airborne contamination of one product by another is a major concern. The question of protection of operators from the physical and physiological effects of the powders, if inhaled/ingested, also arises. Proper installation of air control and extraction systems is therefore crucial. It should go without saying that it is worse than useless to install a dust extraction system which does no more than extract dust at one point in need of protection, only to deposit it at another. Careful consideration needs to be given to the siting of extraction outlets. Filters should be installed within the system to retain dust, rather than to allow it to deposit into another product or area, or to be vented to the general environment. Particularly care is necessary to contain any dust loosened when such filters are removed or replaced.

Unless operated as a closed system, mixing, sifting and blending equipment should be fitted with dust extraction.

Extraction ducting, over say a powder mixer, should be designed so that when the extraction fan is switched off, any powder remaining in the ducting does not fall back into the product. The so-called 'flexible elephant trunk' has a significantly greater capacity for internal dust retention than internally smooth, inflexible ducting.

Control in manufacture

In powder mixing and granulating, critical operating parameters as determined in the product development phase, such as time, temperature, power and rotation speed should be specified in batch manufacturing instructions, monitored during the process, and recorded in the batch records.

Filter bags fitted to fluid bed dryers should not be used for different products without being thoroughly washed between use. In the manufacture of highly potent, or sensitising, products, bags specific to one product only should be used. Such bags should be individually identifiable, and their use recorded. Air entering fluid bed dryers should be filtered, and care is necessary to prevent the air leaving them causing cross-contamination.

Solutions for use in granulating and coating should preferably be prepared freshly, batch-wise. To prepare stock solutions for use in a number of different product batches, over an extended time period, is to risk both chemical and microbial contamination.

Tablet compressing machines should be operated under effective dust control systems, and spaced one from another so as to minimise the possibility of product mix-up. Unless the machines have their own enclosed internal air controlled environment, each machine should be placed in a separate room or cubicle. Calibrated weighing equipment, of suitable accuracy, precision and sensitivity to detect out-of-limits tablets, should be available for in-process tablet weight checks, the results of which should form part of the batch manufacturing record. Tablets removed from a machine for weight- and other in-process checks should not be returned to the bulk batch. The minimal savings are not worth the potential mix-up hazard.

Other in-process controls include periodic checks on tablet hardness, thickness, friability and disintegration. The frequency at which all these should be performed needs to be specified in the batch manufacturing instructions, together with an indication of the method(s) to be employed (e.g. reference to SOPs), and the compliance standards for each test. Results of all in-process tests need to be recorded, and retained as part of the batch manufacturing record.

Punches and dyes must be maintained in good condition, and regularly examined for wear and damage. A chipped punch could well mean a fragment of metal in a tablet. Indeed, special care is necessary to protect against contamination of solid dose forms by fragments of metal, glass or wood. In addition to tablet punches and dyes, screens and sieves should be examined for wear or damage before and after each use. The use of metal detectors on the output of each compressing machine is strongly to be recommended, and the use of glass equipment avoided.

When tablets are coated, the air supplied to the equipment should be filtered. Care is necessary to ensure that air leaving the equipment, perhaps carrying some of the coating material or even traces of the tablet core, cannot cross-contaminate other products.

Similar precautions, as for tablet compression, are necessary in the filling of 'hard' gelatin capsules, to avoid contamination and mix-up. The empty capsule shells should be treated and controlled as for any other starting materials. That is, they should on receipt be awarded lot numbers, tested against a formal test specification, and released and issued to Production in the same manner as for any other starting material. They should be stored so as to prevent drying out, or the effects of moisture. Their use should be recorded on the batch manufacturing record.

Where tablets and capsules are printed, polished and inspected special care must be taken to avoid mix-up. Any printing ink used must also be regarded as a starting material and handled and controlled accordingly, with its use recorded on the batch manufacturing record.

Controlled low levels of humidity may be necessary in some solid form manufacturing areas; e.g. effervescent tablet manufacture, gelatin shell capsule filling.

Liquids, creams and ointments (non-sterile)

Many products of this type are susceptible to microbial contamination and growth. This can lead to product spoilage/breakdown (fermentation of liquids, breakdown of emulsions/creams) and, worse, patient infection (by liquids taken orally, creams applied to broken skin). Some kind of controlled environmental air supply may therefore be necessary, although it may well be of a lower level than that required for sterile products. Creams for application to the unbroken skin surface are also often manufactured to a 'low microbial count' (if not sterile) standard. This can be crucial for patient-protection where the active ingredients (e.g. some steroids) of some creams for application to skin surfaces are known to inhibit the immune response, and thus render the patient particularly susceptible to infection by organisms in the cream. A 'clean', even if not precisely defined, manufacturing environment, preferably combined with 'closed' systems of manufacture, with minimum product exposure and careful cleaning and disinfection of product contact surfaces of equipment is thus often required.

Tanks, containers, pipework and pumps should be designed and installed so that they may be easily cleaned, and as necessary, sterilised. Equipment and pipe installations should be as free as possible from 'dead-legs' and other sites where liquids and residues can accumulate and become the cause of cross-contamination, and/or vehicles of microbial infection. Piping systems used to transfer product or materials (e.g. from bulk manufacture to the packaging line) should be installed and marked so as to minimise the possibility of mix-up through cross-linkage of pipes.

Water used for the manufacture of liquids, creams and ointments should be of at least potable quality, and monitored to ensure a low microbial count. Use of low-count purified water is to be preferred.

Packaging

The packaging operation has tended, at least in the past, to be regarded as a relatively insignificant, Cinderella-like appendage to the main business of production. Such an attitude could hardly be more misguided. A pharmaceutical product is not to be regarded as, say, 50 tablets, 15 g of ointment or 100 ml of liquid, but as a form that is *contained within its package*. The final product is the dosage-form/package unit. The pack, if it is properly designed, and used as specified, contributes important quality features to the product. If it is not properly designed and selected, or if packaging materials are used which are not as specified, the pack can significantly, perhaps seriously, degrade product quality. Furthermore, the packaging operation offers a late (possibly last) opportunity to spot if anything is amiss. That is, it does if all those involved are alert, vigilant and aware. Unfortunately, it also provides a late opportunity to negate all the good quality-preserving work that has gone before.

It is generally considered that there are two main forms, or stages, of packaging:

- *Primary packaging.* That is, filling the product into the package which will immediately surround it, and with which it comes into direct contact. That is, the container itself and its cap, closure, or other seal. These are the primary packaging materials.
- *Secondary packaging.* Often a primary pack is placed in a carton, a box, or a tray, which in turn may be film-wrapped, shrink-wrapped or foil wrapped. Sometimes these secondary packs are further wrapped or packed together (usually in 10s or dozens) using film- or shrink-wrapping or larger cartons or boxes ('outers'). All this is secondary packaging, and the materials used are secondary packaging materials.

(Sometimes primary packaging is called 'immediate packaging', and secondary packaging is referred to as 'outer packaging'.)

With high-speed automatic (or semi-automatic) packaging operations, secondary packaging often follows on directly from primary packaging, without a break, on the same packaging line. The important difference is that, whereas primary packaging materials come into direct contact with the product, secondary packaging materials do not.

Printed packaging material

Another important form of packaging material is printed packaging material. Again, printed packaging materials can be either primary (for example, printed tubes, ampoules or plastic bottles) or secondary (e.g. printed cartons or outers), and the term is usually taken to include labels, and any leaflets which may be included with the product.

As far as the quality of pharmaceutical products is concerned, careful control and use of printed packaging materials is perhaps the most important single factor in packaging operations.

The purpose, or the main functions, of a package could be summarised as follows:

1. To *hold*, or contain, a defined quantity of the product.
2. To *protect* the product from damage, contamination and deterioration.
3. To *identify* the product. (What it is, its batch number, who manufactured it, and so on.)
4. To *indicate* required storage conditions, expiration date or shelf-life.
5. To *instruct* by giving directions for use, dosage, frequency of dose and so on.
6. To *warn* – of any hazards in use or abuse, and give information on side-effects, etc.
7. To *aid* the patient by presenting the product in a form that is easy to use, and if the product is a medicine, to help in ensuring that patients take their medicines as, when and how they should.

Thus, an important function of a package is to give information. This is not *just* a 'good idea', although it *is* a good idea. Particularly where medicines are concerned, much of the information (product identity, batch number, manufacturer, expiry date, storage conditions, etc.) is also required by Law.

Protective packaging

One of the purposes of a package, noted above, is to protect the product inside it. The question thus arises: 'Protect from what?'

Products can be spoiled (and as a possible consequence lose activity, or even become dangerous) through:

- *Mechanical damage.* Shaking, jarring, dropping or other impact can for example break up tablets or capsules within a container, or damage a device, or break or crack a container allowing the product to leak out, or contamination to enter.
- *Heat.* A number of products will break down or deteriorate at raised temperatures. Although protection against heat is largely a matter of storage, the package can help.

- *Light.* A number of products are sensitive to light, which can cause break down and/or discoloration. Opaque, or coloured glass, containers can help protect against this.
- *Humidity.* Moisture can severely damage products. The package must provide protection against the product getting damp.
- *Air.* Exposure to air leads to possible oxidation of product.
- *Contamination.* Exposure to external physical, chemical or microbial contamination sources.
- *Package material or design.* The package itself can also harm a product, if it is a wrong or badly designed pack, or made of inappropriate materials. Obviously the product must not be able to leak, or escape from the package. Packages must also be designed to avoid damage to the product through abrasion caused by vibration in transit. Some materials (for example, many plastics) can absorb substances from the product or allow them to pass through. There is also the possibility that some materials, if used to make containers, can release substances (and what is more, dangerous or poisonous substances) into the product. Some materials used in making containers can react chemically with certain products.

So, any material that has any of the following properties cannot be used to make primary packaging containers and closures:

- Allows the product to seep or leak through it.
- Allows substances (including gases/vapours) to pass through it.
- Releases substances into the product.
- Reacts with the product.
- Adsorbs or absorbs substances from the product.

All these problems have to be resolved by those responsible for the original design and development of the product and its pack, but it is still very important that all possible steps are taken to ensure that in routine packaging operations, only the specified packaging materials, of confirmed specified quality are, in fact, used. The first step is to ensure that each delivery of packaging material, particularly primary and printed material, is sampled and tested against a formal specification before release for use.

What is the reason for secondary packaging, in addition to primary packaging? There are a number of possible reasons and requirements:

1. *Protection of the product.* Secondary packaging can provide an extra layer of protection. A carton, for example, can help prevent breaking of glass or crushing of tubes. It can also provide additional protection from light.
2. *Product identification.* Again, a carton or a box can make available more space for printing the name, the strength, the quantity, batch number and description of the product, plus its manufacturing information and expiry date.

3. *Instructions and information.* A carton or box (printed or labelled) provides the opportunity to print more essential information and instructions for use. This might not be possible on a very small primary pack.

4. *Incorporation of other items.* It is often difficult to include any 'extras' if a primary pack is supplied just on its own. Secondary packs provide the opportunity to do this, for example when a bottle is placed inside a carton. These 'extras' are of two main types:

   (a) *Dosing aids or measures.* For example droppers, applicators, graduated spoons or small plastic measures.
   (b) *Leaflets* which give information about the product and how it should be used.

5. *Security.* A secondary pack can provide an extra level of security against tampering. It can make the primary pack more difficult to get at, or to get at without leaving evidence of having done so. Flaps of cartons or boxes, for example, can be stuck down, or taped over.

6. *Ease of handling.* Orders are often for multiples of 10, rather than single packs. Storage, handling, 'order picking', despatch, loading and unloading are all made easier if primary packs are packed in, say 10s.

7. *Appearance.* Very often a neat secondary pack improves and preserves the appearance of the pack. This may not seem to be as important as some of the other reasons for secondary packaging, but it can have important consequences for acceptability by the consumer, confidence in the product and, indeed, for the company's overall 'image'.

The packaging operation and environment

Thus, secondary packaging can be almost as important as primary packaging. In fact, although the two stages of a packaging operation are often spoken of as if they were quite different, they are often carried out in one continuous operation on a high-speed packaging line. These are much faster and more efficient than simple hand methods, but because things are happening so quickly, it does mean that extra care is necessary to prevent packaging errors, and that is particularly true where printed materials are concerned.

A very important safety factor (in terms both of the safety of the product and of the operators) is the design, layout, maintenance and spatial segregation of packaging equipment and facilities generally.

In addition to the normal premises/environmental requirements (the level of which will depend upon the nature of the product and its degree of exposure), a crucial requirement in the design and layout of packaging rooms or areas is sufficient *space* – space to allow effective separation/segregation of different packaging lines or stations.

Line clearance checks

The biggest cause of contamination or mix-up in the packaging operation are 'left-overs' (product, materials, labels) from a previous batch. It seems very obvious, but it has happened all too often.

Contamination from previously packaged product can occur through:

- Improper cleaning of vessels, hoppers, or other containers of bulk products.
- Unclean (or even 'switched') pipelines.
- Tablets, capsules or pills left behind in hoppers, or in electronic, disc, or slat counters.

Similar, and even worse, hazards can occur through unused packaging materials left on the line, or in label dispensers.

To guard against these problems, before any packaging operation begins, checks should be made to ensure that the work area, line, and equipment are clean and clear of any product, product residues, materials, labels or documents left over, or not required for the packaging run about to begin. This should not be a casual 'once-over' but a thorough and specific check carried out in accordance with written instructions, item by item. These checks should be carried out by people authorised and instructed to do so, who should record on the written instruction (with signature or initials) that each item has, in fact, been checked. The completed checklist should form part of the batch packaging documentation. It may all seem relatively simple, but it would seem that in practice it is not. Over the years, by far the biggest number of recalls of medicinal and similar products have been due to errors in packaging, particularly labelling errors, and there should be no need to emphasise how dangerous a wrongly labelled medicine can be.

As ever, the most important single operational factor is the training and attitude of the people performing the packaging operations. They should not be allowed to think of their work as inferior or of little importance, but be encouraged to take pride in it, and in the contribution they can make to product quality, and consequently patient safety. Operators should be made aware that prevention of packaging errors requires the constant care and attention of all the people working on the packaging line. That is, the operators and checkers and their supervisors. No one should be conditioned to think that quality is someone else's problem or responsibility. It is the responsibility of everyone involved.

The sort of faults which can be detected by visual inspection, and which packaging operators should be trained to constantly look out for include:

- Wrong labels or other printed materials.
- Damaged or torn labels.
- Badly applied labels (crooked or not fully adherent).
- Other damaged or incorrect packaging materials.

- Poor print quality.
- Incorrect or poor quality over-printing.
- Incorrect quantity of product filled.
- Contamination of product.
- Leaking or spilling of product.
- Failure of mechanical and electronic devices such as on-line printers, code readers, missing label detectors, and automatic weight checkers.

Part Seven

Validation

22

Validation: concepts, principles and terminology

*A wealth of corroborative detail, intended to give an air of verisimilitude
to an otherwise bald and unconvincing narrative*

W S Gilbert, *The Mikado*, 1885

Validation has been a dominant, and controversial, topic of discussion over the last twenty years or so, with some of its more fervent devotees seeming almost to have elevated the subject to a mystical/religious status.

There is, in fact, nothing especially new about the concept, or the application, of validation. The first appearance of the word in written English dates from 1648. The general concept (that is, of proving or showing that some thing, statement, argument or activity is sound and well-grounded) is much older. Even the technological application of the concept is hardly new. Since the dawn of technological history, no honest craftsman has made implements, weapons, boats, bridges, machines or dwellings without a belief (based on practical experience) that his work will achieve the desired and intended results. Nor is the application of the concept in the field of *pharmaceutical* technology exactly new. A report of the Society of Apothecaries of London, published in 1832, refers to a 'committee of enquiry' which met every Friday to confirm the quality of raw materials delivered during the previous week. This sounds very much like an early example of materials supply validation. Rather nearer to the present time, heat distribution and heat penetration studies on steam sterilisers, and aseptic 'media fills' (all topics which tend to loom large in current discussions on validation) have been practised in the pharmaceutical industry for over 50 years. (For example, a paper on the use of media fills to validate an aseptic filling process was published in 1948.)

The background to validation

It has been stated that pharmaceutical process validation was first introduced in the USA in the mid 1970s. However, the industry had been practising some forms of validation before then, and in 1971 the first edition of the UK Orange Guide stated:

> Procedures should undergo a regular critical appraisal to ensure that they are, and remain, capable of achieving the results they are intended to achieve.

This, surely, is a statement about validation.

However, in the mid-70s there was a great surge of interest in the concept, often without adequate rational attention being paid to what it all meant. At the time there was a distinct air of 'Validation is a good idea. What is it?' and this precipitated an abundance of wordy definitions, which in many instances, far from clarifying, only served to confuse the issue.

Some writers have attributed the 'invention' of validation to two, at the time, senior FDA officials (E Beyers and B Loftus, who shortly after resigned from FDA to form their own consultancies) on 11 October 1974. Thereafter, the subject was much hyped, to the great joy of conference organisers offering 'intensive seminars', at inflated prices, on 'How to comply with the FDA validation requirements'.

In the generally well-balanced FDA's *Guideline on General Principles of Process Validation* (US FDA, 1987) validation is defined as:

> Establishing documented evidence which provides a high degree of assurance that a specific process will consistently produce a product meeting its predetermined specifications and quality attributes.

The point is made, but not perhaps with the utmost clarity or lack of ambiguity. The early stress placed upon 'documented' should be noted. One of the simplest and best definitions comes from E Fry (at the time a senior official of FDA) who in 1982 at a Pharmaceutical Inspection Convention in Dublin said:

> To prove that a process works is, in a nutshell, what we mean by the verb to validate.

The 1983 edition of the UK Orange Guide (Sharp, 1983), perhaps more formally and comprehensively, defines validation as:

> The action of proving that any material, process, procedure, activity, equipment or mechanism used in manufacture or control, can, will and does achieve the desired and intended result.

The EC GMP Guide (EC, 1992) offers the following definition:

> Validation: Action of proving, in accordance with the principles of Good Manufacturing Practice, that any procedure, process, equipment, material, activity or system actually leads to the expected results (see also qualification).

'Qualification' is defined in this EC Guide as: 'Action of proving that any equipment works correctly and actually leads to the expected results. The word 'validation' is sometimes widened to incorporate the concept of qualification'. More will be said about 'qualification' later in this chapter.

Validation then is the action of proving (and in the more formal context, documenting the proof) that something 'works'. One way of looking at the increasing emphasis on validation is as a stage in the general trend away from regarding end-product testing as the significant determinant of product quality, and it is interesting to note a comment in the FDA validation guideline that:

> Successfully validating a process may reduce the dependence upon intensive in-process and finished product testing. It should be noted that in most all cases, end-product testing plays a major role in assuring that quality assurance goals are met; i.e. validation and end-product testing are not mutually exclusive.

An expression of a well-balanced view, to be contrasted with those which take an extreme either/or position.

The passage from the 1971 UK Orange Guide quoted earlier was perhaps the first statement 'about' validation to appear in an official document, although the word itself is not mentioned in that text. In 1976, the FDA issued proposed CGMP revisions which did use the term, in four different contexts – 'Supplier test results', 'Sterilization processes', 'Manufacturing processes' and 'Computer software'. These references remained in place in the text of the revised US CGMPs when they were published in 1979 [21 CFR, Part 211, Sec. 211.84 (d) (2), Sec. 211.113 (b), Sec. 211.110 (a), and Sec. 211.68, respectively]. These are all quite brief and general statements, and give little hint of the torrent of verbiage that was to follow from a variety of sources.

In 1983, the FDA published its draft guideline on general principles of process validation and, after much discussion, the final version was published (US FDA, 1987). In addition, the FDA's *Guideline on Sterile Drug Products Produced by Aseptic Processing* (June 1987) contains useful guidance on the validation of this type of process. There is an FDA *Guide to Inspection of Computerised Systems in Drug Processing*, issued as reference material for investigators, which contains relatively brief sections on hardware and on software validation. The FDA have also published a *Guide to Inspections of Validation of Cleaning Processes* (July 1993). The FDA *Guide to Inspections of Pharmaceutical Quality Control Laboratories* (July 1993) contains three short paragraphs on 'Methods validation', and their *Guide to Inspections of Microbiological Pharmaceutical Quality Control Laboratories* (July 1993) also contains a short section on 'Methodology and validation of test procedures'. The FDA have also issued a range of guidelines directed at the validation of a range of non-sterile manufacturing processes, and the general regulatory trend worldwide (either by explicit statement or by implication) is to expect at least some level of validation of many types of process, non-sterile as well as sterile.

In addition to the definition quoted above, the 1983 edition of the UK Orange Guide contains four paragraphs (5.9–5.12) on validation, noting that validation should be carried out when any new process, equipment or material is brought into use, or whenever there are any significant changes in materials, procedures or equipment. It adds that 'the extent and degree of the work will depend on the nature and complexity of the product and process'.

The EC GMP Guide (1992) also contains four paragraphs on validation which bear a close resemblance to the four which appeared in the 1983 UK Orange Guide. These are as follows:

> 5.21 Validation studies should reinforce Good Manufacturing Practice and be conducted in accordance with defined procedures. Results and conclusions should be recorded.
>
> 5.22 When any new manufacturing formula or method of preparation is adopted, steps should be taken to demonstrate its suitability for routine processing. The defined process, using the materials and equipment specified, should be shown to yield a product consistently of the required quality.
>
> 5.23 Significant amendments to the manufacturing process, including any change in equipment or materials, which may affect product quality and/or the reproducibility of the process should be validated.
>
> 5.24 Processes and procedures should undergo periodic critical re-evaluation to ensure that they remain capable of achieving the intended results.

It is worth noting that 'validation studies should reinforce Good Manufacturing Practice'; compare this with a passage from the EC *Guidelines on the Quality, Safety and Efficacy of Medical Products for Human Use* (The Rules Governing Medicinal Products in the European Community, Vol. III, Office for Official publications of the European Communities, Luxembourg, 1989):

> ... process validation is intended to establish that the proposed manufacturing process is a suitable one and yields consistently a product of the desired quality. While process validation is generally a concept more closely associated with GMP, and therefore falling into the area of inspections, if a non-standard method of manufacture is used, or if certain aspects of the method of manufacture are crucial for product quality, efficacy or safety but cannot necessarily be detected by analytical means, data on process validation may be required in applications for authorisation to place a proprietary medicinal product on the market. Areas mostly concerned are process environment, process equipment and the manufacturing process itself, the latter being the most important one. Thus data may be required to establish e.g. that:
>
> (i) non-standard sterilisation conditions provide an acceptable level of assurance of product sterility, or
>
> (ii) the manufacturing process for a modified release system will only vary to an extent that will still yield a product of the desired quality and not have any effect on product efficacy or safety.

The value of validation

Not the least of the many surprising things about validation is the way in which such large and arcane semantic structures, such mountains of paper and (as some would argue) such unnecessary effort and expense have arisen from such seemingly slight regulatory bases. This probably has something to do with what has been termed by the author the 'industrial/regulatory interactive spiral staircase effect' (Sharp, 1995). This has already been portrayed in Fig. 3.1 where industry makes a technological advance or develops a new concept; regulatory agencies embrace it in new regulations or guidelines; industry moves to comply, and the more advanced companies (encouraged, possibly, by the opportunity for further technical advance or competitive needs) 'go one better'; regulatory agencies respond to this new state-of-the-art by tightening, or introducing new requirements; industry responds accordingly . . . and so on, ever spiralling upwards on a stairway of increasingly demanding standards, until a empyrean state of TTS (total technological sublimity) is attained. Alternatively, the process may be initiated by the Regulators, but the whole process is often further stimulated by writers, speakers, and seminar organisers who purport to explain 'how to meet the new requirements', and all too rarely fail to consider how all this effects the economics of the industry, and what if any is the benefit to patients.

A few questioning voices have been heard. At the 1982 Dublin seminar, to which we have already referred above, Fry 'presented the only real definition that "to validate" has ever needed' (Akers, 1993). Fry (at the time still a senior official of FDA, and in a paper generally in favour of validation, but with a rational approach) commented *inter alia* that 'a magnificent selling job has been done on the concept of validation . . .'; that it 'is beginning to rank high on our list of sacred concepts, right up there with motherhood, the flag and apple pie'; and that 'the validation requirements have resulted in virtually a new industry to be created, of consulting firms who perform validation studies for pharmaceutical manufacturing clients' (Fry, 1982).

At the same seminar, Witschi (1982) considered the extent to which validation is needed, and suggested a differential approach to the amount of validation effort required, based on such factors as potential hazard in use, mode of administration, criticalness of dose-level and value/reliability of in-process and end-product testing.

Sharp (1986) has attacked a number of the more bizarre manifestations of the validation cult, and suggested that 'the need for validation (is) perhaps inversely proportional to the adequacy of product design, raw material control, in-process control, and end product testing to provide assurance of routine product quality.'

Anisfeld (1993) has questioned the cost/benefit advantages of validation. He noted that 'the annual cost in the US is running at just below a billion dollars' and asked '. . . are we seeing less product failures? . . . less testing? . . . no one seems sure'. He stated that there had been no significant decline in product recalls in the 1980s as compared with the 1970s, and wondered 'How come [if as some validation pundits had suggested validation should ultimately give rise to cost-savings] drug prices keep climbing at three times the rate of inflation?' He declared that we need to 'relate our validation work to the needs of patient safety and product quality'. In 1994, Fry (by then President of FDA) argued that 'Every regulatory document . . . such as the [FDA's] *Guideline on Documentation of Sterilization Validation*

[and] the *Cleaning Validation Inspection Guide* . . . adds to the cost of producing drugs. Many regulatory initiatives are quality-related and make good sense – but when these additional cost burdens do nothing discernible to improve quality, the patient ends up paying more for no good reason.'

Akers (1993) also joined the 'challenge [to] some of the elaborate belief structures upon which validation is based', and expressed the views that 'validation is becoming in many ways a negative force within our industry', that 'outside of sterilisation applications it has become mainly a verbal rather than a technical exercise', and that it is 'evolving into a bureaucratic exercise instead of a scientific one'. He considered that 'validation is conceptually quite simple' but that 'the emphasis, terminology and definition has enabled a few individuals to build empires within their firms or create lucrative side businesses'. He noted an 'increasing tendency towards validation by the pound (i.e. pound weight) where the number of protocols written, and the amount of paper contained therein is equated with success' and urged a 'back to basics' approach of simply demonstrating that 'a process works'.

Although dissenting opinions on validation have been expressed within the pharmaceutical industry, there is certainly a reluctance in some quarters to oppose regulatory bodies, particularly the FDA, on this issue.

The regulatory pressure, particularly from the FDA, to validate *in extensio* will not 'go away', and there is a low probability that the more moderate voices will eventually win the day. Furthermore, despite the confusion that has developed around it (see examples given in Sharp, 1986), it need not be doubted that in basic essence the concept of validation is a sound and valuable one.

The extent of validation

Current validation 'hot topics', particularly insofar as regulatory bodies are concerned, are:

- Validation of sterilisation processes.
- Validation of cleaning procedures.
- Computer systems validation.
- Analytical methods validation.

There can be no doubt that the field in which validation is crucially necessary, and is universally acknowledged to be so, is in the manufacture of sterile products. Because of the limitations of the standard sterility test as a means of giving assurance of the sterility of a batch as a whole and the very serious potential hazards of these products if they are *not* sterile, there is an unquestioned need to validate the processes used to obtain and maintain that condition.

Discussion of process validation has indeed tended largely to focus on sterile products. What of other processes, and of other dosage forms? What, for example, about the validation of the processes used to manufacture tablets, capsules, oral liquids, and non-sterile topical creams and ointments? On these topics distinctly less has been said and written, and on the evidence of what *has* been published, one tends to be drawn to conclude that the writers concerned proceed from an uneasy assumption that since validation is undoubtedly a 'good thing' in sterile processing, it must of necessity be applied with the same formal rigour to other manufacturing processes. Perhaps we should reflect that this is not necessarily so.

It might, perhaps, be more reasonable to suggest that the need for validation is inversely proportional to the adequacy of product design, raw material control, in-process control and end-product testing to provide assurance of the quality of routine batch production. None of these things, alone or in combination, can provide the necessary assurance of the success of a sterilisation process, hence the crucial need, in that context, for validation.

In contrast, consider a simple, non-modified release tablet product. Given a well-designed process, and given that in routine production this process is followed:

- Using materials of confirmed quality;
- Applying appropriate in-process tests and controls;
- Assaying granules to determine even distribution of actives;
- Using modern tabletting equipment (with, for example automatic weight control);
- Applying regular checks on tablet weight, hardness, thickness, friability, disintegration, etc.;
- Performing end-product tests which provide independent checks on these latter parameters, and including for example individual tablet assays.

Given that these things are done, might it not be concluded that each production run is self-validating (or self-invalidating, as the case may be)? Furthermore, may not the same sort of thinking be applied to the manufacture of other non-sterile products?

Perhaps the extent of the need for, and the application of, validation should be determined by a consideration of an interaction between two hierarchies: (a) the critical nature and hazard of the product and (b) the ability of factors other than validation to provide assurance of quality. On this basis, products intended for injection would come top of the list for extensive process validation, on grounds of critical use, potential high hazard, and the absence of any realistic test to confirm a crucial quality characteristic (sterility). On the other hand, a simple liquid preparation intended to soothe hot feet – simple to make, easy to assay, non-critical and unlikely to represent a patient hazard would come well down the list.

To hold such views as these does not, of course, indicate or even imply a disregard for the need for validation, but merely a realisation of the need rationally to evaluate the extent of that need in different contexts.

Terminology and components of validation

Terms commonly occurring in published texts on the subject of validation include:

- Process validation
- Installation qualification
- Operational qualification
- Performance qualification
- Prospective validation
- Retrospective validation
- Concurrent validation.

As already suggested, debate and confusion over validation terminology continues. However, it is necessary to 'know the language' whatever may be one's overall position on the subject of validation.

A possible definition

The following is suggested as a sound, basic, 'working' definition:

> *Process validation:* The action taken to demonstrate, and to provide documented evidence, that a process will, with a high degree of assurance, consistently achieve the desired and intended results.

This definition differs from that of, for example, the EC GMP Guide, in reflecting a current view that validation is a term to be applied only to *processes*, that is, processes are validated, equipment, etc. is 'qualified'. (Recall EC definition of qualification: 'Action of proving any equipment works correctly and actually leads to the expected results'.) It also differs from the US FDA definition in placing the practical demonstration before the documentation, which is both logical, and avoids the unfortunate implication that the be-all and end-all is the production of copious documents.

Pre-validaton

Thus, in this scheme of things, before process validation can commence there must be what may be termed an essential pre-validation phase (or phases). This phase, in addition to such considerations as equipment specification, equipment design and equipment purchase, requires attention to equipment qualification (EQ).

Here we have an example of the creation of a wholly unnecessary terminology. To use a word like 'qualification', already in use in other totally different contexts, when we already have available the perfectly good (and well-understood) word 'commissioning' must strike engineers and others as absurd.

Equipment qualification is in turn considered to have two (at least) main phases:

- *Installation qualification* (IQ), that is the action of demonstrating and certifying that a piece of equipment is properly installed, provided with all necessary (and *functioning*) services, subsidiary equipment and instruments, and is capable of performing in accordance with its basic design parameters.
- *Operational qualification* (OQ), that is, demonstrating that the equipment, as specified and installed, will perform consistently (within pre-defined limits) throughout its operating range (including, some have suggested, operating under 'worst case' conditions).

There have been those who wonder if this distinction between the two phases of qualification (IQ and OQ) is a necessary one, and/or who find it difficult to understand where one ends and the other begins. It has been suggested that it might help to consider IQ in terms of specific static aspects of a piece of equipment or system, and OQ in terms of specific dynamic aspects. On the other hand this distinction might not help at all. To add to the confusion in what is increasingly appearing to be a distinctly *in*-exact science, some have seen the need for DQ ('design qualification') and it has also been recently suggested that IQ stands for 'inspection qualification'. How that differs from 'installation qualification' is not entirely clear.

None of these various phases need to be considered as entirely water-tight compartments. The divisions should exist solely as matters of convenience in discussion. In practice there is likely to be some overlap, or merging, between the various components of validation/qualification. However, as Akers (1993) has noted, there has been 'impassioned and generally useless argument' over where a given activity should be classified in the IQ/OQ/PQ spectrum.

In addition, there are other quite widespread variations in terminology and conception. Some consider 'qualification' and 'validation' as two separate, yet related, activities. Others use the term 'validation' to embrace the overall activity of 'pre-validation'/qualification PLUS process validation.

A possible overall concept of validation

As a simplified illustration of the relationships between these various phases of validation, the concept in Fig. 22.1 is suggested.

A further complication arises from the emergence of a further term – performance qualification (PQ). This has been variously defined. In the 1987 FDA's *Guideline on the General Principles of Process Validation* it was defined as:

Establishing confidence that the process is effective and reproducible.

How this differs, in any substantial way, from 'validation', as defined in the same document ('Establishing documented evidence which provides a high degree of assurance that a specific process will consistently produce a product meeting its pre-determined specifications and quality attributes') is difficult to see. However, if one accepts the need for the term 'performance

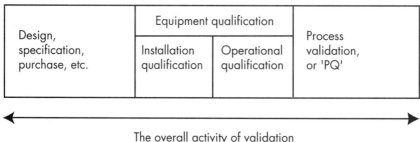

Design, specification, purchase, etc.	Equipment qualification		Process validation, or 'PQ'
	Installation qualification	Operational qualification	

The overall activity of validation

Figure 22.1   A possible concept for validation.

qualification' (as thus defined), then PQ could be substituted for process validation as in Fig. 22.1.

Other validation concepts

Validation has also been considered by some to have a number of possible approaches or strategies. The three most commonly encountered, although others have been suggested, are prospective validation, concurrent validation, and retrospective validation. It is to be noted that the necessity for, or the relevance of, these subsidiary terms is not universally accepted. They have been used to apply either to (a) the process validation phase, or to (b) the complete qualification plus process validation cycle. The following are attempts, digested from the voluminous literature, to give some sort of definition to these, possibly unnecessary, terms:

- *Prospective validation.* This refers to new processes and new equipment, where studies are conducted and evaluated, and the overall process/equipment system confirmed as validated before the commencement of routine production.
- *Concurrent validation.* This applies to existing processes and equipment. It consists of studies conducted during normal routine production and can only be considered acceptable for processes which have a manufacturing and test history indicating consistent quality production. Although lack of suitable records relating to the qualification phases may not necessarily compromise concurrent validation of some processes, evidence of proper machine installation is important in some contexts.
- *Retrospective validation.* This applies to existing processes and equipment, and is based solely on historical information. Unless sufficiently detailed past processing and control records are available, retrospective validation studies are unlikely to be either possible or acceptable. For example, it would be necessary to establish that the process had not been modified and that the equipment was still operating under the same conditions of construction and performance as documented in the historical records. Maintenance records and process change

control documentation would be necessary to support any such claim. Furthermore, the incidence of process failures, and records of rejects and/or reworking would need to be carefully evaluated for evidence of inconsistency in the process. Manufacturing, maintenance, testing and calibration data would all need to unequivocally demonstrate process uniformity, consistency and continuity.

The meaning of 'revalidation' would seem to be self-apparent, but it can in fact refer to the act of repeating all, or part, of a validation study in response to a modification to process or equipment (some would argue that this is validation, not revalidation, since this is now a 'new ball game') or to the regular planned repetition of validation, as for example in the context of regular revalidation of sterilisation processes.

It is worth repeating that there is, worldwide, considerable variation in the understanding and use of the various terms discussed. It would probably be best if both manufacturers and regulators did not confuse or over-concern themselves (or each other) with these semantic niceties. The important issues are that:

- The overall process is understood;
- Equipment is appropriately specified and designed;
- Equipment is properly installed and maintained and is demonstrably operating as specified and designed;
- The process is studied and monitored to ensure that it does achieve the desired and intended result.

To quote Akers (1993) again, perhaps 'the time has come to clear away this terminological debris, and instead focus on what we want our process control programs to achieve in terms of product quality'. But, as already suggested, for the present it is necessary to have at least a grasp of the language.

Validating the validation

For any validation study itself to be valid it is essential that:

- The instruments used in the study are properly calibrated;
- Personnel involved in the study are competent and trained to undertake the work.

Following the study, for the results to remain valid, it is necessary to:

- Maintain all equipment to the same standards as used in the study;
- Ensure that all measuring devices and process controlling instruments remain in calibration;
- Ensure that operating staff remain properly competent to perform the process in routine production;

- Implement a system of change control which will guard against unplanned or inadvertent process changes, and will highlight any change which will require consideration of the need for further validation.

Validation documentation

A further aspect of validation remains to be considered – the need for thorough and comprehensive documentation.

Of the many forms of documentation which may be required, three types may be distinguished as of primary importance:

1.   The validation protocol which defines the procedure.
2.   The report on the validation study.
3.   The supporting documentation presented with the report.

There may be, in addition, a need/requirement for a validation master plan (see below).

Validation protocol

Each major stage in an overall validation process should be conducted in accordance with a detailed, written, pre-established and formally approved validation protocol.

Written change control procedures should also be established, which will prevent unauthorised changes to either the process itself, or to the study protocol, and restrict change during any stage of the study until all relevant data have been formally evaluated for the effect(s) that any change may have on the study, and any conclusions derived from it.

Validation protocols should bear a title, date and unique identification or reference number. They should be formally authorised/approved by person(s) with the competence and authority to do so.

Validation protocols should give in detail:

- The objectives and scope of the study. That is, there should be a clear definition of purpose.
- A clear and precise definition of the process, equipment, system or subsystem which is to be the subject of the study, with details of their performance characteristics.
- Installation and qualification requirements for new equipment.
- Any up-grading requirements for existing equipment, with justification for the change(s) and a statement of qualification requirements.
- Detailed, stepwise statement of actions to be taken in performing the study (or studies).
- Assignment of responsibility for performing the study.
- Statements on all test methodology to be employed, with a precise statement of the test equipment and/or materials to be used.

- Test equipment calibration requirements.
- Reference listing of relevant standard operating procedures (SOPs).
- Statement of requirements for the content and format of the report on the study.
- A statement of acceptance criteria. That is, the criteria against which the results obtained and documented in the course of the study are to be evaluated, in order to determine the success (or otherwise) of the study; to decide whether or not the process is to be considered as validated.
- A statement of the personnel responsible for evaluating, and certifying as acceptable, each stage in the study, and for the final evaluation and certification of the process as a whole, all as measured against the predefined acceptance criteria.

The following is intended as a quick checklist of the basic requirements of a validation protocol:

○ Title

○ Date

○ Unique identification (Ref. No.)

○ Formal authorisation/approval (author, others involved)

○ Objective(s)/scope (clear definition of purpose)

○ Test equipment/materials to be used

○ Calibration requirements

○ Description of procedure to be followed

○ References to any relevant SOPs

○ Report requirements/format

○ Assignment of responsibility

○ Acceptance criteria (i.e. the criteria against which the success, or otherwise, of the study is to be judged).

In developing validation protocols, consideration may also be given to the use of risk, or hazard, analysis (HACCP) to determine the more critical operations within an overall manufacturing process, in terms of the potential risk to quality (and hence to patients) that a failure in any given process step or sub-step would represent, and thus to establish validation priorities.

Validation report

A validation report should bear a title, date and unique identification or reference number. It should include a copy of, or an unequivocal reference to, the validation protocol which was followed in order to generate the report. It should be possible to readily retrieve the protocol and relate it to the report.

The report should contain:

- Outline of procedure followed;
- Copies of, or specific references to, test procedures followed;
- Details of the calibration of test equipment/measuring devices;
- Details of the results obtained in the study;
- Formal assessment of those results against the acceptance criteria;
- Decision, with signature(s).

Supporting data and master plan

Documentation which should be available, as relevant, to support the results and conclusions of the validation report includes applicable SOPs, 'raw' test results, recorder charts/printouts, calibration reports, equipment and work-flow diagrams, full analytical and test reports and environmental monitoring reports.

Some regulatory agents have considered that a company's overall validation policies, plans and programmes should be summarised in a validation master plan (VPM).

Validation data review and evaluation

All information/data generated during the course of a study, as run in accordance with a validation protocol, should be formally evaluated against the acceptance criteria (as defined in the protocol) and judged as meeting or failing to meet those criteria. All decisions thus made should be documented, with written evidence supporting the evaluations and the conclusions drawn.

If any such evaluation shows that protocol criteria have not been met, the study should be considered as having failed to validate the process, and the reasons should be investigated and documented. All necessary corrective action should be taken before the validation study is resumed or recommenced. Any failure to follow the procedure as laid down in the protocol should be considered as potentially compromising the validity of the study itself, and requires critical evaluation of the impact on the study.

Final certification, on completion of a validation study, should be made only and specifically in relation to the predetermined acceptance criteria.

Personnel

All personnel taking part (in any capacity) in validation work should be specifically trained in the tasks assigned to them in the validation protocol.

Documented evidence of the relevant experience and training of all personnel involved in validation studies should be maintained.

Appropriately qualified and experienced supervisory personnel should ensure that the protocol and the testing methodology involved are based on sound scientific and engineering principles and that all studies are properly evaluated and certified. All personnel conducting tests should be trained and experienced in the use of the equipment and measuring devices used. All manufacturing and control operations which are the subject of the study must be conducted in accordance with good manufacturing practice.

Testing facilities and procedures

All tests and measurements (physical, chemical and microbiological) conducted during validation studies should be performed by personnel properly trained and competent to carry out the test procedures assigned to them, using appropriately calibrated equipment, instruments and devices, in suitably equipped laboratories (or other testing facilities). Instrument calibration should be performed in accordance with pre-established and approved programmes and procedures, and calibration records maintained. The calibration status (when calibrated, next due-date, etc.) of any measuring instrument or device should be readily apparent.

Detailed, authorised, written procedures setting out the relevant, validated test methodology should be available for all tests which are to be carried out during the course of a validation study. These written procedures should be referenced in the validation protocol. If external contract laboratory facilities are used in the course of a validation study, the competence of these laboratories to carry out the test(s) required should be determined in advance. This requirement should be stated in the validation protocol. The names and addresses of any contract laboratories used should be documented in the validation report.

Summary

Before leaving the general topic of validation, and moving on to some important specific applications it is perhaps useful to re-emphasise a few general points:

1. It is not to be doubted that the basic concept of validation is, *in essence,* a useful one.
2. It is equally true that some regulatory bodies, and various other self-styled 'authorities' have pushed the concept and its application to extremes.
3. It is also true that the rational practice of validation is an important component of GMP, and hence of quality assurance. The question is:

How much is required? And the answer is that it depends on the nature of the process and the use of the product. Thorough and diligent validation is most crucially needed in the manufacture of products required to be sterile.

4.   If it seems that some of the continuing discussions on the nature, terminology, semantics and philosophy of validation are somewhat redolent of the arcane deliberations of medieval clerics debating the number of angels that could dance on the head of a pin, then that is quite simply because that's the way it is.

References

Akers J (1993). Simplifying and improving process validation. *J Parenter Sci Technol* **47** (6), 281–284.

Anisfeld M (1993). Validation – how much can the world afford? Proceedings of the PDA International Congress, Basel, 1993, pp. 191–197. (See also: Validation – how much can the world afford? Are we getting value for money? *J Parent Sci Technol* **48** (1), 45–48.)

EC (1992). *The Rules Governing Medicinal Products in the European Community, Vol. IV: Good Manufacturing Practice for Medicinal Products*. Luxembourg: Commission of the European Communities. Available from The Office for Official Publications of the European Communities, Luxembourg. Also available from The Stationery Office (HMSO), London, and The EC Information Service, Washington, USA. (Referred to as the EC GMP Guide.)

Fry E (1982). Validation – theory and concepts. Collected papers of PIC Seminar on Validation, Dublin, June 1982. Geneva: EFTA Secretariat.

Fry E (1994). PDA Letter, June 1994.

Sharp J, ed. (1983). *Guide to Good Pharmaceutical Manufacturing Practice*, 3rd edn. London: HMSO. Also stated *verbatim* with guidance on the detailed interpretation of these rules in MCA, 1997. (Referred to as the UK Orange Guide.)

Sharp J R (1986). Problems of process validation. *Pharm J* **236** (11 Jan.), 43–45. (Revised version of a paper presented at a colloquium on industrial pharmacy, Ghent, 1985 and later republished in Sharp (1991).)

Sharp J (1991). *Good Manufacturing Practice – Philosophy and Applications*. Chicago: Interpharm Press.

Sharp J (1995). Validation – how much is required? *PDA J Pharm Sci Technol* **49** (3), 111–118.

US FDA (1987). *Guideline on General Principles of Process Validation*. Rockville, MD: US Food and Drug Administration.

Witschi T (1982). Validation from the inspector's standpoint. Collected papers of PIC Seminar on Validation, Dublin, June 1982. Geneva: EFTA Secretariat.

23

Validation: applications

... nought enters there, of what validity and pitch soe're, but falls into abatement and low price

W Shakespeare, *Twelfth Night*, Act 1, Sc. 1

Chapter 22 was concerned with more general aspects of validation. This chapter considers some of the more important specific applications of the concept. These are:

- Validation of sterilisation processes
- Validation of cleaning procedures
- Computer systems validation
- Analytical methods validation.

In addition to being the most important targets for validation, *per se,* they are also at the time of writing the four regulatory 'hot topics', and are likely to remain so.

Analytical methods validation stands apart from the others in having long-standing acceptance and methodology. It is by no means a 'new wave' issue. It has already been covered in Chapter 17, and will not be further considered here.

Validation of sterilisation processes

It is crucially important that all processes used to sterilise pharmaceuticals, medical devices and the like should be validated, for reasons already discussed. Not surprisingly, different approaches and techniques are employed for each of the major types of sterilisation, namely:

- Filtration (or other bulk sterilisation) with aseptic filling;
- Heat: steam and dry;
- Gaseous (e.g. ethylene oxide);
- Radiation.

Validation of a filtration/bulk sterilisation and aseptic filling process

Discussion of this type of process will exemplify some of the general principles considered in the previous chapter. The treatment of validation of the other types of sterilisation process will be covered in less detail.

Sterile products may be broadly classified into two main categories, according to the manner in which they are produced: those which are sterilised after the product has been filled and sealed in the final container(s) ('terminally sterilised' products) and those where the sterilisation stage (or stages) takes place before the bulk product is filled. In this latter instance, all subsequent processing (typically, the filling and sealing operations) must be conducted aseptically in order to prevent recontamination of the sterilised product. Given a properly sealed container, the integrity of which remains unbreached, terminal sterilisation eliminates the possibility of recontamination. Thus, any product intended, required or purported to be sterile, should be terminally sterilised, unless there are good reasons that dictate otherwise, for example where terminal sterilisation will adversely affect the product. Manufacturers who decide that terminal sterilisation is inappropriate for any given product should be prepared to justify this decision.

The two most common pharmaceutical applications of aseptic processing methods are (a) the filling of liquid products following sterilisation by filtration and (b) the filling of previously sterilised bulk powder products.

The main steps recommended may be summarised as follows:

- As a prerequisite, all studies should be conducted in accordance with a detailed, pre-established *protocol,* or series of protocols, which in turn is/are subject to formal change control procedures.
- Both the personnel conducting the studies, and those running the process(es) being studied should be appropriately trained and qualified and (in all respects) be suitable and competent to perform the tasks assigned to them.
- All data generated during the course of the studies should be formally reviewed and certified, as evaluated against predetermined criteria.
- Suitable testing facilities, equipment, instruments and methodology must be available.
- Suitable clean room facilities should be available, in terms of both the 'local' and 'background' environments.
- Assurance that the clean room environment is, and is maintained, as specified should be secured through initial commissioning ('qualification') and subsequently through the implementation of a programme of retesting, in-process control and monitoring.
- All processing equipment should be properly installed, and maintained.
- When appropriate attention has been paid to the above, the aseptic process may be validated by means of process simulation or ('media fill') studies.

- The process should be revalidated at defined intervals.
- Comprehensive documentation should be available to define, support and record the overall validation process.

Note: Although this present discussion is concerned only with the validation of aseptic processes, it is crucial to the success of any such process that the product, materials, components, etc. that are being handled/processed aseptically (e.g. bulk solution or powder; containers and closures) plus any equipment, vessels or surfaces (e.g. holding tanks, pipework, filling machines) which will or can come into contact with sterilised products/materials have themselves been previously sterilised by appropriate, *validated* sterilisation processes. In any aseptic filling process, assurance of container/closure integrity is also vital. Evidence that *all* this is so should be maintained as part of the overall validation documentation

Protocol development and control

Each stage in the validation of the overall process should proceed in accordance with a pre-established and formally approved, detailed, written protocol, or a series of related protocols. Prior to the commencement of the studies, written change control procedures should also be established, which will prevent unauthorised changes to either the process itself, or to the study protocol, and restrict change during any stage of the study until all relevant data are evaluated.

The protocols should have a title, date and a unique identification or reference number. They should be formally authorised/approved by person(s) with the competence and authority to do so. Protocols should give in detail:

1. The objectives and scope of the study. That is, there should be a clear definition of purpose.
2. A clear and precise definition of the process, equipment, system or sub-system which is to be the subject of the study, with details of performance characteristics.
3. Installation and qualification requirements for new equipment.
4. Any up-grading requirements for existing equipment, with justification for the change(s) and a statement of qualification requirements.
5. Detailed step-wise statements of actions to be taken in performing the study (or studies).
6. Assignment of responsibility for performing the study.
7. Statements on all test methodology to be employed, with a precise statement of the test equipment and/or materials to be used.
8. Test equipment calibration requirements.
9. References to any relevant standard operating procedures (SOPs).
10. Requirements for the content and format of the report on the study.
11. Acceptance criteria against which the success, or otherwise, of the study is to be evaluated.

12. The personnel responsible for evaluating and certifying as acceptable each stage in the study, and for the final evaluation and certification of the process as a whole, all as measured against the predefined acceptance criteria.

Personnel

As with all process validation studies, documented evidence of the relevant experience and training of the personnel involved in conducting the studies should be maintained. Furthermore, the personnel actually performing the aseptic processing (both during the course of any validation studies, and in routine operation) can, and do, inevitably have a crucial effect on the quality of the end product. It is necessary to consider the aspect of the personnel involved in the performance of the validation studies, and of the personnel performing the aseptic processing during both the course of the validation work, and in routine processing. To use a hand-picked elite team of operators to run the process when it is being validated is to defeat the whole objective.

Thus, appropriately qualified personnel should ensure that the protocol and the testing methodology are based on sound scientific principles and that all studies are properly evaluated and certified. All personnel conducting any test procedure should be trained and experienced in the use of the instruments, measuring devices and materials used. Engineering/maintenance personnel too should be fully trained and competent in the operation and maintenance of the machines, equipment, and air control systems involved.

Although automated and barrier techniques may appreciably reduce the contamination risk, the significance of the human factor in all aseptic processing operations cannot be over-stressed. For the results of any validation studies themselves to be valid, it is essential that the risk represented by so potentially random a variable as a human operator is kept as much under control as is possible. That is, steps must be taken to *minimise the variability*. This in turn means that operators performing the aseptic processing operation(s) which are the subject of a validation study should adopt the same techniques, disciplines, and standards of hygiene, clothing and behaviour as they would, and do, in normal routine manufacture. Everything should be done to simulate normal routine processing as closely as possible. Process operators should conduct themselves as in routine manufacture, neither better, nor worse. Furthermore, if the process operators conduct themselves, during routine production, in a manner that is different *in any way* from their behaviour during the validation studies, then conclusions drawn from the validation will themselves be invalid.

It is therefore vital that all personnel involved in aseptic processing operations are trained in, and fully understand, the concepts and principles of GMP, and the relevant elements of microbiology. They must understand the importance of personal hygiene and cleanliness, and be made fully aware of the possible hazardous consequences of product contamination. They should be provided with suitable clean room clothing and trained in the appropriate gowning technique(s). The type of clothing to be worn, and the 'scrub-up' and gowning process, should be defined in written procedures available to the operators and preferably displayed in the changing room(s). The same clothing/gowning standards should be observed during validation studies as in routine production, and *vice versa*.

The maximum number of personnel permitted in the clean room during normal routine production should also be present in the clean room during any validation test runs. At all times, operators should be encouraged to report any infections, open lesions or any other conditions which could result in the shedding of abnormal numbers of particles or microorganisms. As with routine manufacture, no person thus affected should be present in the clean room during validation test runs.

As in routine production, clean room operators involved in validation studies should be microbiologically monitored by taking test samples from gloves, gown and facemasks.

Normal routine process documentation should specify and record the numbers and types of operator interventions that are permitted during processing, and in what circumstances. A similar series of interventions should occur during any validation test runs. Details should be provided as part of the overall validation documentation.

All laboratory tests (including physical, chemical and microbiological determinations) should be performed by a competent laboratory, suitably equipped, and staffed with personnel properly trained and qualified to carry out the test procedures assigned to them. Detailed authorised written procedures defining the relevant validated methodology should be available for all laboratory tests and determinations, which are to be carried out during the course of the study. These procedures should be referenced in the study protocol. If any external laboratory facilities are used, systems should be in place for determining the competence of these laboratories to carry out the tests required. This requirement should be referenced in the study protocol. All measuring/recording/indicating instruments employed in the studies should be adequate for the purpose, in terms of range, accuracy, reproducibility, etc. They must be calibrated in accordance with predefined written procedures before any validation studies are commenced. Records of each calibration should be maintained, and should form part of the overall validation documentation.

It must be clearly understood that for the conclusions drawn from any qualification or validation studies themselves to remain valid during routine production, all controlling and recording instruments must be subjected to a written maintenance and calibration programme.

Clean room standards monitoring

For the results to have valid relevance to routine production, validation studies must be conducted under precisely the same environmental conditions as employed, or intended to be employed, during normal routine production. Confirmation and certification that the room and the workstation(s) used do, in fact, conform to the Environmental Standard specified may be considered as forming part of the 'installation qualification' phase. To this end, the following basic work should be carried out on the initial commissioning (or 'qualification') of a new clean room installation:

- Room air filter integrity tests.
- Determination of air velocity at the face of each air inlet filter.
- Room air change rate.
- Room air particle counts.
- Room air pressure differentials and airflow patterns.
- Lighting, heating, humidity.
- Workstation(s) air filter efficiency tests.
- Determination of air velocity at face of workstation air filters.
- Particle counts within workstation areas.

Following the initial commissioning, a regular retest programme should be adopted, e.g.:

1. Room and workstation air filter tests: repeat at least annually, unless results of normal in-process monitoring indicate a need for more frequent or additional testing.
2. Air velocity and room air changes: repeat at least twice a year.
3. Air particle counts: determine as part of regular in-process monitoring, with formal certification by a competent specialist agency three times per year.

In addition, room air pressure differentials should be monitored on a continuous, ongoing, basis.

Walls, floors, workstations and surfaces generally should be subject to a predetermined programme of cleaning and disinfection. In order to ensure that, during routine manufacture, products remain within the quality parameters established during the overall validation process, it is necessary to design and implement a programme of in-process control and monitoring. Similarly, as part of the overall assurance that process validation studies are conducted under comparably normal processing conditions, *a similar in-process control and monitoring programme should be operated during the process validation runs.*

In-process monitoring and control may be considered under two headings:

- Microbiological
- Environmental particulate.

In addition, where sterile filtration of a liquid product is involved, filter integrity testing of the filter(s) used to sterilise that product should be considered. These filter integrity tests should be conducted *after* each use of the filters, in order to detect any leaks or perforations that may have occurred during the filtration process itself. Often filter integrity testing is also done before the filtration of the product commences, and this is a generally sound practice. It is, however, the integrity test performed *after* the batch, or lot, has been filtered which is critical.

As appropriate to the type of manufacturing process, consideration needs to be given to the following microbiological monitoring and control procedures:

- Bioburden check on bulk solution, prior to sterile filtration.
- Exposure of settle plates at defined critical positions within the general clean room environment and at the controlled workstation(s).
- Use of air sampling devices to determine the number of viable organisms per cubic metre (or cubic foot) of air in the room, and within the workstation(s).
- Use of contact plates, or swabs, to check the microbiological quality of surfaces.

Environmental particulate monitoring should be carried out using appropriate air particle counting devices to check that the general environmental and workstation air remains in conformity with specification. All in-process monitoring and control should be conducted in accordance with a written, predetermined programme, which includes specified test limits and standards, with all results formally reported and evaluated against those limits. This requirement applies as much to validation studies as it does to routine manufacture.

Equipment qualification and maintenance

Various items of mechanised equipment may be used in aseptic processing, for example: ampoule filling and sealing machines; vial, bottle, cartridge, tube or syringe filling, sealing and capping machines; powder fillers, freeze-dryers (lyophilizers) and so on. Before any process validation studies may be commenced, it is necessary that all such equipment should be properly installed and operationally qualified.

The essential requirements are that the equipment is:

1. Confirmed as having been constructed as specified.
2. Properly installed and provided with all necessary *functioning* services, ancillary equipment and instruments.
3. Confirmed as capable of operating consistently, within predetermined limits, over its defined operating range.

Processing equipment must be confirmed as complying with all three above before any subsequent studies can be considered valid.

For the results of any validation studies themselves to remain valid in routine manufacture, a comprehensive routine maintenance programme must be developed, setting out each activity in detail along with the frequency in terms of real time, machine time or other time base. The time base should be clearly defined for each procedure. Unless such a programme is developed and implemented and the manufacturing equipment and attendant instruments remain in the same state of maintenance and calibration as during the validation studies, then any assurance derived from those studies is to be considered as negated.

Media fill studies (solution products)

In the 'media fill', or 'broth fill', technique, a liquid microbiological nutrient growth medium is prepared and filled in a simulation of a normal manufacturing operation. The nutrient medium is processed and handled in a manner which simulates the normal manufacturing process as closely as possible with the same exposure to contamination risk (from operators, environment, equipment, and surfaces) as would occur during routine manufacture. The sealed containers of medium thus produced are incubated under prescribed conditions and then examined for evidence of microbial growth, and thus of an indication of the level of contaminated units produced.

It is important to recognise that, in many instances, media fills are, among other things, a test of the human operators' aseptic techniques. In this test situation the operators can hardly remain unaware that nutrient medium is being filled, and that they themselves are, to an extent, 'under test'. There is, therefore, the possibility that they will take more than their usual care, and thus the normal process will not be precisely simulated. Every effort should be made to ensure that the operators *do* behave normally during the media fills, and conversely (and perhaps more importantly) that during routine production they do not deviate in any way from the high standards adopted during the simulation studies.

A further difficulty, which needs to be noted, is the possibility of contamination of the facility and equipment by the nutrient medium. Some have seen this possibility as a strong argument against the media fill technique. However, if the process is well controlled and the media fill is promptly followed by cleaning and disinfection, and (as necessary) sterilisation of equipment, this should not be a problem. Nevertheless, it *is* important to recognise the potential hazard, and to respond accordingly.

It must also be re-emphasised that the filling of a nutrient medium solution alone does not constitute an acceptable aseptic process validation. The whole manufacturing cycle must be simulated, from the dispensing and reconstitution of the powdered medium under normal manufacturing conditions, to the filling and sealing process itself. Operators (and numbers of operators), numbers and types of filtrations, etc. should all be 'as normal', as should holding times in any mixing vessels, or interim holding tank. General activity should be at a normal level, and no attempt should be made to take any 'special' precautions to ensure that the test run is successful. If any deviation from the normal is permitted, it should only be in the direction of presenting a greater, rather than a lesser, microbiological challenge to the process.

The liquid nutrient medium used should meet the following criteria:

- *Selectivity*: The medium should have *low* selectivity, that is, it should be capable of supporting growth of the widest range of micro-organisms that might reasonably be expected to be encountered. As a minimum requirement it should support the growth of cultures of organisms normally found in the manufacturing environment, and such organisms as:

  — *Escherichia coli*
  — *Pseudomonas aeruginosa*
  — *Staphylococcus aureus*
  — *Candida albicans*
  — *Aspergillus niger.*

- *Clarity*: When made up, the medium should be clear, to allow for the observation of any turbidity (i.e. growth) following incubation.
- *Filterability*: Where the process being simulated includes a filtration stage, the liquid medium should be capable of being filtered through the same grade and type of microbial retentive filter as that through which the actual product is, or will be, filtered.

Liquid soybean casein digest (SCD), also termed 'tryptic soy broth' (TSB) is perhaps the liquid medium most frequently employed. However, other formulations (e.g. liquid tryptone glucose yeast extract, or brain heart infusion) may be used, provided they meet the criteria set out above.

The liquid medium should be sterilised by filtration (if such a stage is part of the normal operation being simulated), in the same way, using the same grade and type filter and housing, and in the same sequence as normal. If it is presterilised by heat, or subjected to any form of heat treatment, it must be *cooled to ambient temperature before proceeding.*

The *number of units* to be filled per run should be sufficient to provide a high probability of detecting a low incidence of microbial contamination. For example, in order to give 95% confidence of detecting a contamination rate of one in a thousand units filled with medium, 3000 units need to be filled. In fact, based on an assumption of a Poisson distribution, or of a binomial distribution of contaminated units, the precise figures are, respectively, 2986 and 2995. Traditionally this is rounded up to 3000. However, see later.

For the initial validation of a new process or facility, or after any major change in the process or the equipment, sufficient consecutive media fill runs should be performed to provide assurance that the results obtained are consistent, meaningful and provide an acceptable level of sterility assurance. At least three separate, consecutive, successful runs per operator-team, or shift, should be performed to provide acceptable initial validation of a given processing line. There is no statistical basis for this 'rule of three'. It just seems like a good idea, and it probably is until somebody thinks of something that is both better, and practicable.

The *volume to be filled per unit* should be the normal production fill volume where possible. In the case of high volume containers, a lesser quantity may be used, provided steps are taken to ensure wetting of all the inner surface of the container, and any closure, by the medium, e.g. by shaking or inversion, and/or by inverting the containers part-way through the incubation period. It is a good practice also to take similar steps to ensure complete inner surface wetting, even when normal full volumes are filled. Immediately following filling, all units filled should be examined for leakages and/or damage. In this context, any leak-test method in which heat is employed must obviously not be used. Any leaking or damaged units should be rejected. The incubation of the filled units should follow immediately after filling and leak testing, and should be for a minimum period of 14 days.

Opinions tend to vary regarding the *incubation temperature* (PDA, 1996; Prout, 1993) to be used, but 25°C to 35°C is a reasonable compromise. Whatever temperature range is chosen, it should be carefully controlled, monitored and maintained throughout the incubation period. For strict comparability between results obtained in different test runs, in practice the incubation temperature should be controlled, on each and every occasion, between tighter limits than the range suggested.

Test controls   To demonstrate the nutritive properties of the medium used, a few filled units from each run should be inoculated with low levels of challenge organisms, and then incubated, suitably labelled, along with the test units. A number of texts appear to suggest that this test-control operation should be conducted almost as something separate and divorced from a main media full run. It clearly makes better sense, and is better science, to randomly select a number of filled units from the run (that means a few extra will need to be filled), inoculate them, mark them carefully and conspicuously to avoid confusion and then incubate them in the same incubator with the other media-filled units. Thus, a suggested control procedure is as follows:

1.   Take six medium-filled units from each run and inoculate in three sets of two with the following organisms, at a level of 100 organisms per unit:

  • 2 × *Staphylococcus aureus*
  • 2 × *Bacillus subtilis*
  • 2 × *Candida albicans*.

2.   Label and incubate these six inoculated control units at 30–35°C along with the test units.

Organisms other than those suggested may be used, provided they represent a similar range of microbial type. An alternative is to use cultures of organisms found in the manufacturing environment. A combination of these environmental isolates and 'standard' organisms such as those listed is much to be recommended.

Reading of results   All units filled and incubated should be visually examined for microbial growth after at least 14 days' incubation. Any contaminated units will be identifiable by the turbidity of the medium. Any contaminated units that are found should be examined in the laboratory, and the con-taminating organisms identified, at least to genus level, so that appropriate preventative action may be taken. For the results of the media fill run to be considered valid, all the inoculated control units should display growth.

Figure 23.1 illustrates the type of process simulation described above, in relation to liquid-filled vial product.

These notes apply to Fig. 23.1:

(a)   Different types of container will require different methods of sterilisation. For example, glass vials are likely to be dry heat sterilised, plastic vials may be sterilised by irradiation or ethylene oxide.

(b)   Any other components, e.g. teats, droppers, will also need to be presterilised by some suitable validated method.

(c)   The process flow for liquid media filling of ampoules will be analogous to the above, without the operations involving stoppers, overseals, etc.

Contamination level   The contamination level found in a media fill run is calculated from the number of contaminated units expressed as a percentage of the number of units incubated.

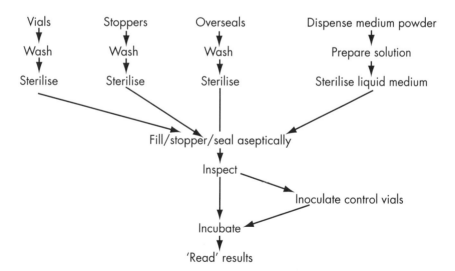

Figure 23.1   Process flow diagram of liquid media filling of vials.

Media fill acceptance criteria

Thus far the process simulation/media fill test may well have seemed a 'good idea'. It has been long accepted, it is widely practised and has regulatory and compendial recognition. Unfortunately it tends somewhat to totter, if not fall, at the last hurdle; that is, when the problem of deciding the criteria by which the success, or failure, of a media fill run is confronted (or not, as the case may be), in the face of some statistical, and very considerable practical, difficulties.

The most widely quoted limit remains not more than 1 in 1000 (0.1%) contaminated media-filled units. This limit was considered acceptable, for example, in the FDA's *Guideline on Sterile Drug Products Produced by Aseptic Processing* (US FDA, 1987), where it is also stated that acceptance of this level in a test does not mean that an aseptically processed lot of product purporting to be sterile may contain one non-sterile unit in every 1000 filled. It is merely a recognition of the scientific and technical limitations of the test procedure itself.

It has, however, to be recognised that a media fill run of 3000 units only gives 95% confidence of detecting a 0.1% microbial contamination level *in those 3000 units*. It does not serve as a direct prediction of a contamination level of 0.1% or less in normal production runs which are normally much, much larger. The fairly common 3000 unit media fill thus represents only a simulated sample of a normal production run, and any % contamination rate calculated from a media fill will therefore be subject to sampling error. Thus three contaminated units found in a media fill of 3000 may well be indicative of a potential contamination rate *in actual production* significantly greater than 0.1%. Although it has been suggested, by various regulatory and other authorities, that a limit of 1 in 10 000 (0.01%), or better, should be the aim, it must be understood that to demonstrate a likelihood of compliance (on a normal production scale) with limits of that order, impractically large numbers of units may need to be filled with medium and incubated. In addition to the time, space and cost implications, there is the not inconsiderable problem of the disposal of the large numbers of broth-filled units after the test.

Table 23.1 indicates the number of units that would need to be media filled, with the respective numbers of contaminated units which could be permitted in order to provide 95% confidence of achieving 0.1% contamination or less in a normal production run of more than 100 000 units (values are rounded-off).

Thus for example, to provide confidence (95%) of complying with the 0.1% limit in a production batch in excess of 100 000 units, 4750 media-filled units would be required with no more than one unit found contaminated, or 6300 units with no more than two, and so on.

Figures relevant to other production batch sizes (less than 100 000) and a 0.1% acceptance limit are given in Table 23.2 (95% confidence, figures rounded).

Thus, for a process in which the normal batch size is 20 000 units, a

Table 23.1 Maximum permitted number of contaminated units, per various media-fill test units, to indicate 0.1% contamination limit in a production run in excess of 100 000 at 95% confidence level

Media fill units	Contaminated units permitted
3000	0
4750	1
6300	2
7750	3
9150	4

media fill of 4340 test units would provide 95% confidence of a limit of 0.1% contamination if no more than one contaminated media-filled unit were found.

It is when the acceptance criterion is tightened that the real problems of scale become apparent. To demonstrate compliance with a contamination limit of one in 10 000 (0.01%) notably larger numbers of units would need to be filled with 'broth'. For example, in relation to a normal production run of 50 000 units, over 46 000 units would need to be filled with medium, with no more than one unit found contaminated on incubation.

These statistical considerations reveal a real practical problem with regard to the number of units which may need to be filled with medium and incubated, particularly in any attempt to demonstrate a probability of a low (for example, less than 0.1%) level of contamination in 'standard' production batch sizes. Although there has been the odd report of media fills (by

Table 23.2 Maximum permitted number of contaminated test units for production runs below 100 000 units to indicate 0.1% contaminated at 95% confidence

Production batch size (units)	Media-fill test units	Permitted contaminated units
5000	2470	0
5000	3680	1
5000	4680	2
10 000	2670	0
10 000	4050	1
10 000	5210	2
20 000	2810	0
20 000	4340	1
20 000	5670	2
50 000	2910	0
50 000	4580	1
50 000	6040	2

automated means) of the order of one million units per run, such numbers are hardly practical for routine use.

And this is where most, if not all, apparently authoritative texts fail to provide any useful guidance to the aseptic process validator, keen to demonstrate contamination rates of, say, no more than 0.001%. The British Pharmacopoeia, for example, while commending the media fill in general terms (Appendix XVII), makes no comment on the number of units to be filled, nor on the acceptance criteria to be adopted. In the circumstance all one can suggest is that, purely on the basis of the practical limitations of the test procedure, a contamination level of 0.1%, detected infrequently in media fills, may be considered to be acceptable. Regular, or common, contamination levels (in media fills) of 0.1% or above should be regarded as unsatisfactory. While it may be statistically unsound to sum in a simple fashion data from a series of discrete events, and then treat these data as if they had been derived from a single event, a series of 'good' media fill results a period of time (assuming reasonable comparability of conditions, etc.) may be regarded as strengthening confidence, if not in any precisely quantifiable fashion. That this is a 'common sense, gut feeling' viewpoint will be apparent. This weakness inherent in the media fill approach to aseptic process validation must, until someone suggests something better, be considered as strengthening the argument that, whenever possible, products intended or purported to be sterile should be terminally sterilised.

Media fills applied to non-solution products

The same general principles, conditions and statistical considerations as set out above apply, but the various types of non-solution sterile product require various adaptations to the approach already described.

Sterile powders   The use of the media fill technique in the validation of the filling of sterile powder products presents certain special problems, arising from the prob-able necessity to employ additional equipment, techniques or manipulations which are different (or additional) to those used in routine production. In such circumstances the media fill cannot unequivocally be said to be a precise process simulation. This inevitable shortcoming may, however, have to be accepted. A number of different approaches have been proposed and used, as follows:

1.   The normal process is simulated as closely as possible, but instead of filling a powder, a sterile liquid medium is filled. This approach is virtually the same as that described above for a solution product and fails to simulate the actual *powder* fill.
2.   The normal process is simulated as closely as possible, with a sterile, dry inert powder filled in place of the normal product or material. Lactose, mannitol and polyethylene glycol 8000 are examples of

'simulation' powders that have been used. There are two possible variations on this approach and in both these variations, a powder fill *is* simulated, but an additional, non-routine step (i.e. the filling of the liquid growth medium) is involved:

(a)   Fill the chosen inert powder into the containers (e.g. ampoules/vials) which are already filled with sterile liquid medium.

(b)   Fill the inert powder first, and then add the sterile liquid medium.

3.   Fill sterile dry powdered medium into the containers, in simulation of the normal powder filling operation, aseptically adding sterile aqueous diluent on-line, to form liquid medium solution. Here a powder fill is simulated, but an additional operation is involved.

Whichever approach is adopted, it is important to ensure that any powder/medium/diluent combination used does not cause growth inhibition through hyperosmolar or other antimicrobial effects.

Suspension products   Simulate the entire normal process as closely as possible, using a sterile inert powder in place of the normal powder ingredient. Micronise, etc. (if this is part of the normal process) and form suspension, using sterile liquid growth medium in place of the normal liquid phase of the suspension product. Fill as normal and incubate.

Freeze-dried product   Simulate the entire normal process (i.e. preparation of bulk solution, filling of solution, loading of freeze-dryer, running of freeze-drying cycle, sealing/ closing of containers and inspection) but use a liquid growth medium (dispensed as a powder, dissolved and sterilised) in place of normal product. Actual freeze drying of the medium solution is not usually practicable, but exposure and holding times in the freeze dryer should be as normal.

Semi-solid products (e.g. sterile ointments and creams)   Simulate the normal process cycle as closely as possible, filling a sterile liquid growth medium made to a similar consistency as the normal product by the addition, for example, of agar (c. 4 g per litre) or carboxymethylcellulose.

For more information on validation, by process simulation, see Prout (1993; see also Prout, 1982).

All the approaches/techniques outlined in this section must be performed in conformity with the general principles of GMP. In all procedures involving the use of growth media it is vital to control any contamination by the media of equipment, surfaces, etc. All media fill studies should be promptly followed by the application of thorough cleaning, disinfecting and sterilisation procedures.

Revalidation

Following initial aseptic process validation, media fills/process simulations should be repeated to an extent, and at a frequency, which will depend on the occurrence of events or changes which may bear upon the potential microbial hazard to the process/product. Significant modifications to equipment or facilities, changes in personnel, undesirable trends in environmental monitoring results, and sterility test failures may all indicate an immediate need to implement a full process validation protocol (i.e. minimum of three consecutive successful media-fill runs) with the facility in question taken out of service until any problems have been resolved, and the results of the three media fills have been evaluated and found acceptable.

In the absence of any significant changes, or of any other events giving cause for concern, then a minimum retest frequency should be twice per year per operator shift or team, for each process line. For single shift operations, the minimum frequency should be three times for each process line per year.

Data review

All information or data generated as a result of implementing the study protocol should be evaluated by authorised persons against the protocol criteria and formally judged as meeting or failing the requirements. Written evidence supporting the evaluation and the conclusions drawn should be available. The evaluation should be made as the information becomes available, and if it shows that protocol criteria have not been met, the study should be considered as having failed to demonstrate acceptability. The reasons should be investigated and documented. Any failure to follow the procedure as laid down in the protocol must be considered as potentially compromising the validity of the study itself, and requires critical evaluation of the impact on the study.

Final certification of the validation study should specify the predetermined acceptance criteria, against which success or failure were evaluated.

Documentation (aseptic process validation)

Documents that should be available to define, support and record the overall validation process include:

1. Protocol(s) covering the overall process, with all relevant written change control procedures and records.
2. Documented evidence that the product, materials, components, etc. that are being handled/processed aseptically (e.g. bulk solution or powder, containers and closures) plus any equipment, vessels or surfaces (e.g. holding tanks, pipework, filling machines) which will or can come into contact with sterilised products/materials have themselves been previously sterilised by appropriate and validated sterilisation processes.

3. Documented evidence of the competence and training of *all* personnel involved in the studies.
4. SOPs defining clothing requirements and gowning procedures.
5. Copies of all relevant SOPs, e.g.

   — Dispensing ingredients.
   — Water quality and supply.
   — Cleaning/disinfection/sterilisation (as appropriate) of all equipment, surfaces and services.
   — Sterilisation of equipment, vessels and pipelines.
   — Filter integrity testing.
   — Machine setup, start-up and adjustment.

6. Written procedures for all laboratory tests.
7. Formally recorded results of all laboratory tests, with a recorded evaluation of those results against criteria established in the study protocol(s).
8. Written calibration programme and procedures covering all controlling, measuring and recording instruments, with the results obtained during those calibrations.
9. Design specifications for major items of mechanised equipment.
10. Written installation qualification procedures, with report confirming successful installation in accordance with those procedures.
11. Written operational qualification procedures, with report certifying that equipment, as installed, will perform consistently within defined limits.
12. Statement of the environmental standards, as designated for each stage of the manufacturing process.
13. Certification of conformity of any controlled environment with the designated standard(s).
14. Environmental retest programme with evidence that this programme is routinely implemented, with a record of the results obtained.
15. Written routine planned machine maintenance programme, with documented evidence of the regular implementation of that programme.
16. Written in-process monitoring and control procedures, with records of results obtained both during process validation and in routine manufacture.
17. Policy/records relating to permitted operator interventions.
18. Full process validation report, including:

    — Medium used.
    — Volume filled.
    — Number of units filled.
    — Number of leakers rejected.
    — Number of units incubated.
    — Incubation temperature.
    — Incubation time.
    — Control organisms used.
    — Filter integrity test results.

— Record of all in-process monitoring and control results.
— Results of examination of incubated units.
— Confirmation of growth in inoculated control units.

19. Final, formal evaluation of results against established criteria, with PASS/FAIL decision.

Validation of steam sterilisation processes

It is commonly averred (e.g. PDA, 1978; Soper, 1994) that there are two main approaches to the design, operation and validation of the steam (i.e. autoclave) sterilisation process:

1. The probability of survival approach.
2. The overkill approach.

Each has two aspects in the context of process validation:

• Physical validation.
• Biological (or microbiological) validation.

As will (hopefully) become apparent, the relative effort demanded in terms of physical, as compared with biological, validation by the two approaches will vary, one to the other.

There could also be said to be a possible third approach, which we will term the 'simplified approach', which eliminates the mental toil of juggling with the kinetics of microbial thermal death-rates (which some, but not all, find difficult and confusing), and reduces the time and effort to be spent on detailed microbiological laboratory studies.

The simplified approach is to 'take as read' the standard compendial cycle, or cycles, and to assume (as seems entirely reasonable) that such a cycle will, if operated properly on a relatively low bioburden load, indeed provide the level of assurance of sterility required. Thus the current (1998) edition of the British Pharmacopoeia states '. . . the reference conditions [for steam sterilisation] of aqueous preparations are heating at a minimum of 121°[C] for 15 minutes'. Assuming the adoption of this time/temperature cycle for routine use, it then simply becomes necessary to ensure in batch production, and to confirm by process validation studies, that the coldest part of the coldest item in the coldest position in the autoclave load attains a temperature of 121°C, and is held at that temperature for at least 15 minutes. It is, of course, necessary to ensure in this, or any other, approach that the product or material is able to withstand this level of heat input without being degraded. It is also necessary to be aware of variations in temperature and heat penetration throughout the load, so as to ensure the attainment of 121°C at the 'coldest part' does not mean that other parts of the load are exposed to heat inputs which would cause degradation. Thus in the simplified approach, as in the others, it is not only necessary to pay attention to autoclave design and operation, and to presterilisation bioburden, but also to determine (a) the heat distribution throughout the chamber load, and (b) the heat penetration into the load.

This simplified approach could be regarded as neither more nor less than an overkill approach, *always provided that an overkill cycle is employed*. Soper (1994) declared that 'compendial sterilisation cycles have been devised using overkill methods'. This is not entirely true. The most commonly cited compendial cycles (with the over-pressure which is required to achieve the corresponding steam temperature) over the years are given in Table 23.3.

The neat progression (10 to 15 to 20 psi) is no coincidence. These cycles were originally derived at a time when it was common to speak of operating an autoclave at so many pounds *pressure*, rather than at a stated *temperature*. Thus, traditional compendial cycles were based more on 'seems like a good idea at nice round pressure numbers', than on overkill concepts. This was all well before today's understanding of thermal death-rates of bacteria. Nevertheless, it is indeed true that 15 minutes at 121°C, in an autoclave, does represent an overkill. To illustrate this point it is necessary to understand something of the F_0 concept, which will be covered in more detail later. For the present F_0 may be simply regarded as an index of the 'heat lethality' delivered by the sterilisation process. The F_0 values have been calculated for the various cycles listed in Table 23.3. This table illustrates two things. It shows the lack of comparability of these historical compendial steam sterilisation cycles. It also shows, in comparison with a common view that a minimum acceptable F_0 value is 8 (Akers & Anderson, 1993), that 121°C for 15 minutes, in delivering an F_0 of 15, does represent an overkill.

The probability of survival approach

This approach originated in the food canning industry (Stumbo, 1973) many years before it became manifest in the pharmaceutical industry, and it is probably worth reflecting on the essential differences between the sterilisation of cans of food and the sterilisation of pharmaceuticals and medical devices.

Cans of food are relatively high volume (in terms both of numbers of

Table 23.3 Typical sterilisation cycles

Temperature (°C)	Pressure (psi)	Holding time (min)	'Heat lethality' F_0
115–118	10	30	7.5–15
121–124	15	15	15–30
126–129	20	10	32–63

units and of space occupied), low-value items. Pharmaceuticals and the like are, by comparison, low volume and high value. All foodstuffs run the risk of 'over-cooking'. By no means are all pharmaceuticals degraded by normal heat sterilisation cycles. It is of particular interest to food processors to determine and apply a minimum acceptable cycle. A powerful motive, in addition to avoiding degrading the food and spoiling its flavour, is to reduce the very considerable time and energy costs of the sterilisation of large numbers of food cans. The food producer is concerned with what is the minimum requirement. Although contaminated food is dangerous, it is probably not as dangerous as a contaminated parenteral, although the point is perhaps debatable. As a function of turnover the cost of sterilisation of parenterals is by no means as great as it is in relation to food. The manufacturer of parenterals will be more concerned with the best possible assurance of sterility. This is not to say that there is anything gravely wrong with the probability of survival approach. It is merely useful to know that it is 'coming from' a different direction.

Some professors at schools of pharmacy, and others, hold that when a population of micro-organisms is exposed to a lethal agent (specifically, lethal heat treatment) the number of surviving organisms decreases exponentially with the extent (or time) of exposure. Thus it is postulated that the process of microbial inactivation is analogous to a first-order chemical reaction, and may be mathematically represented thus:

$$N_t = N_0 e^{-kt}$$

where N_t is the number of surviving organisms after time t, N_0 is the number of organisms at time zero (that is, the pretreatment bioburden) and k is the microbial inactivation rate constant. If the logarithm of the fraction of survivors (N_t/N_0) is plotted against exposure time, the result is a curve (the 'survivor curve') which is linear with a negative slope (Fig. 23.1). The slope of the curve is $k/2.303$, from which k, the microbial inactivation rate constant, can be calculated.

There are those who find some difficulty in accepting that micro-organisms die off in this exponential fashion, especially since the proponents of the view rarely, if ever, present any solid experimental evidence to support it. It may also be of some significance that the 1978 PDA Technical Monograph No.1, shows a 'survivor curve' closely similar to that in Fig. 23.2, with the sub-title '*Hypothetical* microbial death rate (i.e. survivor curve) at a constant experimental temperature' (author's emphasis). It would seem, therefore, that there is some room to wonder if death-rate as an exponential function of time is indeed an absolute proven fact of microbial life, or no more than a convenient hypothesis. The concept is, nevertheless, a cornerstone of the probability of survival approach, and will be assumed in what immediately follows.

D, IF, Z and F values

On the assumption of the log-linear survivor curve, a number of values have been defined.

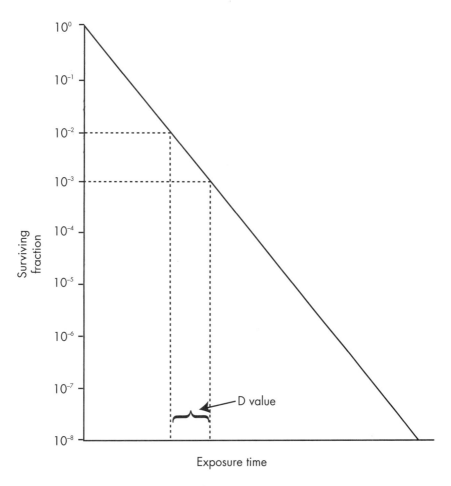

Figure 23.2   Thermal survivor curve.

Instead of k (see above) as a measure of microbial inactivation rate, the **D value** is more often cited and used. This, in the context of a heat sterilisation process, is the time (in minutes), at a given temperature, required to reduce the number of micro-organisms by 90%, that is to 10% of the original bioburden, or a one log cycle decrease in the survivor curve. For an assumed log-linear curve, the D value is equal to 2.303/k. Both are measures of the resistance of an organism to a stated temperature (or other sterilising agent). For heat inactivation, the D value is the time in minutes required to achieve the one log cycle reduction of a population of an organism at a specified temperature, which is usually shown as a subscript, e.g. 'D_{121}'. A D value refers to the resistance (in minutes) of a specific organism. It is meaningless if the temperature is not stated, or understood. (That applies in the context of heat treatment. D values can be, and have been, used in relation to both radiation and gaseous sterilisation, where they are expressed in terms of absorbed dose and time of exposure respectively.)

The **inactivation factor** (**IF**), is a measure of the total microbial inactivation achieved by a given process. It is defined as the reduction in the number of viable organisms brought about by the process. The relationship between inactivation factor and the D value is expressed as:

$$IF = 10^{t/D}$$

where t is the exposure time and D is the D value of the organism at the specified temperature.

If the logarithms of the D values of an organism are plotted against the temperatures at which those D values were determined, the result is a linear curve of negative slope (Fig. 23.3).

The **Z value** of the organism is the negative reciprocal of the slope of this line, and represents the increase in temperature required to reduce the D value of the organism by 90%, that is to produce a one log cycle reduction in the thermal resistance curve. Thus, for a specified organism, a Z value defines the relationship between the time required to achieve a given thermal reduction at one temperature, and the time required to achieve the same effect at another temperature. For all practical purposes it may be considered to be constant, for a given organism, over the relatively small temperature ranges normally used for heat sterilisation (115–135°C for steam and 170–190°C for dry heat). Z values can be determined thus:

$$Z = (T_2 - T_1)/(\log D_1 - \log D_2)$$

where D_1 is the D value of the micro-organism at temperature T_1, and D_2 is the D value of the micro-organism at temperature T_2.

The Z value is a specific characteristic of a species, or type, of micro-organism. Z values vary quite widely from one organism to another. The more heat-resistant organisms (e.g. *Bacillus stearothermophilus*, *B. subtilis* and *Clostridium sporogenes*) have Z values of around 10. Thus, often when a Z value is not known, or has not been determined empirically, a value of 10 is assumed.

An **F value** is a measure of heat sterilisation efficiency. It may also be defined as a measure of the overall lethality of a process. It equates a heat treatment at any temperature (with regard to its ability to destroy micro-organisms) with the time in minutes required, at a defined reference temperature, to destroy a reference organism of a stated Z value. For steam heat at a reference temperature of 121°C, and in relation to an organism with a Z value of 10°, the F value is termed the F_0 value, usually articulated as either 'eff-owe' or 'eff-sub-zero'. Thus, to say that a steam sterilisation process has an F_0 of 8 means that the sum of all the effects of the process, in terms of lethality in relation to an organism with a Z value of 10, is equivalent to 8 minutes at 121°C. F_0 may be expressed mathematically as:

$$F_0 = D_{121}(\log N_0 - \log N) = D_{121} \log IF$$

where D_{121} is the D value of the reference organism at 121°C; N_0 is the initial number of the reference organism; N is the final number of the organism, and IF is the inactivation factor.

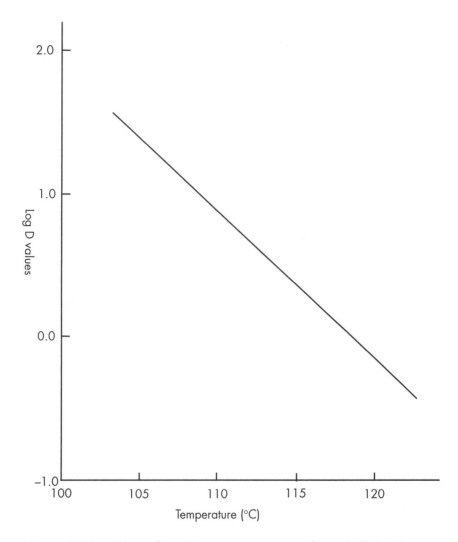

Figure 23.3 Values of log D against temperature from which Z values are calculated.

In most steam sterilisation processes the reference organism is usually taken to be *B. stearothermophilus*, with an assumed Z value of 10 and a D_{121} of 1.5 minutes in aqueous systems. However, components of a formulation can affect thermal resistance of organisms, and if sterilisation cycles are to be designed and validated based upon F_0 concepts, it would become necessary either to show that the formulation does not increase thermal resistance above the assumed value(s), or to determine the D_{121} value of a reference organism in the product to be sterilised.

Usually, heat sterilisation protocols (compendial and otherwise) define a temperature and a holding time at that temperature, and take no account of the heating-up and cooling-down phases of the overall cycle.

But the heat (say above 100°C) imparted to the load can contribute significantly to the overall lethality of the process (and, potentially, to product degradation). Application of the F_0 concept permits integration of the total lethality of a process, including the heating-up and cooling-down phases, and forms the basis for the microprocessor control of autoclaves, and for the commercially available multipoint thermocouple, with automatic printout integrator sets.

Application of F_0 to the validation of a steam sterilisation process

As an important preliminary, it is worthy of re-emphasis that it is meaningless to think, or talk, of the validation of an autoclave cycle, or of an autoclave load, in isolation. It is the validation of a defined time/temperature cycle, when applied to a defined (in terms of both content and loading pattern) load, in a specified autoclave, which is crucially important. It is not possible to extrapolate results obtained with one cycle, applied to one load, in one autoclave to any other cycle, load or autoclave. It is, however, not unreasonable to argue that a cycle validated for a maximum load in a given autoclave will be more than adequate for a smaller load, of the same product or material, in the same autoclave.

Although the theoretical basis for the design and validation of steam sterilisation processes, based upon the probability of survival and the F_0 concept, is derived from studies on, and hypotheses about, the thermo-kinetics of microbial death rates, the main emphasis in practice is usually on *physical* (as distinct from *biological*) validation. Physical validation is aimed at ensuring a defined, reproducible F_0 value throughout a load, and specifically at the coolest part of that load. However, the use of biological indicators (BIs) in addition to temperature-sensing devices is often recommended for validation studies. The use of BIs as monitoring devices in routine manufacture is generally not to be recommended, on the common sense grounds that, if it can be avoided, it is far from a good idea to knowingly introduce heat-resistant spores into a sterile products manufacturing area.

Currently, with regard to BIs, there would appear to be a difference both in practice and in regulatory requirements in Europe as compared with the USA. Thus, in the USA, the FDA seem to expect manufacturers to use BIs in the validation of autoclave cycles, and on occasions to require their use to monitor routine production cycles. In Europe, the tendency has been rather to limit the use of BIs in validation studies, and for regulatory agencies to actively discourage their routine production use on grounds of the potential for microbial contamination.

There have been suggestions that not only the design and validation, but also the routine operation of steam sterilisation cycles, should be based upon the determination of the thermal resistance of organisms found (a) in the manufacturing environment and/or (b) in or on the product, immediately prior to sterilisation. Such a position presents both theoretical and practical difficulties. True, it is important to carry out microbiological monitoring of the manufacturing environment, and to perform batch-wise checks on presterilisation bioburden. However, a knowledge of 'typical' environmental microflora will not necessarily predict the bioburden of any one specific product batch. Furthermore, while a knowledge of presterilisation bioburden is an essential element in making a final product release decision, it is hardly a practical or sensible proposition to determine a presterilisation bioburden, and then delay sterilisation (with the bioburden multiplying all the while) until laboratory studies on the thermal resistance of that bioburden have been completed, and a sterilisation cycle tailored to suit. In practice, test organisms of known heat resistance (e.g. *B. stearothermophilus*) are used, with a Z value of 10 assumed (Haberer & Wallhaeusser, 1990).

For any attempt at the validation of a steam sterilisation process to yield meaningful and reliable information, it is an essential prerequisite that the steriliser (autoclave) has been properly designed and built, has been properly installed, been supplied with all necessary services (including steam of the required quality), is fitted with instruments (temperature and pressure gauges) of known accuracy and precision, and is functioning as desired and intended. That is, it must be qualified in terms both of installation and operation. It is also essential that it is subject to a programme of planned preventative maintenance (PPM), aimed at ensuring that it remains at the same operational standard as at the time of process validation. Data acquired during process validation are invalid in relation to a steriliser which has subsequently been modified, or which has deteriorated operationally.

It is crucial to the success of steam sterilisation processes that instruments and devices used to control a process and to measure critical process parameters are regularly calibrated in accordance with a predetermined calibration programme, and that the autoclave and all attendant equipment, instruments and devices are all subject to a planned preventative maintenance (PPM) programme.

The calibration programme should concentrate particularly on instruments and devices used in the measurement and control of:

* Time
* Temperature
* Pressure.

Calibration records should be maintained, for each instrument or device, that include:

* The make and serial number of the instrument.
* The autoclave to which it is related, or on which it is installed.
* Date of calibration.
* Date of previous calibration.
* Reference to procedure followed.
* Calibration standard instruments used, and their certification.

- Tolerances applied, and any adjustments made.
- Result.
- Signature.
- Calibration interval and next calibration due-date.

The programme for PPM should specifically define daily, weekly, quarterly, half-yearly and yearly maintenance activities.

Heat distribution and heat penetration studies

These are performed by using heat-sensing probes, normally thermocouples, connected to an electronic recording instrument. The most commonly employed thermocouples are Teflon-coated copper/constan (Type T). Resistance temperature detectors (RTDs) have been used. They are sensitive, but are not sufficiently corrosion-resistant for regular use in autoclaves. Before and after each use, it is essential that the thermocouples be calibrated. This can be done by immersing the probe tips in a water and/or heating bath along with a certified reference standard thermometer immersed to the same depth. The use of two reference temperatures is recommended: 0°C (ice/water bath) and around 120–125°C (oil or glycerol bath). Calibration equipment, designed for just this purpose is also commercially available. The recorder readings at the reference temperature(s) are compared with those of the reference thermometer, and the recorder adjusted to bring the temperature sensed by each probe in line with the reference thermometer. The accuracy of the thermocouples should be ±0.5°C. Thermocouples which do not display that level of accuracy, as compared to the reference thermometer reading, should be checked for bad connections, shorts and the like. If the problem cannot be resolved they should be discarded.

Initial heat distribution studies are often performed on an empty chamber, to investigate if and where any cold spot or spots are to be found. Between 10 and 20 thermocouples should be used per cycle, distributed throughout the chamber in a predetermined (and recorded) pattern. The probes can be temporarily fixed to the chamber walls by means of adhesive tape capable of withstanding the sterilising conditions. (Rightly or wrongly, autoclave tape is often used.) Great care is necessary to ensure that the thermocouple tips make no contact with the chamber wall, or with any other metallic object. Around 10 to 20 thermocouples should be used per cycle. It has been suggested (Akers and Anderson) that two probes from the set should remain, for reference, outside the chamber, each immersed in one of the two temperature baths.

Following the empty chamber studies, further cycles are run with full, half and minimum loads in order to study the effects of chamber loads on the location of the cold spot(s). The difference between the temperature at the coldest spot and the mean chamber temperature should not exceed ±2.5°C.

Following the heat distribution studies, heat penetration studies should be performed. The successful validation of a steam sterilisation cycle depends upon being able to demonstrate the delivery of the desired F_0 to the coldest part of the coldest article located at the cold spot(s) determined in the heat distribution studies. To this end, thermocouple probes are inserted into containers of liquid products, or into packages of devices or dressings, or deep into items of equipment. Further probes located in the chamber close to the articles with probes inserted should also be used. The crucial issue is whether or not the F_0 achieved in the coldest part of the coldest item in the coldest location is equal at least to the value required to ensure the desired level of probability of micro-organism survival (or its inverse 'sterility assurance level'). If it is not then it is necessary to redesign the time/temperature cycle.

The use of BIs, in addition to physical methods, is fairly common, and, as noted, some regulatory authorities have required it as a component of the process validation of steam sterilisation. The most commonly used are preparations of the heat-resistant spores of *B. stearothermophilus*. It is necessary that, before use, the D_{121} and Z values, and the number of organisms present be accurately known. Because of potential changes in storage, it is necessary to experimentally determine D values, whether the BIs have been purchased, or prepared in-house.

Similar heat distribution and heat penetration studies to those outlined above are performed on cycles based upon overkill, compendial or simplified approaches, without the need to become over-concerned with thermal death-rates and F_0 values. But it is, of course, necessary to ensure that the time/temperature cycle employed does not degrade the product or article being sterilised.

Validation of dry heat sterilisation cycles

Dry heat sterilisation takes two main forms: sterilisation using the conventional hot air oven, and sterilisation by means of a sterilising tunnel. A major difference from a validation aspect is the additional variable introduced by the conveyor system in the tunnel, which may operate at different speeds, either by intention or inadvertence. The basic validation objectives are the same as for steam sterilisation. That is to ensure that, repeatably, under all normal conditions of use, all items being treated reach the required temperature (which as we have seen will be higher than for steam sterilisation) for the required time, and thus to render them sterile. Often there is the ad-ditional objective of rendering them pyrogen-free.

As ever an essential prerequisite is that the oven or tunnel has been properly designed and built, has been properly installed, been supplied with all necessary services, fitted with instruments of known accuracy and precision, and is functioning as desired and intended. It is also essential that the equipment is subject to a programme of planned preventative maintenance (PPM), aimed at ensuring that it remains at the same operational standard as at the time of the process validation. Data acquired during process validation are invalid in relation to equipment which has subsequently been modified, or which has deteriorated operationally. Examples of engineering aspects which need to be investigated, specified, and maintained under control before, during and after the process validation are:

- Hot air oven

    — Air intake system and filtration.
    — Air exhaust system and filtration.
    — Fan speeds and internal air circulation.
    — Stability of current to fan(s) and heaters.
    — Functioning of heaters.
    — Temperature sensing/measuring/indicating devices.
    — Integrity of door seals.

- Sterilising tunnel

    — Relative air pressures at entrance and exit.
    — Filtration of cooling and exhaust air.
    — Current to heaters and fans.
    — Functioning of heaters.
    — Control of conveyor speed.
    — Particulate control (in tunnel and on exit to clean room).

In a hot air oven, heat distribution and heat penetration studies can be performed in a manner similar to that employed in relation to steam sterilisation. Temperature variation throughout a load should not exceed $\pm 5°C$. If biological validation is performed, in addition to physical methods, the indicator organisms commonly used, and recommended by the pharmacopoeias, are spores of *B. subtilis* var. *niger*.

Validation of a sterilisation tunnel, although based upon the same principles, presents some additional challenges. There is the question of the airflow within the tunnel, which must be carefully balanced to ensure that validation and routine use conditions remain constant. It must be possible closely to control, and maintain under control, conveyor speed, and hence time of exposure. Heat distribution and penetration studies are performed using calibrated thermocouples, with leads sufficiently long to allow transportation (and subsequent recovery) along the entire length of the tunnel. To avoid a 'bird's nest' of wires some form of harness will probably be necessary to keep things neat and tidy.

Validation of ethylene oxide sterilisation

The success, or failure, of an ethylene oxide (EtO) sterilisation process is dependent on the interaction of five physical variables – EtO concentration, humidity, temperature, time and pressure/vacuum – in addition to such biological variables as bioburden and EtO resistance of bioburden. That is why considerable emphasis needs to be placed upon equipment qualification, maintenance and control, and also why microbiological monitoring by use of BIs is usually considered necessary both in process validation, and in routine manufacture.

An EtO cycle must be designed taking into account the chemical and physical nature of the product or material to be sterilised, and the nature and EtO-permeability of its packaging. Careful attention needs to be given to the calibration of the instruments used to monitor the conditions within the sterilising chamber – heat-sensing thermocouples and recorders, humidity sensors and recorders, pressure gauges and recorders, gas chromatography instrumentation for determination of EtO concentration within the chamber, and timer controls.

Preliminary heat distribution studies should be performed on the empty chamber, in order to determine cold spot(s) and thus the crucial locations for subsequent loaded chamber heat penetration runs. The final step is to perform a series of cycles (minimum of three) on a fully loaded chamber (load defined as for routine manufacture) using both thermocouples and BIs. In the validation of EtO sterilisation, the use of BIs is usually considered mandatory, and not an optional extra. (Note that the pharmacopoeias require, for EtO sterilisation, the use of BIs in each routine manufacturing load.) The recommended BI is spores of *B. subtilis* var. *niger*. These should be placed within the load (with emphasis on the previously determined cold spots), at a rate of around 10 BIs per 100 cubic foot of chamber space, at the same locations as the thermocouples. Throughout the test runs the temperature(s), humidity, gas concentration, and pressure should all be carefully monitored and recorded. The process may be considered validated if it can be shown that, in all the test runs, the desired conditions were achieved throughout the load, and that all the indicator organisms were destroyed.

Validation of radiation sterilisation processes

The dose of sterilising radiation delivered to a load depends upon the strength of the source, the distance of the load from the source, the density (in radiation penetration terms) of any material between the load and the source, and the total exposure time. In Britain and in Europe generally, the minimum required dose is 25 kGy, although some other countries have specified higher doses. Physical process validation consists of performing test runs with calibrated dosimeters inserted throughout the load so as to ensure that the required lethal dose is delivered to the entire load. Biological indicator organisms of a suitable D value may also be used. In the context of radiation sterilisation, D value is defined as the dose of radiation required to produce a 90% reduction in the number of organisms. The pharmacopoeias recommend spores of *Bacillus pumilus*, each indicator preparation to carry at least 1×10^7 viable spores.

Validation of cleaning procedures

Unless otherwise stated the term 'cleaning procedures' is generally taken to mean, in the context of validation, procedures for the cleaning of equipment.

The FDA's *Guide to Inspections of Validation of Cleaning Processes* (US FDA, 1993) quite clearly refers only to equipment cleaning. The prime motive is to ensure that procedures used for cleaning are adequate to ensure the very minimum possibility of contamination of one product by another. Along with mix-ups with printed packaging materials, cross-contamination is one of the major reasons for product recall, and the major cause of cross-contamination is product residues inadequately cleaned from manufacturing equipment.

The essential preliminary is that there are authorised written procedures. It is totally impossible to validate procedures that are conceptual, all in the mind, *ad hoc* or rule of thumb. Written procedures are needed for each piece, or type, of equipment. If different approaches are adopted for cleaning between batches of the same product, as compared with cleaning between batches of different product, then these both should be clearly covered in the written procedure(s), as should the measures taken to remove traces of any agents (detergents, solvents) used in the cleaning process. The validation of the cleaning processes, implemented in accordance with these written cleaning procedures, should be subject to the same documentation requirements as outlined in Chapter 22. It is generally considered that equipment cleaning between batches of the same product may be considered adequate if the equipment is visibly clean, with no further validation required, a view endorsed by the FDA (see US FDA, 1993).

A traditional method for measuring the effectiveness of a cleaning process has been to sample the final rinse liquid and examine the sample in the laboratory for traces of the previous product or material. While still used, this method has of late encountered some disfavour.

Currently the more favoured method is direct surface sampling, using swab samples taken from defined areas (say 100 cm^2) at defined locations. The advantage of swab sampling (which can also be used to evaluate surface microbial contamination) is that it enables the targeting of the more obviously difficult-to-clean surfaces. The disadvantages are that the more difficult-to-clean surfaces may well be the most inaccessible, and may require a level of disassembly which would not occur in routine manufacture (thus introducing variables not encountered routinely). The very use of swabs may, in itself, also introduce chemical and/or microbial contamination.

A third method, which some manufacturers have employed, is to manufacture a placebo batch in the cleaned equipment, under the same conditions as normal, and then examine samples of the placebo for contamination. This is hardly a very good idea, not least from the aspect of the cost in terms of time, effort and money.

Acceptance criteria

Not for the first time, a problem is encountered when it comes to the determination of acceptance criteria for validation studies. (It seems strange that, in the context of all the fuss and noise that has been made about validation, in at least two major validation areas – aseptic process validation and cleaning process validation – there is a notable degree of indeterminacy over the criteria to be adopted for deciding whether or not a process has been validated.) The FDA avoids the issue by declaring that it 'does not intend to set acceptance specifications . . .' (US FDA, 1993). Suggestions that have been offered (Cook, FDA, McCormick and Cullen) include levels of contamination which would consistently ensure no more than 10 ppm of the contaminant in subsequent batches of product, or to not more than 1/1000th of the minimum daily dose of the contaminant in the maximum daily dose of subsequent products.

Computer systems validation

Although the expression 'computer systems validation' is commonly used and heard it needs to be realised that it is not only mainframe computer hardware and software which needs to validated, but all computer/microprocessor control systems. Thus, better expressions would be 'validation of automated systems' or 'validation of computer-related systems'.

The validation process should establish documentary evidence which provides a high degree of assurance that an automated system will consistently function as specified and designed, and that any manufacturing process involving the automated system will consistently yield a product of the required and intended quality.

User specifications for both the hard- and software which comprise an overall system should be subject to design review and qualification, to ensure that the system will be, and remain, fit for the purpose intended. This design review/qualification should include a careful consideration of potential system failures, and of the possibility (and the consequences) of any undetected system failure which could adversely affect product quality.

Hardware must be:

1. Suitable, and of sufficient capacity, for the tasks required of it.
2. Capable of operating, not merely under test conditions, but also under worst case production conditions (e.g. at top machine speed, high data input, high or continuous usage).

Hardware should be tested to confirm the above, with the tests repeated enough times to ensure an acceptable level of consistency and reproducibility. Hardware validation and revalidation studies should be documented, in accordance with the basic documentation requirements outlined in Chapter 22.

Software should be validated to ensure that it consistently performs as intended. Test conditions should simulate worst case production conditions, e.g. of process speed, data volume and frequency. Tests should be repeated a sufficient number of times to ensure consistent and reliable performance. Software validation and revalidation studies must be documented as for hardware validation.

Much of the necessary microprocessor/computer hardware and software validation may well be performed by the machine, hardware or software supplier. However, it must be stressed that the final responsibility for the suitability and reliability of any automated system used in pharmaceutical manufacture must rest with the pharmaceutical manufacturer.

Manufacturers should obtain (and retain) from the relevant third party sufficient data (specifications, programmes, protocols, test data, conclusions, etc.) to satisfy themselves, and any enquiring regulatory body, that adequate validation work has been carried out to assure system suitability.

For those involved, or interested, in automated systems in pharmaceutical manufacturing, see *GAMP (Good Automated Manufacturing Practice) Supplier Guide for Validation of Automated Systems in Pharmaceutical Manufacture* (GAMP, 1998) and the PDA's *Validation of Computer-Related Systems* (PDA, 1995).

References

Akers M, Anderson N (1993). Sterilisation validation of sterile products. In: Berry and Nash (eds), *Pharmaceutical Process Validation,* 2nd edn. New York: Dekker.

Cook R S (1994). Validation. In: Lund W (ed.), *The Pharmaceutical Codex: Principles and practice of pharmaceutics,* 12th edn. London: Pharmaceutical Press.

GAMP (1998). *GAMP Supplier Guide for Validation of Automated Systems in Pharmaceutical Manufacture,* Version 3.0. The Hague: GAMP Forum.

Haberer K, Wallhaeusser K-H (1990). Assurance of sterility by validation of the sterilization process. In: Denyer and Baird, eds, *Guide to Microbial Control in Pharmaceuticals.* New York: Ellis Horwood.

McCormick P, Cullen L (1993). Cleaning validation. In: Berry and Nash, eds, *Pharmaceutical Process Validation,* 2nd edn. New York: Dekker.

PDA (1978). Validation of steam sterilisation cycles. *PDA Technical Monograph No. 1.* Philadelphia: Parenteral Drug Association.

PDA (1995). Validation of computer-related systems. Technical Report No. 18. *PDA J Pharm Sci Technol* 49 (Suppl).

PDA (1996). Process simulation testing for aseptically filled products. Technical Report No. 22. *PDA J Pharm Sci Technol* 50 (Suppl 1).

Prout G (1982). Validation and routine operation of a sterile dry powder filling facility. *J Parenter Sci Technol* 36 (5), 199.

Prout G, ed. (1993). The use of process simulation tests in the evaluation of processes for the manufacture of sterile products. Technical Monograph No.4. Swindon: Parenteral Society.

Soper C J (1994). Sterilisation. In: Lund W (ed.), *The Pharmaceutical Codex: Principles and practice of pharmaceutics,* 12th edn. London: Pharmaceutical Press.

Soper C, Davies D (1990). Principles of sterilization. In: Denyer and Baird (eds), *Guide to Microbial Control in Pharmaceuticals.* New York: Ellis Horwood.

Stumbo C (1973). *Thermobacteriology in Food Processing,* 2nd edn. New York: Academic Press.

US FDA (1987). *Guideline on Sterile Drug Products Produced by Aseptic Processing.* Rockville, MD: US Food and Drug Administration.

US FDA (1993). *Guide to Inspections of Validation of Cleaning Processes.* Rockville, MD: US Food and Drug Administration.

Part Eight

Self-inspection/quality audit and
other techniques

24

Self-inspection and quality audit

Thou turn'st mine eyes into my very soul
W Shakespeare, *Hamlet*, Act 3, Sc. 4

Why audit? There are two very good reasons for performing quality audits. These are because:

- It is a regulatory requirement.
- It is a good and sensible thing to do.

Definitions

The International Standards Organisation has defined a quality audit thus (ISO 8402: 1986 'Quality vocabulary'):

Quality audit

A systematic and independent examination to determine whether quality activities and related results comply with planned arrangements, and whether these arrangements are implemented effectively and are suitable to achieve objectives.

In addition to its appearance in the ISO 'Quality vocabulary', this definition is also repeated in a number of other ISO documents, e.g. the ISO 9000 series. It is rather vague and makes no mention of the crucial issue of what is to be done as follow-up to the audit.

By comparison, a definition offered by the European Organisation for Quality (EOQ) was relatively laconic:

Quality audit

A systematic and independent examination of the Quality System or of its parts.

The use of the definite article ('the') is odd. What is *the* Quality System one might ask; is there only one?

The UK Department of Health's publication *Quality Systems for Sterile Medical Devices and Surgical Products* (the 'Blue Guide'; 1990), contains the following, which is similar to the ISO definition:

Internal quality audits

The supplier shall carry out a comprehensive system of planned and documented internal quality audits to verify whether quality activities comply with planned arrangements, and to determine the effectiveness of the quality system.

The second edition (1985) of the French national GMP Guide ('Bonnes Pratique de Fabrication' or BPF, since superseded by the Euro-harmonised third edition) provided the following two definitions (author's translation):

Self-inspection consists of a periodic detailed examination of conditions and working procedures by a team from the production site, with the aim of verifying that good pharmaceutical manufacturing practices are being applied and to propose any necessary corrective measures to responsible management.

and

A *quality audit* consists of an examination and an evaluation of all or part of a system of quality assurance. It must be carried out by a specialist or a team designated for this purpose. It may be extended, as necessary, to suppliers and sub-contractors.

These two, taken together, are useful definitions which do make the important point that one of the objectives is to propose corrective methods. It is not, however, explicitly stated that there is a need to ensure that the proposed corrective steps are, in fact, taken – and that if they are not, the whole point of the exercise is lost. A perhaps inappropriate distinction is also drawn between a 'self-inspection' and a 'quality audit'. It is more logical to consider 'self-inspection' as a sub-class of the more general class 'quality audit', and thence derive the following classification of audit types:

1. Imposed *upon* manufacturer or supplier

    (a) Regulatory
    (b) Customer, or potential customer
    (c) Third-party (on behalf of customer).

2. Performed *by* manufacturer

    (a) Internal (i.e. self-inspection)

        — overall
        — departmental
        — product-orientated
        — system-orientated.

    (b) External, e.g.

        — of supplier
        — of contract manufacturer

— of contract packager
— of contract warehouse/distributor.

Some have variously drawn a distinction between an inspection and an audit, but it is difficult to see why any such distinction is necessary. The exercise can vary in length, depth and intensity as circumstances dictate, and the only distinction necessary is 'internal' vs 'external', and even then the ultimate objectives are similar.

Regulatory requirements

The regulatory requirement for the performance of *internal* quality audits is clear and unequivocal in both the European GMP Directive (91/356/EEC, Article 14) and the EC GMP Guide. The issue does not appear to be addressed in the US CGMPs for either drug products or for medical devices. The European GMP Directive (91/356/EEC, Article 14) states:

> *Self-Inspection:* The manufacturer shall conduct repeated self-inspections as part of the quality assurance system in order to monitor the implementation and respect of Good Manufacturing practice, and to propose any necessary corrective measures. Records of such self-inspections and any subsequent corrective action shall be maintained.

It is unclear what is meant by 'repeated' (every hour, or once every 50 years?), but that is what the directive says.

The EC GMP Guide states in its first chapter ('Quality management', 1.2) that the system of quality assurance should ensure that:

> ix   There is a procedure for self-inspection and/or quality audit which regularly appraises the effectiveness and applicability of the quality assurance system.

Again, 'regularly' is ambiguous, and the intended meaning of 'applicability' unclear. There also would appear to be only the one ('the') quality assurance system.

EC GMP Guide, Chapter 9, 'Self-inspection'

In addition to the above statement, the EC GMP Guide devotes a whole short chapter to self-inspection, thus:

> Principle: Self-inspections should be conducted in order to monitor the implementation and the respect of Good Manufacturing Practice (GMP) principles and to propose necessary corrective measures.

> 9.1   Personnel matters, premises, equipment, documentation, production, distribution of the medicinal products, arrangements for dealing with complaints and recalls, and self-inspection, should be examined at intervals following a pre-arranged programme in order to verify their conformity with the principles of Quality Assurance.

9.2   Self-inspections should be conducted in an independent and detailed way by designated competent person(s) from the company. Independent audits by external experts may also be useful.

9.3   All self-inspections should be recorded. Reports should contain all the observations made during the inspections and, where applicable, proposals for corrective measures. Statements on the actions subsequently taken should also be recorded.

This short chapter from the EC GMP Guide embraces a number of important, key, auditing issues, namely:

- 'Pre-arranged programme' (i.e. *planned* not impromptu).
- 'Independent' (presumably means *unbiased*).
- Conducted 'by competent persons'.
- 'Record'.
- 'All observations'.
- Make 'proposals for corrective measures'.
- 'Record all actions subsequently taken'.

Regulatory statements on *external* audits in EC/UK guidelines are sparse, but there are passages where the need to perform external quality audits is inferred, as in the following examples.

UK Orange Guide (1983)

Appendix 4 ('Identity of Starting Materials'), 1c, should be based on:

... purchasing company's own assessment of [the supplier's] QA systems and procedures.

Appendix 5 ('Avoidance of mislabelling and similar errors') states:

2.   Measures which will help to avoid labelling errors include:

(c)   An understanding (from first-hand knowledge) by the pharmaceutical manufacturer of his printer's facilities and procedures, and of the precautions taken in the print-shop to avoid mix-up ...'

EC GMP Guide

5.25   The purchase of starting materials ... should involve staff who have a particular and thorough knowledge of suppliers.

5.26   Starting materials should only be purchased from approved suppliers ...

5.40   The purchase of ... packaging ... materials should be accorded similar attention.

The reasons for quality auditing

These may be summarised as follows.

1.   Internal – in order to:

- Determine the level of compliance.
- Build confidence (one hopes) in GMP and the QA system.
- Build inter-departmental trust, understanding and communication (if the audit is done properly and tactfully).
- Determine measures necessary to improve, e.g.

    — premises, equipment, environment
    — operations, actions, procedures
    — personnel/training.

- Provide a stimulus for improvement.
- Recommend corrective action.
- Monitor improvement.

2.   External – in order to:

- Establish and monitor capability of supplier and/or contractor to deliver goods and services that are fit for purpose (and on time, and in the quantity required).
- Build mutual confidence.
- Promote understanding and communication between the parties involved (both sides can learn).
- And, generally, as listed for 'Internal'.

Steps to performing a quality audit

A fundamental prerequisite for the successful performance of any quality audit is the availability of competent, trained auditors. Given their availability, the key steps are:

- Plan/prepare
- Arrange/announce (?)
- Arrive at site of audit/meet/explain purpose
- Perform audit
- Sum up
- Formal report, with recommendations
- Follow up.

The only one of these steps against which there is a question mark is the issue of whether or not the auditor(s) should announce, in advance to the auditee, their intention to audit at a stated time. In general, the only good reason to spring an audit would be when a regulatory body wants to try to catch a manufacturer suspected of improper practices. For non-regulatory audits (internal or external) it can be said that there is more to be gained from announcing intentions in advance (availability of key staff, co-operative attitude, etc.) and, potentially much is to be lost (possible non-availability of staff, lack of cooperation and resentment) by failing to do so.

The tools of the auditor

In planning and preparing to audit, certain tools are available (or should be) to the auditor:

1.   Documents:

   •   Quality/GMP regulations, standards and guidelines (local, national and international).
   •   Previous audit and follow-up reports.
   •   Auditee's own documents and records.
   •   Audit checklists/*aides-mémoir*.

2.   The auditor's own faculties and abilities – eyes and ears, thoughts and expressions, character, etc.
3.   The auditing plan, its preparation and its quality.

To consider some of these 'tools' in a little more detail, examples of the 'quality regulations, standards and guidelines' are:

1.   Local (or 'corporate') e.g.

   •   Audited company's own internal regulations, codes of practice and guidelines.
   •   Their quality manual (if one exists).
   •   Their site master file (if there is one).

2.   National, e.g.:

   •   UK Medicines Act and Regulations
   •   UK Orange Guide (medicinal products)
   •   UK Blue Guide (sterile devices)
   •   US CGMPs
   •   French BPF.

3.   International, e.g.

   •   WHO GMP Guide
   •   EC GMP Directive (91/356)
   •   EC GMP Guide
   •   EC Devices Directive
   •   PIC GMP Guide
   •   ISO 9000 Series
   •   the Pharmaceutical Supplier Codes of Practice.

The important thing here is to determine and agree, on all sides, the guideline, regulation or standard against which the audit is, or will be, performed. An audit which is performed against a vaguely notional, general concept of quality is hardly likely to be successful, or of any great use.

Checklists

Another possible auditing tool is the checklist. A number of 'off the peg' examples have appeared in both commercial and official publications. Some include a points-scoring system, with scores being accumulated to make a pass or fail decision.

There are both advantages and disadvantages to the use of checklists. The advantages are that they keep the auditor's mind on the job in hand, and force a structured approach. They provide a way of making notes, in short form and in a structured manner. They also can provide a prop for the tyro auditor who, under pressure, may become uneasy about what to ask, or look at, next. The disadvantages are that they tend to be inflexible, and the audit (because of a company's geographical, functional and administrative structure) may not 'happen' in the same order as the checklist. That is, the structure of the checklist may not reflect the structure on the ground. The checklist may also become the auditor's master rather than his servant. There is a danger of spending more time on completing the checklist than on looking, seeing and listening, and thus failing to see the quality 'wood' for the checklist 'trees'.

The awarding of marks for each item on the checklist, which are then added together in order to make a 'pass' or 'fail' decision is a dubious activity unless appropriate weightings are given to the specific elements. For example, the presence of litter on the factory surrounds, although indicative, is clearly not as critical as an inadequately validated sterilisation cycle.

If a prop is felt necessary, any checklist should be as brief and as simple as possible. Form 24.1 gives an example of part of a simple checklist.

The auditor

In the achievement of the objectives of an audit, and to ensure that it is well and effectively conducted, the most important of the tools listed above is the auditor himself, and his eyes, ears, brain, character and communication skills. It is thus worth asking the question: 'What sort of person makes a good quality auditor or inspector?'

Some people have a natural talent for the job, while others will never be any good at it. In the middle there is a fair-sized group of people who, if they put their minds to it and have the relevant knowledge, *and* gain the relevant experience, will make a reasonable job of it. The essential qualities of a good auditor are:

- An appropriate range and depth of knowledge, both of QA/GMP and of the relevant technology.
- Range and depth of relevant experience.
- Good powers of observation.
- An enquiring, yet open, mind.
- Ability to think on his or her feet.
- Articulate – good communication skills.

GMP AUDIT NOTES

DISPENSARY

Area/Site Audited .... By .... Date ....

(A+ = Good, A = Acceptable, B = Unacceptable, C = Immediate Action)

	Rating	Comments
Gen. Cleanliness & Good Order – Written Cleaning Procs.?		
Security/ Controlled Access		
Materials/Goods stored/handled/ identified so as to prevent damage, contam., deter., loss or mix-up?		
Protection of goods against: – Weather – Vermin – Pilferage		
Personnel – Adeqt. Number? – Dress – Training/ Awareness		
Written Procs. (Receipt/Storage Issue/Recording)		

Page 1 of 2

	Rating	Comments
Are Procs. Followed?		
"Safety Manual"		
Can only Appvd. Materials be Dispensed?		
Resealing/security of Bulk after disp.		
Control of bulk-balance after disp.		
Double check on Weigh/measure.		
Recording: – Dispensary Recs. – B.M.R.		
Containers for Dispd. Mats. (Suitable/clean/labelling)		
Calibration/Checking of balances and measures		
Dust. Extractn. & Cont. of X-CON		
Dispensing Tools (scoops/spatulas/measures) Condition/Cleanliness/Storage		

- 'Unflappability' – able to stay cool.
- Ability to take a constructive approach.
- Able to make sound judgements on the matters observed.
- Able to be persistent, yet patient and diplomatic, in pursuit of the objectives of the audit.
- Able to *listen.*
- Of good health.

Many of these are obvious. It is important for an auditor to understand that there may well be ways for a manufacturer to achieve the desired quality objectives, other than those with which he/she (the auditor) is familiar. He/she should be prepared to listen patiently and sympathetically to explanations offered, and to make a sound, open-minded judgement on the validity of those explanations. Whatever happens he/she must be able to stay calm, and not enter into contentious argument. Quality auditing can be both mentally and physically demanding. It is not a job for the unfit or infirm.

The personal skills and qualities required of an auditor are thus extensive, although many of them, if not innate, can be acquired or developed. It is important, however, that no person who is entirely unsuited to the job, or to whom it is anathema, should be coerced into doing it. An unwilling auditor is a bad auditor. Possibly even worse is the type of person who sees the job as a means of satisfying their appetite for power.

Audit planning and preparation

Given a competent auditor, or auditing team, the success (or failure) of an audit in achieving its objectives much depends on the quality of the advance planning and preparation. It is vital that all concerned are aware of type and objectives, and the date and time, of the audit, and of the areas and/or systems to be covered. If the audit is to be performed by a team, then the team leader or lead spokesman should be decided in advance.

It is important to learn as much as possible (and to think as much as possible) about the site/area to be audited, in advance.

Audit preparation checklist

Taking these various points together the following audit preparation checklist may be set down:

○ Agree date and time of audit.

○ Clarify and communicate objectives and the standard, regulation or guideline against which audit will be performed.

○ Decide type of audit and auditing strategy (see below).

○   Define areas/systems to be covered.

○   Inform auditee.

○   Obtain and review details of site/area to be audited, e.g.

— site/area plans or drawings;
— personnel organisation charts;
— products manufactured;
— quality manual, or site master file (if available);
— any available records of complaints and recalls;
— any reports of previous audits and follow-up records.

○   Prepare a structure for note-taking, or devise a checklist.

○   Hold final team briefing meeting.

Auditing strategies

A number of different possible approaches to conducting an audit, or audit strategies, have been proposed. These may be summarised as follows:

- Forward trace, i.e. following production flow from receipt of goods or materials to despatch, or delivery to next department.
- Backward trace i.e. the reverse of the above.
- Product-orientated audit.
- Documentation-based audit.
- Problem-orientated (e.g. centred around complaints or recalls, and any corrective action taken).
- System-based audit.
- Completely random (??).

Mixes of strategies are entirely possible. By far the commonest, and most simple and logical approach is the first ('forward trace'). It can be applied to an entire manufacturing site, or to a single department. A normal logical workflow is followed from where it starts to where it ends. Doing things in reverse ('backward trace') has had its advocates, but it is difficult to see any advantages, and it surely makes the task more difficult for the auditor(s). There is absolutely no merit in a completely random approach, unless the main objective is all-round confusion.

A product-orientated approach is a perfectly viable option. Here the focus is on just one product, or family of similar products. It leads to an intense, in-depth concentration on the manufacture of just that one product (or family), but it is vitally important to remember that it is also necessary to evaluate other, more general, departments or functions (e.g. stores, dispensary, laboratories, data processing) for their impact on the quality of that product.

An audit can be documentation-based, as favoured by the FDA. Such an approach is easy on the feet, but of limited value in terms of getting to grips with the whole quality picture. Other workable audit types can be problem-orientated (a special case, when a known problem needs to be investigated to discover causes and to propose corrective action), or directed at a system (e.g. water supply and quality, air supply, engineering, computer systems).

Arriving and starting

All necessary arrangements and preparations having been made, back-ground information gathered and strategies determined, auditors arrive at the site or the department to be audited. They should arrive:

- On time
- Well organised
- Well prepared.

They should aim to look smart in appearance, with a well-mannered, pro-fessional style and approach that is sensitive to the thoughts, feelings, atti-tudes, procedures, safety/security requirements, and indeed the 'culture', of the people to be audited.

The opening meeting

There will be, or should be, some form of opening meeting. This is likely to be more formal at an external than at an internal audit. A suggested agenda for this meeting is:

- Introductions (audit team/the auditees).
- Auditors explain purpose/objectives.
- Meet those who will be escorting the auditors/responding to their questions.
- Auditors enquire of company rules, work practices and the like (if this is an unfamiliar site).
- Agree programming/timing.

Here is also the chance to establish good working relationships between the two sides, and also to gather general information (e.g. site size and geogra-phy, manufacturing capability/capacity, product types and range, any con-tract work or services used or supplied), if this is not already known.

Style and conduct of audit

The manner and style in which the audit is conducted bears heavily on the success (or failure) of the audit. Auditors should be themselves and not act out a role. It can be fatal to pretend to know more than you do, and then be caught out. Although an essential air of seriousness should pervade, a little leavening of humour can help things along. But it should be remembered that what sounds funny to some people could be offensive to others. Under no circumstances should an auditor mock or ridicule any person, system or institution, no matter how ludicrous they, or it, may seem to be.

Within the bounds of normal politeness, and while keeping as far as possible to the agreed programme, auditors should aim to lead, rather than be led. That is, they should persistently but patiently seek to see what they came to see, and not just those things the escort(s) want to show them.

Questions asked should be pointed, probing, specific and precise, and require a specific answer. Questions in the form 'No doubt you . . .' invite, almost demand, the response 'Yes we do'. Auditors should not necessarily avoid asking the obvious question. They should never think 'Nobody could be that daft or careless'. Unquestionably, someone somewhere could. Where appropriate, evidence should be required of the veracity of responses made to questions asked, or statements made. For example:

Q.   'How often do you check the quality of the water in your ring-main supply?'
A.   'Twice a week.'
Q.   'May I see your record of the results over the past year?'

The value of silence should be remembered. Auditors should wait patiently for the response to their questions. They may not get an adequate answer, but the urge to fill an oral vacuum is a powerful one, and the auditor may well hear something else of interest. A golden rule for auditors is to *listen* harder than they talk. As the audit proceeds, the auditor should make careful notes, and record all relevant data.

A few more points on the personal approach of auditors. They should aim to be constructive, and certainly avoid destructive or personal criticism. An auditor should stay cool and, no matter the provocation, avoid any heated arguments. If an auditor makes a mistake, or misunderstands something, they should admit it, and seek to understand better – rather than cover-up. Under the stress of an intense audit, it is entirely possible to misunderstand something, but this is no crime or slur upon the auditor's competence. Better to clarify things at once, rather than jump to possibly false conclusions. However, it is worth following up hunches, which may well prove not to be as chancy and irrational as at first they may seem. Potentially hazardous malpractices may be unearthed by acting upon a hunch.

Novice auditors will probably have preconceived ideas, based on their own particular training, as to the way things should be done, and in which order. Auditors must be flexible, and not necessarily expect everybody to be doing things in their preconceived way, and in their preferred order. (See the point made above regarding the rigid approach, which can be imposed by checklists.) It is important to remember that it is the end result that matters and be prepared to consider alternative means of achieving the desired quality result.

An interesting and constructive light is shed upon the auditing style and approach outlined above in a recent statement from the European Commission (EC Working Party on Control of Medicines and Inspections, January 1995):

> The task of an inspector is not limited to the disclosure of faults, deficiencies and discrepancies. The inspector should connect an observation with assistance in making the necessary improvements. An inspection should normally include educational and motivating elements.

It is not possible to say whether the inspectorates of all the member states of the EU fully adhere to these precepts, which exemplify the approach of the UK Medicines Inspectorate. It also seems that investigators of the US FDA act differently; their task seemingly being to find, and collect evidence of, 'violations' of the US regulations.

Audit observations

So, what are auditors looking for on an audit? What do they need to see, to learn, to observe, to investigate and take note of? These may be classified under three main headings:

1. Basic general company information.
2. Departmental conditions and practices.
3. Management systems.

General company information

The basic general information that auditors need to have, or acquire, includes plant location and the immediately surrounding environment. For example:

- Are the factory surrounds kept neat, clean and tidy? (Such things may not directly affect product quality, but scruffy grounds are indicative of an attitude.)
- Are there any undesirable activities (sewage works, rubbish tips, etc.) in the immediate vicinity?
- How is the company managed?
- Is the technical, manufacturing and quality management on-site, or is the site managed from afar, and merely an outpost of a large industrial empire?
- Is there a clear and explicit chain of command, made clear in organisation chart(s), with written job descriptions for supervisory and management positions?
- What is the company's training policy, and how is it implemented, programmed and recorded, both in relation to induction and continuing training?

- Where does the company obtain its starting and packaging materials from?
- Does it use contractors to manufacture and/or supply any of its products, or to provide any services (analytical, engineering/maintenance)?
- Does it provide, under contract, any goods or services to other organisations?

Departmental practices

Most medicinal and other healthcare products are manufactured in a series of different departments or sections. Some of the things that auditors need to note are common to all (or most) departments and sections, e.g. security, cleanliness and good order, the physical measures taken to avoid cross-contamination and mix-up, the availability of written procedures, and whether these are being followed. Other departmental points to be noted will be specific to the work of a given department or section, e.g. stores, tablet/capsule manufacture, sterile products, packaging, testing laboratory. Here the auditor's knowledge and understanding of the relevant science, technology and techniques is crucial.

Despite the departmentalised manner in which manufacture tends to proceed, it is important for auditors to avoid a compartmentalised attitude, and to think in terms of the overall picture. In all but the very simplest and smallest of operations, production does tend to progress by the movement of materials, products, and documents from one department to another. Each of the individual departments or sections may be fine in isolation, but how do they all fit together? Is one department supplying the next with what it really wants? And is this second department getting what it thinks it is getting? The auditor should probe the interfaces between departments and attempt to evaluate how the things that one department does, or produces, impacts upon the others.

Systems

The 'systems' that may, or should, be examined include:

- Quality system (of course)
- Overall documentation and document control
- Change control systems
- HVAC (heating, ventilation and air-conditioning)
- Water supply system
- Engineering maintenance
- Plant services generally.

'Diversionary tactics'

It is not unknown for manufactures to attempt to waste auditors' time, so that they become rushed to complete the audit and thus less observant and perceptive, or even to indulge in diversionary tactics. Techniques which have been employed include:

- Delaying the start through prolonging the opening discussion, and requesting an early finish.
- Prolonged tea and coffee breaks.
- Variably timed staff breaks, making it time consuming to summon 'the one who knows the answer'.
- Conducting the auditor the long way round the site.
- Confusing the auditor by surrounding him with many escorts/experts giving lengthy and elaborate explanations which over-exaggerate the complexity of the operation.
- Deliberate planting of minor faults, on the theory that auditors feel that they must justify their existence by finding *some* faults, and having done so, they will then relax.
- Strategically timed fire alarms or drills.
- Taking auditors out for a lavish lunch, by the scenic route.

These, of course, largely apply to external audits, but they do serve to remind potential auditors that they need to beware of deliberate delays and diversions, which some auditees may see as in their short-term interests. The good auditor should stick firmly to the matter in hand.

The concluding summary session

Most audits, of whatever type, conclude with a summary session, which should greatly benefit both parties. This will be the opportunity for auditors to outline their findings, and to make their recommendations; for the auditees to comment and offer explanations (or to challenge as appropriate); and for both parties to agree any necessary corrective action.

The time for the summary session should be agreed in advance, and auditors should strive to keep to that timing, in order to ensure that key auditee personnel will be available and present. Auditors should allow time to organise their notes, so as to be in a position to make a structured presentation of the audit findings. Note that this does not have to be a highly polished performance; it will, inevitably be somewhat off the cuff, but it should be in a logical sequence, with the right degree of emphasis placed upon the most important issues. If the audit has been a team effort, then the auditors should agree a lead spokesman, in advance of the session. There is no reason why the other auditors should not join in, but this should be done in a controlled fashion, with one speaker at a time. The presentation of the audit findings should be factual rather than conjectural. It should be as concise as possible and trivialities avoided. Efforts should be made to reach agreement, on both sides, of the justice of the findings, and on any corrective action which needs to be taken. The auditors should be ready and willing to offer constructive advice.

The audit report

After the audit comes the business of writing the report. This is something that few people like doing, but it must be done, and it is better (and in the end easier) that it is done as soon after the audit as possible, while the experience is fresh in the mind. The report is the auditor's formal record of what was seen, done, heard and agreed. Whether a copy of the full report is sent to those audited, or just a summary of findings and recommendations for corrective action, will be a matter of judgement, depending on circumstances. Thus, the report should written, and a copy (whole or in part) sent to the auditee without delay. It should include all significant, non-trivial findings. It should be well-structured, and be compatible with the oral summary given at the concluding summary session. That is, it should contain no surprises.

A suggested structure for an audit report is:

1. Site/area audited.
2. Date/time of audit.
3. Auditor(s).
4. Objectives/purpose of audit.
5. Personnel encountered (names and positions).
6. Changes since any previous audit (organisation, premises, equipment, procedures, products etc.).
7. Observations – in logical order.
8. Corrective measures requested.
9. Oral responses of auditee.
10. Final conclusions.

Follow-up

The final phase of the audit is the follow-up. It is at least as important as any of the other stages, since there is no point in quality auditing unless any necessary corrective action is taken *and confirmed*. The follow-up could be said to have commenced at the concluding summary session, with the oral requests made and the assurances given. These should be confirmed by written requests, and written assurances from the auditee that the requested corrective actions have been taken. For full and final confirmation a further on-site meeting may be held, combined with a partial or total re-audit.

Corrective action form

For internal audits (and perhaps some external audits) the use of a simple corrective action report (see Form 24.2) is a simple and easy way of requesting action, receiving information on action taken, and keeping track of any follow-up required.

CORRECTIVE ACTION REPORT   Ref. No. ....

To ....   Date ....

During an audit of .... the following
was/were rated as unacceptable/immediate action required:

The following corrective action is recommended:

Signed ....   Date ....

Corrective action taken/comments:

Signed ....   Date ....

Auditor review of corrective action:

Problem resolved .... Action unsatisfactory ....
Follow-up necessary ....

Comments:

Signed ....   Date ....

25

SPC, HACCP and other techniques

We are just statistics, born to consume resources
Horace (65–8 BC)

Statistical process control

Statistical process control (SPC) is currently something of an 'in' topic, apparently seen by some quality experts as a brave new concept. However, it is in essence all rather similar, if not identical, to the more traditional statistical quality control, which some of the same experts hitherto regarded as having now been superseded by quality assurance and then by total quality management.

As its name implies, SPC is about the application of statistical methods to monitor and control processes. Only a brief outline is given here, and for more detailed information see Caplen (1988) and Oakland (1986).

Control charts

A classic application of SPC is the use of control charts. Such charts are based on a reasonable assumption that in any process there will be random variation; that is, it cannot be expected that every item produced by a process will be right on specification. Even when the process is well under control, measurements made on units of a product will vary within a range that is characteristic of the process. The other assumption (also reasonable, but not always warrantable) is that the variations from the process average are distributed in accordance with the normal, Gaussian distribution curve.

In setting up such a control chart for a process, it is first necessary to study the process in detail, to make measurements on the product of that process, to analyse the variation in those measurements, and thus to establish the parameters of the curve which describes the variation in the particular numerical quality (e.g. weight, volume, length, hardness, capacity) which is being studied.

Control charts based on standard deviation, σ

In a normal distribution 68.3% of all readings will fall within ±1 standard deviations (σ) from the mean, 95.5% within ±2σ and 99.7% within ±3σ, the standard deviation being calculated from the square root of the mean of the squared deviations from the mean value, that is:

$$\sigma = \sqrt{\frac{\Sigma(x - \bar{x})^2}{n}}$$

where $(x - \bar{x})$ is the deviation of individual readings (x) from the arithmetical average or mean $(\bar{x})$ and n is the number of readings. Thus, a control chart on which to plot the results of readings (or measurements) taken at intervals of time can be constructed from three parallel lines – the process average, the upper control (or action) limit, and the lower control (or action) limit. Typically, upper and lower control (or action) limits are fixed at ±3σ (Fig. 25.1).

Note that the very act of constructing the chart can have quality assuring implications. For example, the process average may not necessarily be the desirable 'target'. The study may thus reveal a need to revise the process, or re-adjust the equipment. The ±3σ range may be wider than the specification for the product allows, or which has hitherto been considered tolerable. Again, some form of revision or adjustment will be necessary to tighten the limits to say 2.5σ.

A chart constructed in this way is used to plot results of measurements against time. Any result falling within the upper and lower control limits can be considered to result from normal process variation. The process is under control and no action is necessary. If results fall outside these limits, then the process is considered to be out of control. It needs to be adjusted,

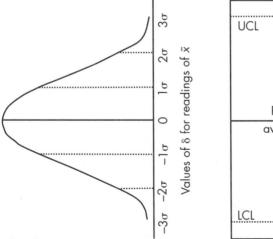
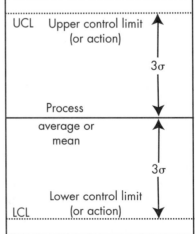

Figure 25.1   Relationship between control limits and a normal distribution curve.

the cause of the abnormal variation determined, and any necessary corrective action taken.

For some purposes, a further pair of control lines is drawn on the chart, say at 2σ deviation from the mean value. The two sets of control lines are called the upper and lower warning limits. A series of results falling between a warning and an action limit may be an indication that the process, while still nominally in control, may be heading out of control.

Control charts based on cumulative sum deviations

Other types of charts have been described and used for different purposes, for example 'CUSUM' (CUmulative SUM) charts on which data are plotted as cumulative sums. Such charts can be useful in highlighting small but persistent changes.

Consider, for example, a filling line set up to fill bottles with 100 ml of liquid. Samples are taken from the line at intervals, the fill volume checked, and the deviation from the required fill recorded (99 ml = −1.0; 102 ml = +2). The cumulative difference is calculated for each sampling interval and recorded as in Table 25.1.

If the cumulative differences, collected over rather more intervals than suggested, are plotted against time, the result will be a cumulative sum curve. If it is a horizontal straight line, it means that the fill is being maintained at an average value equal to the required value. A straight line of positive slope means that the fill has changed to a new steady average level, above the required fill. The steeper the slope the greater the difference. If the slope is negative, the new steady average is below the required level. A curved line (positive or negative) means that the average fill is not steady but is either increasing or decreasing.

In general, these concepts and techniques were largely developed for use in the engineering and parts manufacturing type of industry. Their broad, general application to medicines manufacture is debatable, and is perhaps a field requiring further investigation. There are, however, obvious

Table 25.1   Statistical method of process control using CUSUM values

Observed value (ml)	Standard (ml)	Difference (ml)	Cumulative difference (CUSUM) (ml)
101	100	+1	+1
100	100	0	+1
102	100	+2	+3
101	100	+1	+4
100	100	0	+4
101	100	+1	+5
103	100	+3	+8
102	100	+2	+10
99	100	−1	+9
103	100	+3	+12

applications of control charts in the control of the ongoing manufacture of numbers of discrete units, all of the same nature and type, rather than of bulk masses of material, such as powders, liquids, creams and ointments. Control charts are widely used in tablet and capsule manufacture (tablet and capsule-fill weights) and in packaging (fill weights, numbers and volumes).

Process capability

In this technique, statistical principles are applied in order to determine how capable a process is of producing a product within its specification limits. Not least of its merits is the way it can reveal the folly of setting limits with which a process is incapable of complying.

A process capability index (C_p) indicates the relationship between the variations about a process average (of a process producing a succession of discrete objects, where the variations around that mean can be assumed to be distributed normally) and the difference between the upper and lower tolerance limits predetermined for the products of that process. It may be calculated as:

$$C_p = \frac{(U - L)}{6\sigma}$$

where (U – L) equals the total tolerance, that is the upper minus the lower specification limit, and σ is the standard deviation calculated from values measured on the product of the process.

If (U – L) is greater than 8σ, the process is said to have a high relative capability, with a C_p value greater than 1.33. For consistent quality from a repetitive process a C_p of 1.33 or more is desirable.

If (U – L) is between 6σ and 8σ, corresponding to a C_p of 1.00 to 1.33 the process is said to be of medium relative capability. It will only be possible to remain within specification if the process mean can be held constant and central throughout the run.

If (U – L) is less than 6σ, giving a C_p of less than 1.0, the process is of low relative capability, that is the distribution curve is too wide to fit within the specification limits, and out-of-specification products are inevitable. There are two possible courses of action to take in this unsatisfactory situation: (a) reduce the process variability by improving (or installing new) equipment, improving materials, or method of manufacture, or some other aspect of the process (e.g. training of operators), or (b) widening the specification limits.

Again the concept is more applicable to the engineering industry, for example, to the machining of a series of metal cylinders, with defined tolerances for diameter. Assuming that measurements of diameter are normally distributed and thus fall within $\pm 3\sigma$ of the mean (i.e. the process average), if the required product tolerance range (or 'specification-width') is equivalent to 6 of those standard deviations, then the process capability is 6/(2 × 3) = 1; there is therefore no room for slipping of the mean. If the tolerance-range is 8σ then the process capability factor is 1.33 (8/6). If 10σ it is 1.67 (10/6), and so on. Thus, this is a useful concept when applied to the control of dimensional variables of serially manufactured machine parts and the like. It has little or no relevance to much of pharmaceutical manufacture, but it has been used in relation to tablet and capsule fill weights, and the control of fill volumes or weights on packaging lines. There are obvious applications in the manufacture of a number of devices.

Parametric release

Parametric release has been discussed, in relation to sterile products, in Chapter 20. It may be wondered to what extent is the concept applicable to the manufacture and release of other types of product.

 This is an issue which has been much debated. It would be difficult to argue against the essential 'rightness' of so-called parametric release in the context of terminally heat-sterilised products, and in the knowledge of the fundamental weakness of the traditional sterility test. However it does need to be noted that we are here talking of a single characteristic (sterility) of just one very specific type of product (terminally heat-sterilised sterile products). Even so, only relatively few manufacturers of such products have as yet adopted this 'parametric release' approach and abandoned sterility testing altogether. Other manufacturers are more cautious, and whilst they no doubt comply with the preconditions specified for parametric release (see Chapter 20), they continue to carry out sterility testing. A number of major manufacturers have explored the extension of the concept to other areas of manufacture, and for a period it provided a lucrative topic for some seminar organisers. Currently (late 1998), it seems to have gone rather quiet, and although, in the UK for example, the MCA have indicated their willingness to consider applications to approve the release of products (of any type) 'parametricly', the response has apparently been minimal.

 At the time of writing, the European Agency for the Evaluation of Medicinal Products (EMEA) has announced, by means of a concept paper, plans for the development of European Guidelines on parametric release, probably in the form of a new annex to the EC GMP Guide (Ref. CPMP/QWP/2431/98).

 Whatever ultimately happens, one pitfall will need to be avoided; that is, making an assumption that this is an either/or, or all-or-nothing situation. There has been, in the pharmaceutical industry, a tendency to create unnecessary antitheses (e.g. materials testing vs supplier audit and/or certification; in-process control vs end-product testing; validation vs product testing, and so on). There is no reason or need for these things to be antithetical. All are components of, and techniques for, achieving the ultimate objective: the quality of the product and the safety, well-being and protection of the patient. Supplier audit and certification, materials testing, process validation, in-process control, end-product testing and parametric release should all be regarded as potential elements of a rational, mutually supporting, synthesis, with the extent of the application of any one element depending on the nature, type, and use of the product, and on the extent to which the other elements of the synthesis are employed.

Hazard analysis critical control points (HACCP)

HACCP (often pronounced 'hass-ip') stands for hazard analysis critical control points. It is a tool for evaluating the steps in a manufacturing process in terms of the potential risk, or hazard, to the quality of the product represented by each of those steps. This analysis is then followed by the determination of the steps where, critically, control is required to prevent, or minimise, the hazard(s). The technique was first conceived and developed in the food industry in the early 1970s. To date it has not been universally adopted in the pharmaceutical industry, but interest appears to be increasing.

In the formal application of HACCP to an overall manufacturing process, seven steps or elements are involved:

1. Analysis and identification of the potential risk (hazard) represented by each step in the process.
2. Determination of the critical control points (CCP) where it is necessary to control the hazards.
3. Definition of the limits within which each critical parameter should be controlled.
4. Establishment (and validation) of in-process control methods and tests to be used to determine, for each critical control point, whether or not the potential hazard is maintained within the defined limits.
5. Establishment of corrective measures designed to correct any out of control situation at each and every CCP.
6. Confirmation that the HACCP regime (and hence the manufacturing process adopted) is indeed functioning as intended (i.e. a sort of self-inspection of HACCP).
7. Document the entire system, in terms both of HACCP steps to be followed, and of the results obtained.

Some may wonder 'What's new?' It must nevertheless be conceded that following such a structured thought process does concentrate the mind on essentials.

For further information, with a detailed example, see Jahnke (1997).

Just-in-time materials ordering system (JIT)

Just-in-time (JIT) is a technique (or set of techniques) the major aim of which is to reduce space required for storage, and concomitantly to reduce inventory holding costs by arranging things so that materials are delivered 'just-in-time' for them to be used in manufacture, and that the products produced from those materials are delivered to the customer just at the time they are required. The concept is of Japanese origin, and is not in essence a QA technique. Its implementation does however have significant quality implications, making considerable demands and imposing additional strains on any pre-existing quality systems. Although it has been given some thought it does not seem to have been introduced with any success into the pharmaceutical industry in Britain. Other industries have however adopted JIT.

References

Caplen R (1988). *A Practical Approach to Quality Control*, 5th edn. London: Hutchinson Business Books.

Jahnke M (1997). Use of the HACCP concept for the risk analysis of pharmaceutical manufacturing processes. *Eur J Parenter Sci* 2 (4), 113–117.

Oakland J (1986). *Statistical Process Control, a Practical Guide.* Oxford: Heinemann.

Index

Page numbers in **bold** indicate main discussions; those in *italics* indicate figures, tables and forms.